Osteosarcoma

Takafumi Ueda • Akira Kawai
Editors

Osteosarcoma

A Multidisciplinary Approach to Treatment

Springer

Editors
Takafumi Ueda
Osaka University
Osaka, Japan

Osaka National Hospital
Osaka, Japan

Akira Kawai
National Cancer Center Hospital
Tokyo, Japan

ISBN 978-4-431-55695-4 ISBN 978-4-431-55696-1 (eBook)
DOI 10.1007/978-4-431-55696-1

Library of Congress Control Number: 2016930103

Springer Tokyo Heidelberg New York Dordrecht London

Printed on acid-free paper

Springer Japan KK is part of Springer Science+Business Media (www.springer.com)

Preface

Among a variety of bone and soft-tissue sarcomas, osteosarcoma is one of the most difficult to treat, affecting adolescent and young adult patients with a survival rate of less than 10–15 %, even after amputation, because of the development of pulmonary metastasis. However, following the introduction of effective chemotherapy, including doxorubicin, high-dose methotrexate, cisplatin, and ifosfamide, in the late 1970s and 1980s, the prognosis of osteosarcoma improved dramatically, and it has now become a treatable disease after a long history of inevitable fatality. The "giants" of osteosarcoma treatment, including Dr. N Jaffe, Dr. G Rosen, and Dr. R Marcove, played a major role in this revolution in the United States, and thereafter the treatment was introduced in Japan and quickly adopted, pioneered by a number of notable Japanese specialists including Dr. S Yamawaki, Dr. H Fukuma, and Dr. N Kawaguchi.

Now, 40 years later, over 60 % of patients with osteosarcoma can survive the disease with multidisciplinary treatment including neoadjuvant chemotherapy for about 1 year and wide local excision of the primary tumor. Additionally, aggressive pulmonary metastasectomy for patients with lung metastasis has contributed to this improvement in survival. Limb-salvage surgery is now the gold standard for more than 90 % of patients with localized extremity osteosarcoma.

In addition to the original treatment methods developed in Western countries, several unique and effective methods of reconstruction/limb-salvage surgery have been developed in Japan as a result of the limited availability of allografts. Moreover, carbon-ion radiotherapy for patients with unresectable osteosarcoma, such as that in the pelvis and spine, has been developed exclusively in Japan. Here we describe our experiences and ongoing efforts to develop multidisciplinary treatment for osteosarcoma. Leading experts in their various fields have contributed to this book by detailing their research efforts over many years. We believe this book will provide a unique and universal perspective on osteosarcoma treatment in Japan in the early twenty-first century.

Part I focuses on basic research and experimental therapy for osteosarcoma. In Chap. 1, Dr. Toguchida overviews current knowledge of genetic alterations in osteosarcoma. In Chap. 2, Dr. Itoh reviews recent developments in osteosarcoma metastasis research, and in Chap. 3, Dr. Tsukahara et al. describe their many years of dedicated research work on immunotherapy for osteosarcoma.

Part II focuses on the clinical features and prognostic factors of osteosarcoma. In Chap. 4, Dr. Ogura et al. describe the results of treatment for stage IIB osteosarcoma in the extremities at referral hospitals. In Chap. 5, Dr. Nishida describes the clinical features of osteosarcoma in elderly patients, and in Chap. 6, Dr. Kaya reviews the prognostic factors of patients with osteosarcoma.

Part III focuses on chemotherapy for osteosarcoma in Japan. In Chap. 7, Dr. Hiraga reviews the history of osteosarcoma chemotherapy in Japan including the results of the first multicenter clinical trial of neoadjuvant chemotherapy for osteosarcoma (NECO). In Chap. 8, Dr. Kakunaga et al. describe ongoing multicenter efforts to develop specific chemotherapy regimens (OOS) for osteosarcoma.

Part IV focuses on surgery for osteosarcoma. In Chap. 9, Dr. Matsumine describes the outcomes of endoprosthetic reconstruction, a gold-standard technique following resection of osteosarcoma. In Chap. 10, Dr. Futani reviews a specific type of endoprosthesis, the extendible endoprosthesis for skeletally immature children. In Chap. 11, Dr. Kunisada et al. describe the results of treatment for osteosarcoma in the pelvis, one of the disease sites presenting the most difficult challenges. In Chap. 12, Dr. Morii discusses the management of postoperative infection after limb-salvage surgery for osteosarcoma.

To achieve safe, long-standing limb function after treatment of extremity osteosarcoma, several original and useful methods of reconstruction have been developed in Japan. These pioneering approaches are discussed in Part V, "Biological Reconstruction", which makes this book unique. In Chap. 13, Dr. Araki reviews the long-term results and current concept of intraoperative extracorporeal irradiated bone grafts. In Chap. 14, Dr. Ae discusses the long-term outcomes of treatment with pasteurized autogenous bone grafts, and their optimal indications. In Chaps. 15 and 16, Dr. Tsuchiya describes two original methods of reconstruction: liquid nitrogen-treated tumor-bearing bone grafting and the distraction osteogenesis technique. In Chap. 17, Dr. Matsumoto describes a method of in situ preparation that makes it possible to dissect a tumor without danger of contamination by tumor cells during surgery.

Part VI focuses the treatment of unresectable/metastatic osteosarcoma. In Chap. 18, Dr. Imai et al. review the results of carbon ion radiotherapy for unresectable osteosarcoma, and in Chap. 19, Dr. Iwata et al. describe the results of treatment for osteosarcoma with pulmonary metastasis.

Part VII focuses the quality of life of patients who have undergone treatment for osteosarcoma. In Chap. 20, Dr. Yonemoto et al. describe the quality of life of pediatric and adolescent survivors of osteosarcoma.

We are indebted to all of the authors and our distinguished colleagues for completing this e-book. Without their assistance and expertise, this project would not have been possible. We also express our appreciation and gratitude to all doctors and medical staff who have been involved in the treatment of osteosarcoma patients, to whom this e-book is dedicated. We hope and anticipate that this e-book will make a valuable contribution to the further improvement of treatment for patients with osteosarcoma.

Osaka, Japan Takafumi Ueda
Tokyo, Japan Akira Kawai

Contents

Part I

Basic Research and Experimental Therapy

Genetics of Osteosarcoma

1

Junya Toguchida

Abstract

Osteosarcomas (OSs) are functionally defined tumors, and the function may be affected by two endogenous factors: cell-of-origin and genetic alterations. Since the identification of mutations of two tumor suppressor genes, RB1 and p53, a large number of studies have been conducted to identify genetic alterations of OS. Finally the whole-genome sequencing analyses provided us with the landscape of genetic alterations of OS, which confirmed the previously known features of OS such as anomalous structural variations. In addition to p53 and RB1, ATRX and DLG2 genes were identified as candidates of new driver genes in OS. Animal models provided us with the role of each driver mutation. Therefore now we are able to illustrate the basic molecular machineries to drive OS cells. However, it seems that the additional genetic alterations may endow OS cells with phenotypic heterogeneity and also tools to protect them from the molecular target therapy, which should be considered for the development of new therapeutic modalities.

Keywords

RB1 • p53 • Mutation • Whole-genome sequence • Gene expression profile

J. Toguchida (✉)
Institute for Frontier Medical Sciences, Kyoto University, 53 Shogoin-Kawahara-cho, Sakyo-ku, Kyoto 606-8507, Japan

Center for iPS Cells Research and Applications, Kyoto University, 53 Shogoin-Kawahara-cho, Sakyo-ku, Kyoto 606-8507, Japan

Department of Orthopaedic Surgery, Kyoto University Hospital, Kyoto University, 53 Shogoin-Kawahara-cho, Sakyo-ku, Kyoto 606-8507, Japan
e-mail: togjun@frontier.kyoto-u.ac.jp

T. Ueda, A. Kawai (eds.), *Osteosarcoma*, DOI 10.1007/978-4-431-55696-1_1

1.1 Introduction

Osteosarcoma (OS) is defined as a primary malignant tumor with mesenchymal cells producing osteoid and/or bone [1, 2]. Thus OS is a tumor defined by its function, although the level of function may be variable, because the amount of osteoid and/or bone differed considerably among tumors, ranging from extensive mature bone formation to minimum amount of immature osteoid [1, 2]. As for the cell-of-origin of OS, cells on the osteogenic lineage in bone marrow stromal cells are reasonable candidates, which include various types of cells [3]. Also it is well known that OS tumor cells exhibit karyotypes with a high degree of complexity, which may contribute to the biological heterogeneity [4]. Therefore it is reasonable to speculate that OSs diagnosed under the current criteria cover various tumors with heterogeneous cellular and genetic background. Despite such factors potentially contributing biological heterogeneity, clinical features of OS are remarkably homogeneous, in terms of their aggressive phenotype and response to chemotherapy, suggesting the common molecular pathway for the development of this type of tumors [5]. Investigation for molecular genetics of OS started when the mutation of retinoblastoma gene (RB1) and p53 gene was found in OS in 1986 and 1987, respectively [6, 7]. Since then a large amounts of efforts have been devoted to understand OS at the molecular level [8]. Recent progresses in the field of genome analyses and animal models gradually have disclosed the molecular architecture of OS. The general feature is, however, not remarkably different from what we have expected after the discovery of RB1 and p53 mutation in OS, and still we need a progress to understand this ominous disease. In this chapter, by reviewing the progress in the past decades, the road to be followed is discussed.

1.2 Genetic Alterations of OS

There are two types of genetic alterations in any type of cancers: driver mutations and passenger mutations [9]. The driver mutations are causally related to the development of each type of tumors and indispensable for the principle features of tumor cells endowing unlimited growth ability, invasiveness, and escaping from apoptosis. In contrast, the passenger mutations are simply accumulated over the course of development and cell growth and may be redundant and dispensable. Although these definitions are clear, it is not easy to distinguish between them from the information obtained by classical genetic analyses. Recent innovations in whole-genome analyses using next-generation sequencing machines, however, have opened a novel world of cancer genetics and made it possible to overlook the landscape of genetic events in each type of tumors [10, 11]. Based on the complete information of genetic alterations such as structural variations (SVs), copy number variations (CNVs), and single-nucleotide variations (SNVs), driver mutations for each cancer can be identified by sophisticated mathematical analyses [9]. In the case of OS, two reports were published using next-generation sequencing

Table 1.1 Genetic alteration identified by the next-generation sequencing analyses

Reference	[12]	[13]
No. of samples	34 primary tumors	10 primary tumors
Type of samples	Whole-genome sequencing	Whole-exome sequencing
Total number of mutation/tumor	1483.1	NA
No. of mutations in exon	1017	202
No. mutations in exon/tumor	25.5	15.5
No. mutated genes	932	195
No. of mutated genes in common	19	
No. of mutated genes found in more than two tumors	20	1

technology, of which one performed the whole-genome sequencing (WGS) [12] and the other described the whole-exome sequencing (WES) [13] (Table 1.1).

1.2.1 General Features of Genetic Alterations

1.2.1.1 Structural Variation (SV)

It is well known that karyotype of OS exhibits extreme aneuploidy with a large number of aberrant chromosomes [4]. The chromosomal instability of OS cells was also demonstrated by the frequent occurrence of loss of heterozygosity (LOH) [14]. In agreement with these previous data, the WGS by Chen et al. showed a high incidence of SVs in OS [12]. The study identified 10,806 SVs in 34 tumors, of which 377 produced in-frame fusion genes. RNA-sequencing data were available for 64 predicted fusion SVs and among them 15 fusion genes were expressed. Using the previously reported data of other tumors (embryonal rhabdomyosarcoma, acute T cell lymphocytic leukemia, and medulloblastoma), the basal mutation rate and the number of SNVs, SVs, and CNVs of OSs were compared with those of these tumors, and the number of SVs was significantly higher in OS compared with other tumors. LOH was also detected with high frequency; 10 out of 13 tumors showed more than 7 LOH, indicating again the high incidence of SVs in OS. Chromothripsis, literally "chromosome shattering," is a recently discovered phenomenon by which thousands of clustered chromosomal rearrangements occur by a single mutation event in the localized and confined genomic region [15]. The WGS of OS found four cases showed chromothripsis in the region of chromosomes 6q, 13q, 14q, and 17q in each case.

1.2.1.2 Single-Nucleotide Variation (SNV)

The WGS of 34 OS samples by Chen et al. identified 1483.1 SNV/tumor, and this frequency (1.15×10^{-6}) was comparable with the standard mutation rate in the human genome [12]. Among these SNVs, 25.2 mutations/tumor (ranging 5–103) resulted in either missense, nonsense, or splicing mutations, and the total number of genes showing these types of mutations were 932. Among them 20 genes were found in more than two cases, but only four genes (*p53*, *RB1*, *ATRX*, and *DLG2*) were identified by the statistical analyses as significantly mutated genes, and these genes were described as driver mutations in the next section.

Joseph et al. performed the WES using ten primary samples and three cell lines [13]. The number of mutations in the exon regions resulting in amino acid changes was 195, and surprisingly only one gene (the *p53* gene) was mutated in more than two cases. Therefore the p53 gene was the only gene which showed mutations in more than two cases both in the WGS and WES studies. The difference between two studies may be caused by the difference in the sequencing method, but may reflect the heterogeneity of OSs.

1.2.2 Driver Mutations

As described in the previous section, the WGS isolated four genes as the driver mutation of OS, of which two (the *RB1* and *p53* gene) were previously recognized as the driver mutation because of their involvement of hereditary cases and the result of mouse models, and the remaining two genes (the *ATRX* and *DLG2* gene) were novel candidates for the driver mutation of OS.

1.2.2.1 The *p53* Gene

The involvement of p53 in OS was first demonstrated by somatic mutations [7], and LOH on the chromosome 17p [16], and further confirmed by the identification of its mutant as the causative for a familial cancer syndrome, Li-Fraumeni syndrome, which is characterized by a high risk for various cancers including breast, brain, and adrenal grand cancers and osteosarcomas [17, 18]. The p53 protein is responsible for monitoring the integrity of the genome and the control of cell cycle checkpoints after DNA damage [19]. The number of mutations in the *p53* gene identified by the WGS was 28/34 (82.5 %), in which 19 were SVs and 9 were SNVs. Although some tumors were free from the *p53* gene mutation, mutations of genes directly regulating the p53 such as the *MDM2* gene were found in such tumors [20], and therefore it is acceptable to consider that almost all OSs have abnormalities in genes on the p53 pathway.

The driver function of mutant p53 in osteosarcomagenesis was further confirmed by animal models (Table 1.2). p53 knockout mice were fertile and developed a number of tumors including osteosarcoma [21]. Conditional knockout mice using the expression of genes in osteogenic lineages such as the *Prx1*, *Osterix*, and *Col1A1* genes developed OS with a high frequency, almost 100 % in some cases [22–26]. Although the precise mechanism of how the loss of p53 can induce OS so frequently is not yet known, it might be related to the function of p53 as a guardian of genome [19], because the high incidence of SVs is the hallmark of OS.

Table 1.2 Tumor incidence of genetic engineered mice

Predicting target cells	Cre-driver gene	Target gene	Predicted genotype	Incidence of OS	Reference
Mesenchymal stem cells	Prx1	p53 and RB1	p53$^{-/-}$	61 %	[22]
			p53$^{-/-}$:RB1$^{-/-}$	18 %	
		p53 and RB1	p53$^{-/-}$	62 %	[23]
			p53$^{-/-}$:RB1$^{+/-}$	92 %	
			p53$^{-/-}$:RB1$^{-/-}$	29 %	
Pre-osteoblast	Osterix	p53 and RB1	p53$^{-/-}$	87.8 %	[24]
			RB1$^{-/-}$	0 %	
			p53$^{+/-}$:RB1$^{+/-}$	50 %	
			p53$^{+/-}$:RB1$^{-/-}$	90 %	
			p53$^{-/-}$:RB1$^{+/-}$	(207 days)	
			p53$^{-/-}$:RB1$^{-/-}$	(147 days)	
		p53 and RB1	p53$^{-/-}$	100 %	[25]
			RB1$^{-/-}$	0 %	
			p53$^{+/-}$:RB1$^{+/-}$	30.0 %	
			p53$^{+/-}$:RB1$^{-/-}$	77.8 %	
			p53$^{-/-}$:RB1$^{+/-}$	(292 days)	
			p53$^{-/-}$:RB1$^{-/-}$	(127 days)	
	Col1A1 (3.6 kb)	p53	p53$^{-/-}$	60 %	[26]
Osteoblast	Col1A1 (2.3 kb)	p53	p53$^{-/-}$	85 %	[22]
		Notch	Exogenous NICD	100 %	[63]
	Osteocalcin	Ptc	Ptc$^{+/-}$:p53$^{+/-}$	70 %	[65]

1.2.2.2 The *RB1* Gene

Retinoblastoma (RB) is a malignant tumor that develops in the eyes of infants, and approximately 25 % of patients show bilateral and multiple tumors, which are caused by germline mutations of the *RB1* gene [27]. The *RB1* gene is a ubiquitously expressed gene, the encoded protein of which regulates the cell cycle through the control of cyclins [28]. The loss-of-function mutations of *RB1* induce abnormal cell growth, and therefore this gene is called a tumor suppressor gene [28]. Patients with germline mutations of the *RB1* gene have a high risk of developing other malignant tumors during their lifetime, with OSs most frequently encountered [29]. The mutation search in sporadic OS revealed a loss of functional RB protein in approximately 60 % of sporadic OSs, suggesting that RB1 plays a critical role in the development of not only RB but also OS [30]. Thus the *RB1* gene is the first gene mutated in OS with a high frequency, although it is not yet clear why the loss of RB protein predisposes the high risk of OS.

The WGS by Chen et al. discovered ten mutations of the *RB1* gene among 34 cases, of which seven were SVs and three were SNVs [12]. The frequency of mutation was lower than those of the p53 gene, but the function of RB1 was also inhibited by mutations of RB-associated genes such as the amplification of the CDK4 [31] and cyclin D [31] genes and the functional loss of the p16 gene by promoter methylation [32], and therefore the loss of RB function is also an important driver mutation in OS.

The mice model story of the RB1, however, was not as simple as in the case of the p53 (Table 1.2). Simple knockout mouse of the RB1 gene was embryonic lethal, and the heterozygous mice, which represented hereditary patients of RB, developed pinealomas but not retinoblastomas or osteosarcomas [33]. As same as the p53 gene, several lines of conditional knockout mice have been generated using the expression of genes on the osteogenic lineages. In contrast to the *p53* gene, the loss of RB1 in these cells failed to produce OS in most of cases [24, 25]. The effect of loss of RB1 was only manifested when these mice were crossed with p53 knockout mice, in which loss of RB1 accelerated the tumor formation and reduced the survival time [24, 25].

It is not yet known that why the loss of RB1 preferentially induces osteosarcomas, even though the function of RB1 is important in any types of cells. One of the hypothetical explanations is that RB1 protein has some specific roles in osteogenic differentiation. However, conflicting results were reported by in vitro and in vivo studies as for the effect of loss of RB1 on osteogenic differentiation [34–36]. This issue should be further investigated to understand precise role of RB1 mutations in the development of OS.

1.2.2.3 The *ATRX* and *DLG2* Gene

The mutations of the *ATRX* (ATP-dependent helicase ATRX) gene was found in 10/34 cases (five as SV and five as SNV) [12]. ATRX is involved in ALT (alternative lengthening of telomere) [37], which is the main mechanism for the maintenance of the telomere length in sarcomas [8]. The mutations of *DLG2* (disc, large homolog 2) was found in 18/34 cases, all of which were SVs [12]. DLG2 is a member of the membrane-associated guanylate kinase family with multiple PDZ domains and involved in epithelial polarity during cell division [38]. In *Drosophila*, DLG is a tumor suppressor, but the tumor suppressor function was not yet confirmed in human cancers.

1.2.3 Genes Involved in the Hereditary Predisposition

1.2.3.1 DNA Helicase Genes

DNA helicases consist of family of enzymes catalyzing the separation of double-strand DNA in several cellular processes such as DNA replication and DNA repair [39]. There are several hereditary diseases caused by the mutation of DNA helicase genes including Bloom syndrome (caused by the mutation of the *RECQL2* gene) [40], Werner syndrome (*RECQL3* or *WRN* gene) [41], and Rothmund-Thomson syndrome (*RECQL4* or *RTS* gene) [42]. Patients with genetic defects in these genes manifest a number of disorders and are predisposed to cancers including OS [39]. Among these helicase genes, mutations of the *RECQL4* gene seem to be most closely linked with the development of OS [43]. The important differences between the *RB1* or *p53* genes and DNA helicase genes in terms of the involvement of OS are that the former genes were frequently mutated in sporadic cases as somatic mutations, whereas almost no somatic mutations have been reported in the latter genes [44]. Although the hereditary involvements of DNA helicase genes are clearly observed in human cases, no definite observation was found in mice models of these genes. Homozygous *Recql4* mutant mice developed variable phenotype depending on the type of mutations, but the incidence of OS development was very low [45]. Therefore, although the extreme aneuploidy of OS suggested the link between the DNA repair systems and tumor development, it is not yet known how the mutations of DNA helicase genes were involved in the development of OS.

1.2.3.2 Single-Nucleotide Polymorphism Associated with OS

The genome-wide association study (GWAS) has been performed to find genetic factors contributing the development of each disease in various fields including sarcomas [46, 47]. In the case of osteosarcoma, two SNPs were found to be associated with the risk for the development of osteosarcoma [48]. One of them is in the *GRM4* gene that encodes a metabotropic glutamate receptor, which involves c-AMP signaling cascade. The glutamate signaling is best characterized in the central nervous system, and its role in the bone metabolism is not known, although bone tissues expressed the GRM4 gene [49]. The effect of identified SNP for the regulation of the GRM4 gene is also not known. However, from the standpoint of recent focus in cancer research, the identification of a gene involving metabolic pathway as a risk factor is an interesting matter. The expression of the GRM4 gene is expressed in OS cells [50] and is associated with aggressive phenotypes of several cancers [51, 52]. Functional analyses of the GRM4 gene in OS cells may provide a key to answer this association.

1.2.4 Genes on the Signal Pathways Involved in OS

Studies of the molecular mechanisms of growth and progression in OS have identified more than 20 genetic alterations (Fig. 1.1). Most of them, however,

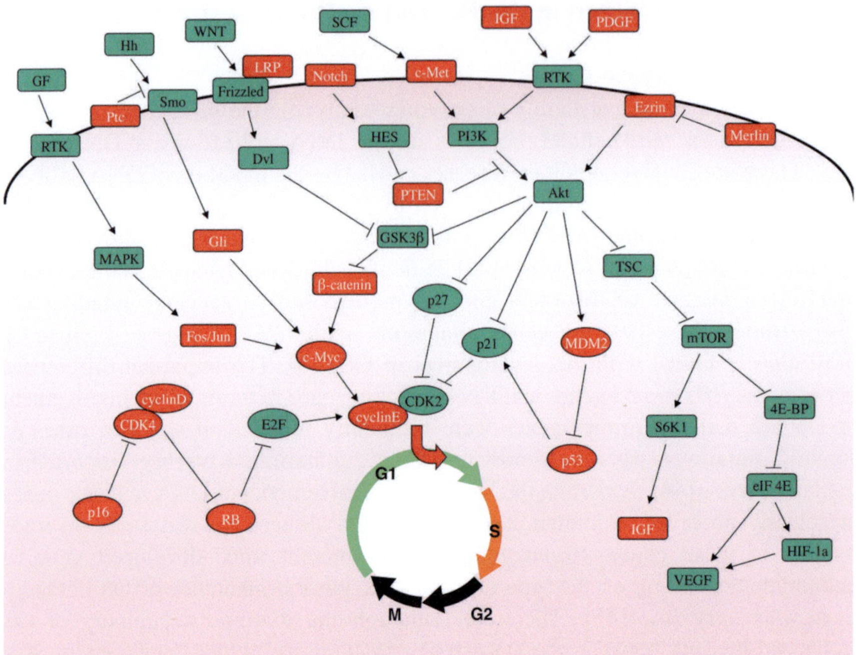

Fig. 1.1 Genetic alterations in osteosarcoma. Genes with mutations (DNA and/or RNA level) are indicated with *red*

were dysregulation in mRNA or protein level, and few mutations were found in genomic DNA level. The most striking feature was their redundancy in the growth signals. OSs expressed the receptors for IGF, VEGF, HER2, ErbB-4, PTHR, and HGF, and many of them are redundant [53–59]. This imposed the difference in the development of molecular target therapy for OS. One of typical examples was the recent clinical trial of mTOR inhibitor. Several signal pathways on OS are connected to the Akt kinase through the activation of PI3K. Activated Akt then activates mTOR via inhibition of TSC, which then activates S6K and eIF4E, resulting in the activation of invasion-related protein such as VEGF. Activated Akt also inhibits the function of GSK-3, resulting in the nuclear accumulation of β-catenin, which then drives target such as c-myc. These data suggested that Akt is a hub molecular for growth signaling in OS, and the inhibition of mTOR function seemed to be a promising molecular approach to the treatment of OS. The result of clinical trial using novel mTOR inhibitors, however, showed minimum responses possibly due to the activation of other signal pathways [60]. Although this illustrated the difficulty to apply the molecular target therapy for OS, several clinical trials using chemical targeting following signal pathways are currently ongoing.

1.2.4.1 The Notch Pathway

The Notch pathway is one of the evolutionally conserved pathways and manifests various functions in the development and homeostasis [61]. Involvement of the Notch pathway in OS was reported in several studies, in which the Notch signal was upregulated in tumor samples and the inhibition of this pathway suppresses tumor cell activity [62]. Transgenic mice containing the activating domain of Notch (Notch intracellular domain, NICD) driven by the *Col1A1* promoter developed human OS-like tumors with complete penetrance, and combination with p53 knockout mice accelerated the tumor formation [63]. Although no definite mutations were found in molecules on the Notch sigal pathway, inhibition of this pathyway will be one of therapeutic targets.

1.2.4.2 The Hedgehog Pathway

Hedgehog signal is known to be involved in the human OS, although no definite genomic alteration on this signal pathway is found [64]. Patched is the repressive receptor of Hedgehog signal, and the loss of patched resulted in the acceleration of Hedgehog signal. Homozygous knockout mice of the *Patched* gene was lethal, and heterozygous mice develop OS when there were crossed with $p53^{+/-}$ mice [65].

1.2.4.3 The Wnt Pathway

The Wnt signal is one of the critical signal pathway for the development, maintenance, and regeneration of bone tissues [66]. Nuclear accumulation of the beta-catenin protein in OS was reported [67], and the inhibition of WNT signal suppressed the aggressive phenotype of OS cell lines [68].

1.3 Expression Profiles of OS

In addition to the genomic information, the information of gene expression profiles of tumors have been used to identify genes for predicting features of tumors such as the aggressive phenotype and the sensitivity for chemotherapeutic drugs.

1.3.1 Prediction for Aggressive Phenotype

Several groups have tried to evaluate gene expression profile of OS to elucidate the specific features of OS. Leonard et al. compared gene expression profile of OS with those of mesenchymal stem cells, their putative precursors, and isolated several genes expressed highly in OS, one of which was the Ezrin encoding a cytoskeleton-associated molecule [69]. The Ezrin gene was also identified in the independent study of canine OS [70]. Khanna et al. compared the gene expression profiles of canine OS with and without distant metastasis and identified the Ezrin gene as metastasis-predicting gene [70]. Because the Ezrin activates Akt, which in turn activates mTOR signal, the clinical trials have been conducted as described in the previous section [60]. Although the data was negative, the gene expression profiling is one of the powerful strategies to isolate the phenotype-related genes.

1.3.2 Prediction for Drug Sensitivity

It is a general agreement that the response to neoadjuvant chemotherapy is the most reliable prognostic factors, and therefore the identification of genes predicting the sensitivity for each chemotherapy provides important information for selecting the strategy. Searching literatures identified four articles regarding this issue [71–74]. All of them used basically similar protocols consisted of MTX, CDDP, and ADR, and the number of samples were comparable (Table 1.3). The response ratio of each study showed similar results, and each study identified a number of genes up- and downregulated in poor responders. Unfortunately, very few genes were commonly up- or downregulated among four studies, and no particular signal pathways were detected to be involved in the chemosensitivity. This may be caused by the difference in the platform of expression analyses, the preparation of samples, and/or the method for the evaluation but also may reflect biological heterogeneity of OS. Interestingly, the genes detected as commonly up- or downregulated were those related to basic cellular metabolisms. NAD(P)H dehydrogenase genes were identified as the only gene upregulated in all four studies, and the upregulation of the hydroxyacyl-coenzyme A dehydrogenase gene was identified three of four studies. Considering the redundancy in growth signal pathways in OS, these results suggest that basic components of metabolic process might be better targets for future therapies. Larger samples with a unified chemotherapeutic protocol may be required to answer this question.

1.4 Conclusion

Accumulation of genetic, molecular, and cellular information on OS enables us to illustrate the hypothetical processes during osteosarcomagenesis (Fig. 1.2). Cell of origin may be broad among cells on several steps in the osteogenic differentiation. Apparently the loss of function of p53 gene is the key driver mutation, and the most important role of mutant p53 in OS tumorigenesis may be induction of chromosomal instability. Osteogenic property of tumors cells should not be inhibited, because the production of osteoid/bone is critical to be diagnosed as OS and the loss of RB function may contribute to accelerate the tumorigenesis with maintaining the osteogenic property. Therefore the loss of function of these two factors may be indispensable events in OS. The function of two newly identified genes, *ATRX* and *DLG2*, in OS may add new insights of molecular signature of OS. Therefore now we are able to illustrate the basic molecular machineries to drive OS cells. However, from the therapeutic view point, the redundancy of growth signal of OS is a tough obstacle to be overcome. OS cells seem to be driven in the automatic mode without the control of driver, of which the content may be different

Table 1.3 Identification of genes predicting response for chemotherapy

References	[71]	[72]	[73]	[74]
No. of samples	13	30	20	20
Type of samples	Pre-Cx biopsy	Post-Cx resection	Post-Cx resection	Pre-Cx biopsy
Content of Cx	CDDP, DPX, MTX, IFO	CDDP, DOX, MTX	CDDP, DOX, MTX	CDDP, DOX, MTX, IFO
Response (good:poor)	6:7	15:15	7:13	9:11
No. of probes	23,010	12,625	9216	5776
No. of predicting genes	60	99	45	44
No. of genes upregulated in poor cases	48	59	41	28
No. of genes downregulated in poor cases	12	40	4	16

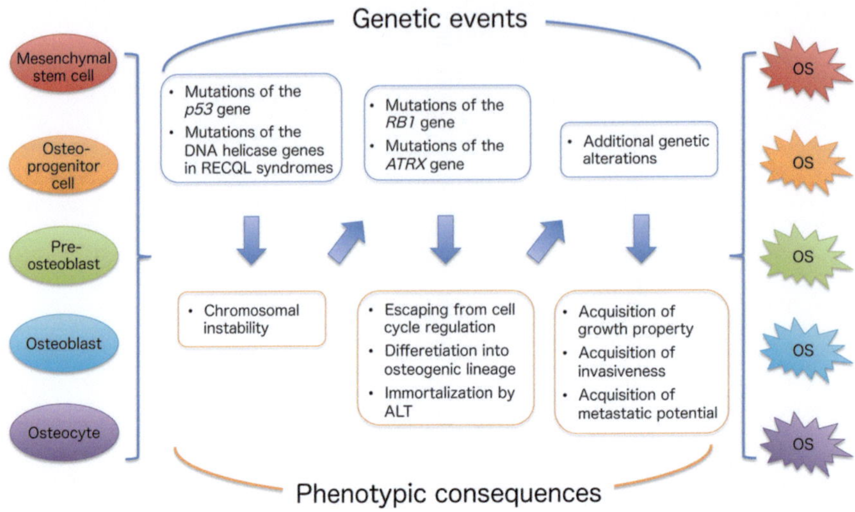

Fig. 1.2 Hypothetical consequence of the development of osteosarcoma

in each tumor. If it is the case, the future therapeutic will be either general approach to shut off the energy of tumor cells targeting the molecules of basic cellular metabolism or super-personalized therapy based on bioinformatics on each tumor. Because of the limitation of space, the recent topics in cancer research such as epigenetic abnormality and micro-RNA were not covered in this chapter, both of which may have important roles in OS, and should be discussed in the next opportunity.

References

1. Dorfman HD, Czerniak B. Bone cancers. Cancer. 1995;75:203–10.
2. Unni KK, Inwards CY. Dahlin's bone tumors: general aspects and data on 10,165 cases. 6th ed. Philadelphia: Lippincott Williams & Wilkins; 2010.
3. Rubio R, Abarrategi A, Garcia-Castro J, et al. Bone environment is essential for osteosarcoma development from transformed mesenchymal stem cells. Stem Cells. 2014;32:1136–48.
4. Sandberg AA, Bridge JA. Updates on the cytogenetics and molecular genetics of bone and soft tissue tumors: osteosarcoma and related tumors. Cancer Genet Cytogenet. 2003;145:1–30.
5. Meyers PA, Gorlick R. Osteosarcoma. Pediatr Clin N Am. 1997;44:973–89.
6. Friend SH, Bernards R, Rogelj S. A human DNA segment with properties of the gene that predisposes to retinoblastoma and osteosarcoma. Nature. 1986;323:643–6.
7. Masuda H, Miller C, Koeffler HP, Battifora H, Cline MJ. Rearrangement of the p53 gene in human osteogenic sarcomas. Proc Natl Acad Sci U S A. 1987;84:7716–9.
8. Helman LJ, Meltzer P. Mechanisms of sarcoma development. Nat Rev Cancer. 2003;3:685–69.
9. Garraway LS, Lander ES. Lessons from the cancer genome. Cell. 2013;153:17–37.
10. Baca SC, Prandi D, Lawrence MS, et al. Punctuated evolution of prostate cancer genomes. Cell. 2013;153:666–77.

11. Lawrence MS, Stojanov P, Polak P, et al. Mutational heterogeneity in cancer and the search for new cancer-associated genes. Nature. 2013;499:214–8.
12. Chen X, Bahrami A, Pappo A, et al. Recurrent somatic structural variations contribute to tumorigenesis of pediatric osteosarcoma. Cell Rep. 2014;7:104–12.
13. Joseph CG, Hwang H, Jiao Y, et al. Exomic analysis of myxoid liposarcoma, synovial sarcoma, and osteosarcoma. Gene Chromosom Cancer. 2014;53:15–24.
14. Yamaguchi T, Toguchida J, Yamamuro T, et al. Allelotype analysis in osteosarcomas: frequent allele loss on 3q, 13q, 17p, and 18q. Cancer Res. 1992;52:2419–23.
15. Stephens PJ, Greenman CD, Fu B, et al. Massive genomic rearrangement acquired in a single catastrophic event during cancer development. Cell. 2011;144:27–40.
16. Toguchida J, Ishizaki K, Nakamura Y, et al. Assignment of common allele loss in osteosarcoma to the subregion 17p13. Cancer Res. 1989;49:6247–51.
17. Malkin D, Li FP, Strong LC, Fraumeni Jr JF. Germ line p53 mutations in a familial syndrome of breast cancer, sarcomas, and other neoplasms. Science. 1990;250:1233–8.
18. Toguchida J, Yamaguchi T, Dayton SH, et al. Prevalence and spectrum of germline mutations of the p53 gene among patients with sarcoma. N Engl J Med. 1992;326:1301–8.
19. Lane DP. Cancer. p53, guardian of the genome. Nature. 1992;358:15–6.
20. Lonardo F, Ueda T, Huvos AG, Healey J, Ladanyi M. p53 and MDM2 alterations in osteosarcomas: correlation with clinicopathologic features and proliferative rate. Cancer. 1997;79:1541–7.
21. Jacks T, Remington L, Williams BO, et al. Tumor spectrum analysis in p53-mutant mice. Curr Biol. 1994;4:1–7.
22. Lin PP, Pandey MK, Jin F, et al. Targeted mutation of p53 and Rb in mesenchymal cells of the limb bud produces sarcomas in mice. Carcinogenesis. 2009;30:1789–95.
23. Calo E, Quintero-Estades JA, Danielian PS, Nedelcu S, Berman SD, Lees JA. Rb regulates fate choice and lineage commitment in vivo. Nature. 2010;466:1110–4.
24. Berman SD, Calo E, Landman AS, et al. Metastatic osteosarcoma induced by inactivation of Rb and p53 in the osteoblast lineage. Proc Natl Acad Sci U S A. 2008;105:11851–6.
25. Walkley CR, Qudsi R, Sankaran VG, et al. Conditional mouse osteosarcoma, dependent on p53 loss and potentiated by loss of Rb, mimics the human disease. Genes Dev. 2008;22:1662–76.
26. Lengner CJ, Steinman HA, Gagnon J, et al. Osteoblast differentiation and skeletal development are regulated by Mdm2-p53 signaling. J Cell Biol. 2006;172:909–21.
27. Abramson DH. Retinoblastoma: saving life with vision. Annu Rev Med. 2014;65:171–84.
28. Burkhart DL, Sage J. Cellular mechanisms of tumour suppression by the retinoblastoma gene. Nat Rev Cancer. 2008;8:671–82.
29. Wong FL, Boice Jr JD, Abramson DH, et al. Cancer incidence after retinoblastoma. Radiation dose and sarcoma risk. JAMA. 1997;278:1262–7.
30. Wadayama B, Toguchida J, Shimizu T, et al. Mutation spectrum of the retinoblastoma gene in osteosarcomas. Cancer Res. 1994;54:3042–8.
31. Wei G, Lonardo F, Ueda T, et al. CDK4 gene amplification in osteosarcoma: reciprocal relationship with INK4A gene alterations and mapping of 12q13 amplicons. Int J Cancer. 1999;80:199–204.
32. Maelandsmo GM, Berner JM, Florences VA, et al. Homozygous deletion frequency and expression level of the CDKN2 gene in human sarcomas – relationship to amplification and mRNA levels of CDK4 and CCND1. Br J Cancer. 1995;72:393–8.
33. Jacks T, Fazeli A, Schmitt EM, Bronson RT, Goodell MA, Weinberg RA. Effects of an Rb mutation in the mouse. Nature. 1992;359:295–300.
34. Gutierrez GM, Kong E, Sabbagh Y, et al. Impaired bone development and increased mesenchymal progenitor cells in calvaria of RB1-/- mice. Proc Natl Acad Sci U S A. 2008;105:18402–7.

35. Berman SD, Yuan TL, Miller ES, Lee EY, Caron A, Lees JA. The retinoblastoma protein tumor suppressor is important for appropriate osteoblast differentiation and bone development. Mol Cancer Res. 2008;6:1440–51.
36. Gündüz V, Kong E, Bryan CD, Hinds PW. Loss of the retinoblastoma tumor suppressor protein in murine calvaria cells characterized by low expression of N-cadherin. Mol Cell Biol. 2012;32:2561–9.
37. Clynes D, Gibbons RJ. ATRX and the replication of structured DNA. Curr Opin Genet Dev. 2013;23:289–94.
38. Roberts S, Delury C, Marsh E. The PDZ protein discs-large (DLG): the 'Jekyll and Hyde' of the epithelial polarity proteins. FEBS J. 2012;279:3549–58.
39. Brosh Jr RM. DNA helicases involved in DNA repair and their roles in cancer. Nat Rev Cancer. 2013;13:542–58.
40. Ellis NA, Groden J, Ye TZ, et al. The Bloom's syndrome gene product is homologous to RecQ helicases. Cell. 1995;83:655–66.
41. Yu CE, Oshima J, Fu YH, et al. Positional cloning of the Werner's syndrome gene. Science. 1996;272:258–62.
42. Kitao S, Shimamoto A, Goto M, et al. Mutations in RECQL4 cause a subset of cases of Rothmund-Thomson syndrome. Nat Genet. 1999;22:82–4.
43. Wang LL, Gannavarapu A, Kozinetz CA, et al. Association between osteosarcoma and deleterious mutations in the RECQL4 gene in Rothmund-Thomson syndrome. J Natl Cancer Inst. 2003;95:669–74.
44. Nishijo K, Nakayama T, Aoyama T, et al. Mutation analysis of the RECQL4 gene in sporadic osteosarcomas. Int J Cancer. 2004;111:367–72.
45. Mann MB, Hodges CA, Barnes E, Vogel H, Hassold TJ, Luo G. Defective sister-chromatid cohesion, aneuploidy and cancer predisposition in a mouse model of type II Rothmund-Thomson syndrome. Hum Mol Genet. 2005;14:813–25.
46. Pillay N, Plagnol V, Tarpey PS, et al. A common single-nucleotide variant in T is strongly associated with chordoma. Nat Genet. 2012;44:1185–7.
47. Postel-Vinay S, Véron AS, Tirode F, et al. Common variants near TARDBP and EGR2 are associated with susceptibility to Ewing sarcoma. Nat Genet. 2012;44:323–7.
48. Savage SA, Mirabello L, Wang Z, et al. Genome-wide association study identifies two susceptibility loci for osteosarcoma. Nat Genet. 2013;45:799–803.
49. Cowan RW, Seidlitz EP, Singh G. Glutamate signaling in healthy and diseased bone. Front Endocrinol (Lausanne). 2012;3:89.
50. Kalariti N, Lembessis P, Koutsilieris M. Characterization of the glutametergic system in MG-63 osteoblast-like osteosarcoma cells. Anticancer Res. 2004;24:3923–9.
51. Chang HJ, Yoo BC, Lim SB, Jeong SY, Kim WH, Park JG. Metabotropic glutamate receptor 4 expression in colorectal carcinoma and its prognostic significance. Clin Cancer Res. 2005;11:3288–95.
52. Brocke KS, Staufner C, Luksch H, et al. Glutamate receptors in pediatric tumors of the central nervous system. Cancer Biol Ther. 2010;9:455–68.
53. Burrow S, Andrulis IL, Pollak M, Bell RS. Expression of insulin-like growth factor receptor, IGF-1, and IGF-2 in primary and metastatic osteosarcoma. J Surg Oncol. 1998;69:21–7.
54. Ferracini R, Renzo MFD, Scotlandi K, et al. The Met/HGF receptor is overexpressed inhuman osteosarcomas and is activated by either a paracrine or autocrine circuit. Oncogene. 1995;10:739–49.
55. Gorlick R, Huvos AG, Heller G, et al. Expression of HER2/erbB-2 correlates with survival in osteosarcoma. J Clin Oncol. 1999;17:2781–8.
56. Kaya M, Wada T, Akatsuka T, et al. Vascular endothelial growth factor expression in untreated osteosarcoma is predictive of pulmonary metastasis and poor prognosis. Clin Cancer Res. 2000;6:572–7.

57. Hughes DP, Thomas DG, Giordano TJ, Baker LH, McDonagh KT. Cell surface expression of epidermal growth factor receptor and her-2 with nuclear expression of her-4 in primary osteosarcoma. Cancer Res. 2004;64:2047–50.
58. Jung ST, Moon ES, Seo HY, Kim JS, Kim GJ, Kim YK. Expression and significance of TGF-beta isoform and VEGF in osteosarcoma. Orthopedics. 2005;28:755–60.
59. Yang R, Hoang BH, Kubo T, et al. Over-expression of parathyroid hormone Type 1 receptor confers an aggressive phenotype in osteosarcoma. Int J Cancer. 2007;121:943–54.
60. Chawla SP, Staddon AP, Baker LH, et al. Phase II study of the mammalian target of rapamycin inhibitor ridaforolimus in patients with advanced bone and soft tissue sarcomas. J Clin Oncol. 2012;30:78–84.
61. Tao J, Chen S, Lee B. Alteration of Notch signaling in skeletal development and disease. Ann N Y Acad Sci. 2010;1192:257–68.
62. Zhang P, Yang Y, Zweidler-McKay PA, Hughes DPM. Critical role of Notch signaling in osteosarcoma invasion and metastasis. Clin Cancer Res. 2008;14:2962–9.
63. Tao J, Jiang MM, Jiang L, et al. Notch activation as a driver of osteogenic sarcoma. Cancer Cell. 2014;26:390–401.
64. Warzecha J, Göttig S, Chow KU, et al. Inhibition of osteosarcoma cell proliferation by the Hedgehog-inhibitor cyclopamine. J Chemother. 2007;19:554–61.
65. Chan LH, Wang W, Yeung W, Deng Y, Yuan P, Mak KK. Hedgehog signaling induces osteosarcoma development through Yap1 and H19 overexpression. Oncogene. 2014;33:4857–66.
66. Chen Y, Alman BA. Wnt pathway, an essential role in bone regeneration. J Cell Biochem. 2009;106:353–62.
67. Haydon RC, Deyrup A, Ishikawa A, et al. Cytoplasmic and/or nuclear accumulation of the beta-catenin protein is a frequent event in human osteosarcoma. Int J Cancer. 2002;102:338–42.
68. Hoang BH, Kubo T, Healey JH, et al. Dickkopf 3 inhibits invasion and motility of Saos-2 osteosarcoma cells by modulating the Wnt-beta-catenin pathway. Cancer Res. 2004;64:2734–9.
69. Leonard P, Sharp T, Henderson S. Gene expression array profile of human osteosarcoma. Br J Cancer. 2003;89:2284–8.
70. Khanna C, Wang X, Bose S, et al. The membrane-cytoskeleton linker ezrin is necessary for osteosarcoma metastasis. Nat Med. 2004;10:182–6.
71. Ochi K, Daigo Y, Katagiri T, et al. Prediction of response to neoadjuvant chemotherapy for osteosarcoma by gene-expression profiles. Int J Oncol. 2004;24:347–55.
72. Mintz MB, Sowers R, Brown KM, et al. An expression signature classifies chemotherapy-resistant pediatric osteosarcoma. Cancer Res. 2005;65:1748–54.
73. Man T, Chintagumpala M, Visvanathan J, et al. Expression profiles of osteosarcoma that can predict response to chemotherapy. Cancer Res. 2005;65:8142–50.
74. Salas S, Jezequel P, Campion L, et al. Molecular characterization of the response to chemotherapy in conventional osteosarcomas: predictive value of HSD17B10 and IFITM2. Int J Cancer. 2009;125:851–60.

Basic Research for Osteosarcoma Lung Metastasis (LM8)

2

Kazuyuki Itoh

Abstract

Fifteen to 30 % of OS patients present with lung metastasis at diagnosis, and their 5-year survival rate is still only 20 %, regardless of therapy. Thus, the control of metastasis is still quite hard, and new effective therapy against the metastasis diseases is strongly needed. In this chapter, I would like to summarize the present status of OS metastasis research, especially using our established excellent OS mouse lung metastasis model LM8. Employing this model, we reported several popular candidate molecules as targets for OS lung metastasis, including MMP, motility, VEGF, etc. I also discuss new targets, tissue stiffness, and Twist-1 as future candidates against OS metastasis.

Keywords

Lung metastasis • Molecular target therapy • MMP • Motility • VEGF • Dendritic cell therapy • Stiffness

2.1 Introduction

The majority of osteosarcoma (OS) patients suffers from localized disease, and up to 70 % survive with state-of-the-art treatments including local surgical control of primary sites combined with neoadjuvant multidrug chemotherapy. However, 15–30 % of OS patients present with metastasis at diagnosis, and their 5-year survival rate is still only 20 %, regardless of therapy [1]. The control of metastasis is still quite hard, and new effective therapy against the metastasis diseases is

K. Itoh, M.D., Ph.D. (✉)
Department of Biology, Research Institute, Osaka Medical Center for Cancer and Cardiovascular Diseases, 1-3-2 Nakamichi, Higashinari-ku, Osaka 537-8511, Japan
e-mail: itou-ka@mc.pref.osaka.jp

T. Ueda, A. Kawai (eds.), *Osteosarcoma*, DOI 10.1007/978-4-431-55696-1_2

strongly needed. In this chapter, I would like to summarize the present status of OS metastasis research, especially using our established OS mouse model LM8.

2.2 LM8: Excellent Animal Model for Osteosarcoma Lung Metastasis Research

It is quite crucial to establish the excellent experimental animal model for medical scientific research. Especially for the metastasis research, the two most important factors are syngeneic and orthotopic. Syngeneic means the same species of animal, which reduce immune reaction of host animal after transplantation of the tumor. Using syngeneic model, we could investigate the metastatic spread in the wild-type host background. By contrast, in the case of xenografting model of human osteosarcoma transplanted to the immune-competent mouse (i.e., nude or SCID), it is hard to analyze the tumor-host interaction with immune reactions. Next, orthotopic means the site of transplantation. Metastatic cascade consists of long travel from the primary site to the final colonized organ; thus, OS cells should be injected to the sites, where it arises in the human subjects.

LM8 is a subclone from the original mouse osteosarcoma Dunn cells. Dunn cells were chemically induced male osteosarcoma cell line, firstly reported by female veterinarian Dr. Dunn in NCI [2]. This osteogenic osteosarcoma was quite important for the bone formation research, since mouse BMP4 was originally cloned from this cell line. However, it could not metastasize to the distant organs after transplant to the subcutaneous orthotopic regions. In order to establish the lung metastasis-seeking subclones from Dunn cells, Drs. Ueda and Aoki followed Fidler and Poste's method for B16 melanoma lung metastatic model [3]. They repeated the eight cycles of tail vein injection-prepare lung nodules-in vitro culture-tail vein injection (Fig. 2.1). During this procedure for the enrichment of lung metastasis-seeking cells, LM8 clones could make lung metastasis colonies at 4–5 weeks after transplantation into the subcutaneous region at 100 % efficiency [4]. We deposited this LM8 into the Riken Cell Bank in Japan in 1998; since then, more than 100 papers were published worldwide in PubMed, and LM8 became the most popular osteosarcoma cell line for the metastasis research.

2.3 Candidate Target Molecules

When we compared the expression of some of the proteins related to the cancer metastasis, most of the metastasis-related genes (proteins) MMP, VEGF, etc. are upregulated in LM8 compared to the parental Dunn cells, as expected (Table 2.1).

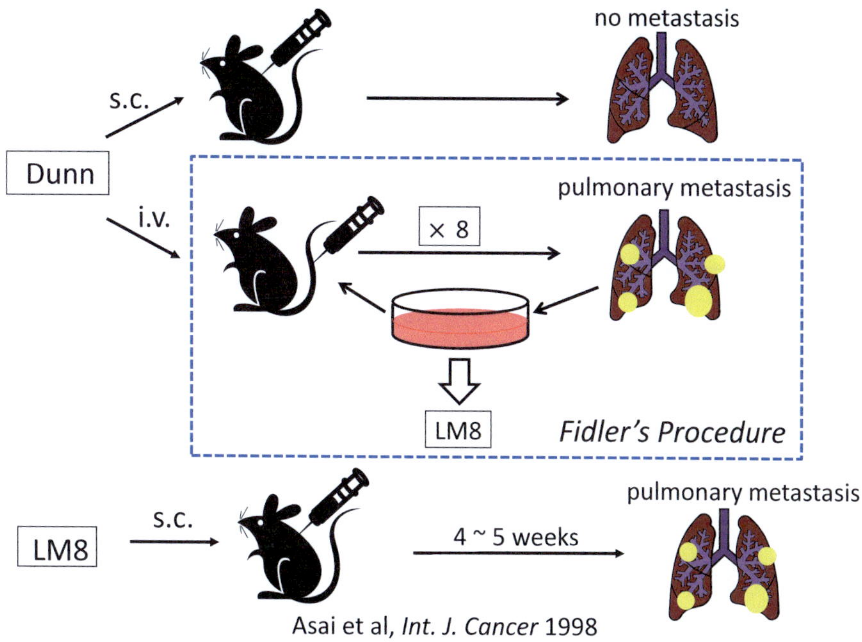

Fig. 2.1 Establishments of highly metastatic OS cell line, LM8

2.3.1 MMP

Since MMP played several important biological roles in metastatic spread, a number of pharmaceutical companies tried to develop specific inhibitors for clinical trials. Indeed, several compounds were undertaken for the phase III clinical trials in the late 1990s; however, no drug has been approved so far. A number of reasons were pointed out, including inappropriate clinical protocols, no surrogate markers, heterogeneity of cancer cells, etc. [5]. We also tried several MMP inhibitors for the LM8 animal experiments, but no positive effect was found for the lung metastasis.

2.3.2 Motility

When we established LM8 cells from parental Dunn cells, we already recognized the clear morphological difference between the two. LM8 cells acquired fibroblastic morphology with striking filopodia on the cell surface. Immunostaining showed faint stress fiber formation and peripherally localized integrin beta 1, and biochemical analyses present the activated Cdc42 and autophosphorylation of focal adhesion kinase (FAK) in LM8 cells when compared to Dunn cells. LM8 cells had activated motility in single-cell migration mode. LM8 migration was increased by a

Table 2.1 Comparison of several biological characters between LM8 and Dunn

			LM8		Dunn
Metastasis	Subcutaneous transplantation		Massive pulmonary metastasis in 4 weeks		No pulmonary metastasis
Morphology	Filopodia formation		2.2 filopodia/cell		1.4 filopodia/cell
	Stress fiber formation		Few	<	Numerous
	Focal adhesion	Integrin β1, paxillin, vinculin	Localized in cell edge		Cell edge and cytoplasm
		FAK Y397 phosphorylation	High	>	Low
Motility	Vertical migration		20 % of applied cells	>	12 % of applied cells
	Horizontal migration		Fast	>	Slow
			Fibroblastic shape		Rounded shape
VEGF	RNA and protein expression		High	>	Low
MMP	MMP-2 secretion		High	>	None
Cdc42	GTP-Cdc42		High	>	Low
	Cdc42 siRNA		20 % → 12 %		No change
Rho-ROCK-myosin	Myosin II phosphorylation		Low	<	High
	Y-27632 (10 μM)		20 % → 32 % (haptotaxis)		Slightly decrease (haptotaxis)
			MLC-P↓		
	Blebbistatin (2.5 μM)		20 % → 28 % (haptotaxis)		No change

Rho-associated protein kinase (ROCK) inhibitor, Y-27632, while it was decreased by Cdc42 silencing using RNA interference system (Table 2.1) [6].

We also found that a clinically approved camptothecin analog irinotecan suppressed the migration, Cdc42 activity, and autophosphorylation of FAK and attenuated integrin beta 1 distribution selectively in LM8 cells. Daily oral administration of irinotecan significantly reduced the rate and size of pulmonary metastasis in syngeneic C3H mice (Fig. 2.2). The concentrations of irinotecan-active metabolites SN38 were equivalent to in vitro experiments to inhibit motility of LM8. The fibroblastic morphology and activated cell migration with the dependency on Cdc42 but not Rho-ROCK signaling pathway argued that LM8 moved in mesenchymal mode of cell migration. This activated mesenchymal migration was a key component of the pulmonary metastasis of LM8 cells. The inhibition of mesenchymal migration by irinotecan, in addition to its cytotoxic effects, might be effective in preventing pulmonary metastasis of osteosarcoma [6].

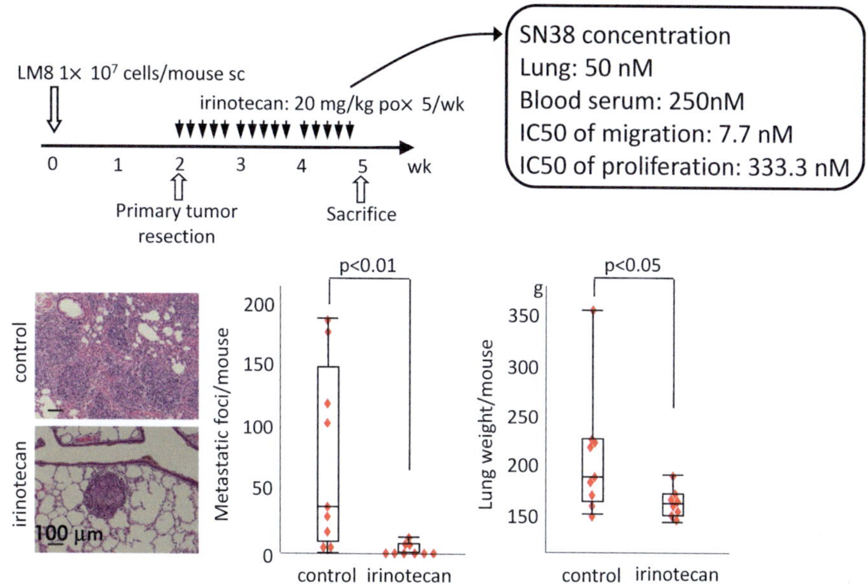

Fig. 2.2 Irinotecan suppressed lung metastasis by LM8 using primary tumor resection model

2.3.3 VEGF

Anti-VEGF therapy was the first approved clinical therapy for the metastatic tumor (firstly colorectal cancer liver metastasis, [7]). VEGF is a multifunctional growth factor showing a number of biological functions besides neovascularization. And, thus, the inhibitions of angiogenesis reduced primary tumor growth and microvessel density in keeping with many earlier reports, but strikingly accelerated invasion and metastasis [8]. In this chapter, I describe our findings for the novel functions of VEGF for the OS lung metastasis. We firstly analyzed the multiple steps of metastatic cascade one by one as follows.

We firstly investigated the chronological detection of circulating tumor cells (CTCs) from mice with either cell line. LM8 CTCs appeared faster, at a higher rate and with a greater number compared to Dunn CTCs (Fig. 2.3). Cultured cells from CTCs of LM8 showed higher proliferative ability than cells from the primary site in suspension culture, which mimicked the environment of the bloodstream for CTCs. The proliferative ability of LM8 cells was also higher than that of Dunn cells in 3D collagen culture with low stiffness (~150 Pa; close to conditions in the lung) (Fig. 2.4). We next focused on the extravasation step. LM8 showed higher migration ability compared to Dunn with transendothelial migration assay (Fig. 2.5). We also found a disruption in endothelial barrier function throughout co-culture with LM8 using time-lapse imaging. In addition, LM8 secreted high levels of vascular endothelial growth factor (VEGF), while VEGF signal inhibition with a small molecule tyrosine kinase inhibitor (pazopanib) decreased disruption of the vascular

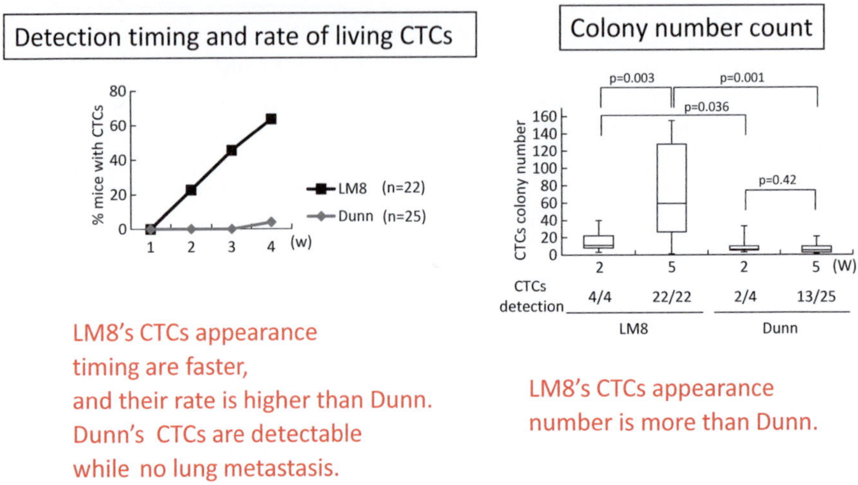

Fig. 2.3 Chronological detection of living circulating tumor cells from LM8 and Dunn

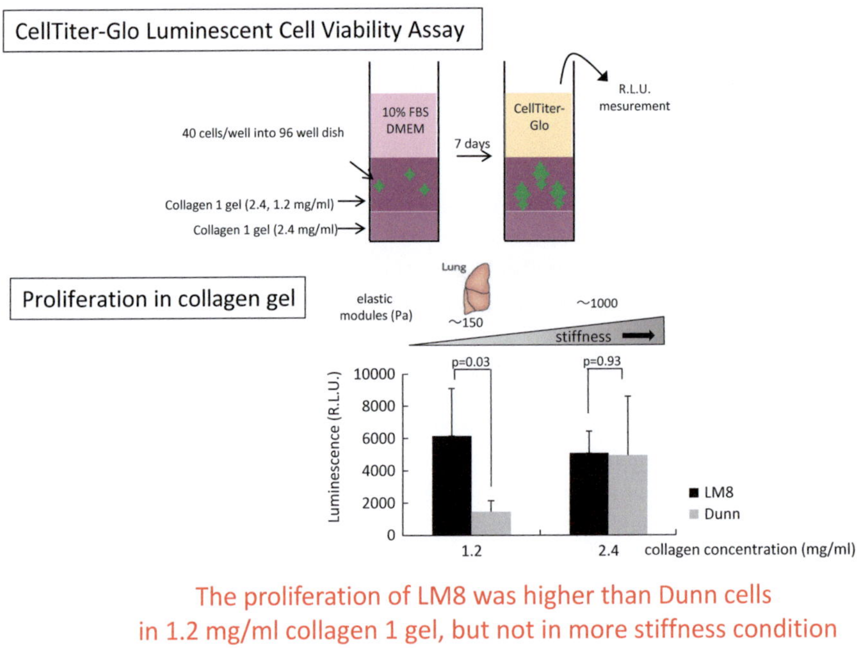

Fig. 2.4 Growth of LM8 and Dunn in the different stiffness conditions

barrier and transendothelial migration of LM8 (Fig. 2.6). Finally, daily oral administration of pazopanib reduced the rate and size of pulmonary metastasis in vivo (Fig. 2.7). Collectively, these results show anti-VEGF therapy as a candidate for pulmonary metastasis of OS [9].

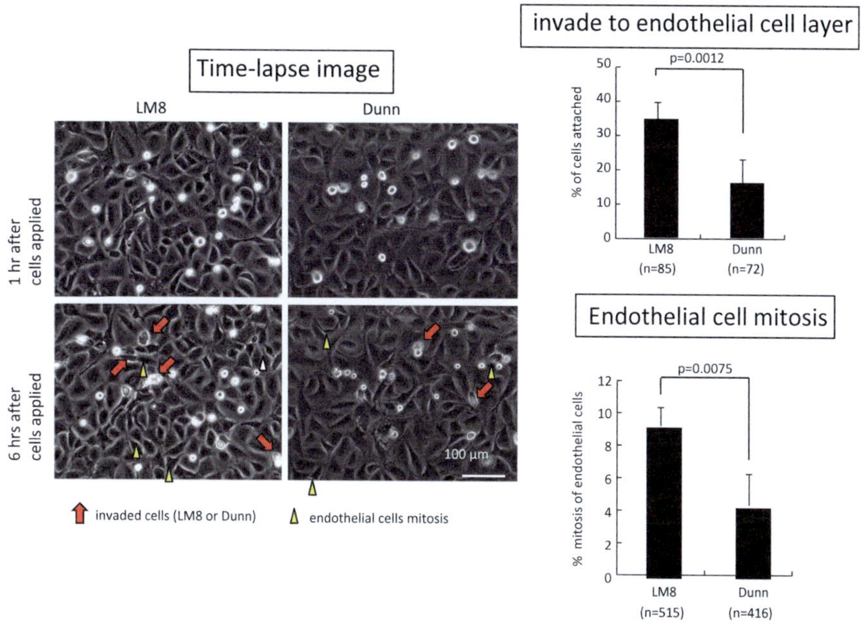

Fig. 2.5 Extravasation ability of LM8 and Dunn using transendothelial invasion assay

2.3.4 Dendritic Cell Immunotherapy

We also examined the efficacy of dendritic cell immunotherapy for lung metastasis using LM8. Vaccination of dendritic cells generated from syngeneic mice increased lymphocyte interferon-γ production, particularly when dendritic cells were pulsed by tumor antigens, and induced lymphocyte proliferation and cytotoxicity against LM8 cells. We performed three animal experimental protocols. Dendritic cell vaccination before tumor inoculation prevented tumor development. Dendritic cell vaccination after developing the primary tumor suppressed growth of subcutaneous tumors and lung metastases (Fig. 2.8). Dendritic cell vaccination after surgical resection of the primary tumor also produced suppression of lung metastases. In addition, in vitro Boyden chamber assay revealed dendritic cell-treated lymphocytes attenuated tumor invasiveness (Fig. 2.9). Our findings suggest dendritic cell-based immunotherapy may be an effective postoperative therapeutic approach to prevent metastasis in patients with osteosarcoma [10].

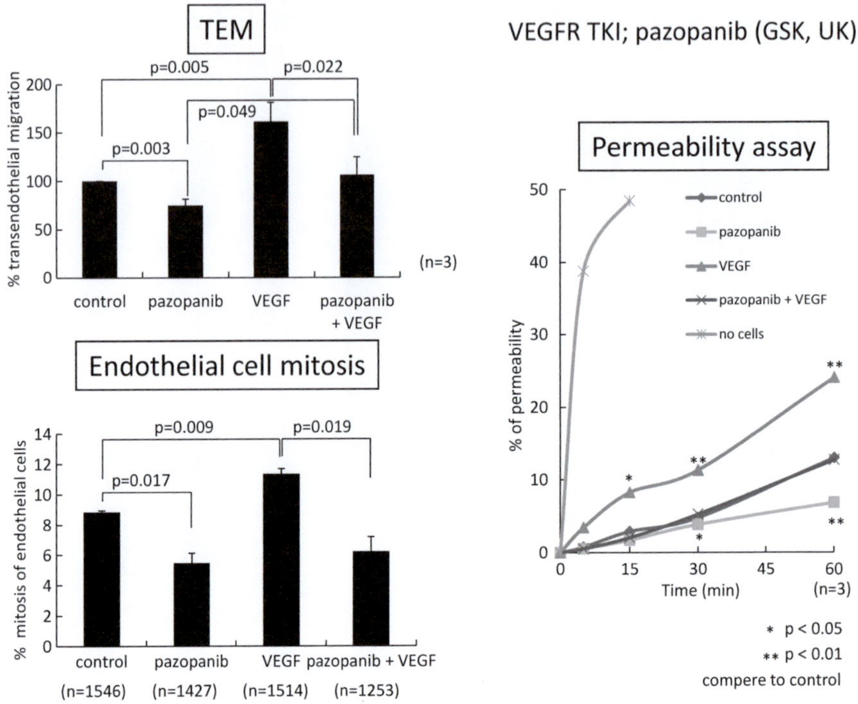

Fig. 2.6 Effects of blockage of VEGF-VEGFR on transendothelial migration and endothelial mitosis

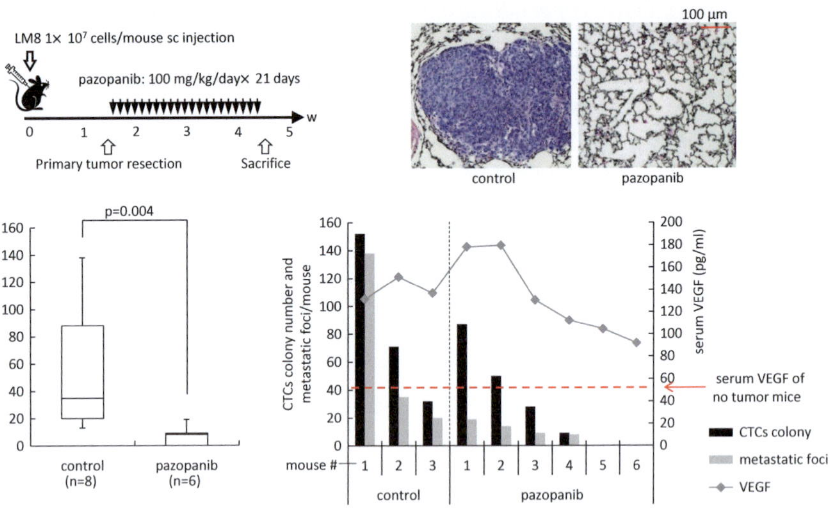

Fig. 2.7 Pazopanib (VEGFR-TKI) inhibited lung metastasis by LM8

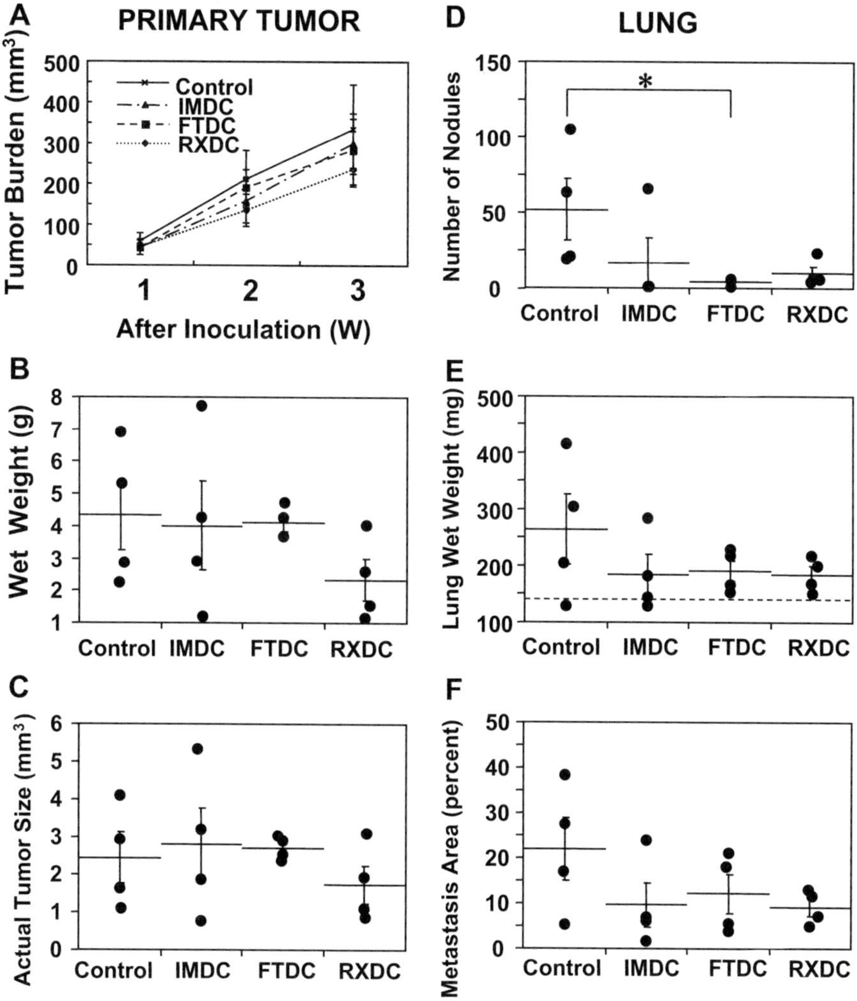

no pulsing (immature dendritic cells [IMDC]),
in vitro pulsing with freezethawedtumor lysate (FTDC),
in vitro pulsing with irradiatedtumor (RXDC).

Fig. 2.8 Effects of dendritic cell vaccination on established primary tumors and lung metastases by LM8

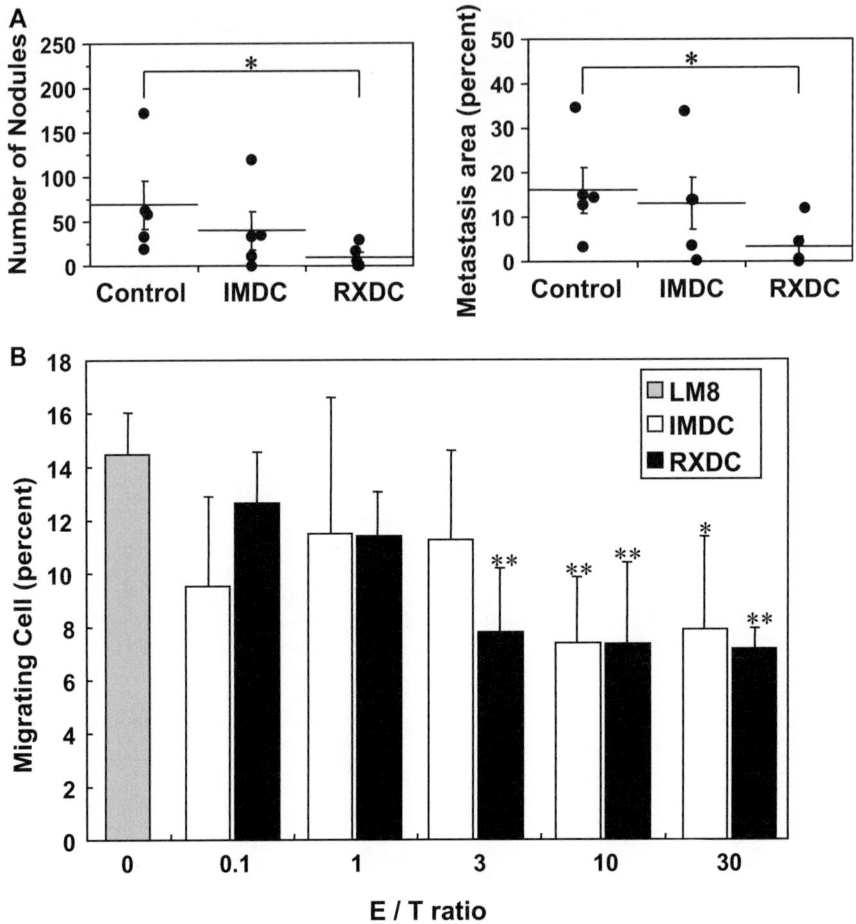

Fig. 2.9 Effects of dendritic cell vaccination after tumor resection and tumor cell motility using Boyden chamber assay

2.4 Future Candidates

2.4.1 Stiffness

As mentioned above, tissue mechanics modulates the growth of tumor at different sites, such as distant metastatic lung. Indeed, LM8 could grow at the similar speed at both primary and metastatic sites, while Dunn could not. How the tissue mechanics affected tumor growth is of great concern. Dr. Yui moved from my lab to Valerie Weaver's group at UCSF to establish the model to investigate the mechanism. Most recently, her group reported that mechanical force (stiffness) controlled the expression of PTEN via miRNA-18a level [11]. This opens a new venue to search candidate molecules to suppress tumor metastasis at the distant metastatic sites.

2.4.2 Twist-1

We seek the driver gene, which regulates the metastasis of OS. Most recently, we found the strike difference in the expression level of master regulator gene, Twist-1, between Dunn and LM8. Since Twist-1 has been reported to regulate multiple biological function in a number of tumors, it would be a good candidate to control the OS metastatic spread.

References

1. Klein MJ, Siegal GP. Osteosarcoma: anatomic and histologic variants. Am J Clin Pathol. 2006;125:555–81.
2. Dunn TB, Andervont HB. Histology of some neoplasms and non-neoplastic lesions found in wild mice maintained under laboratory conditions. J Natl Cancer Inst. 1963;31:873–901.
3. Poste G, Fidler IJ. The pathogenesis of cancer metastasis. Nature. 1980;283:139–46.
4. Asai T, Ueda T, Itoh K, Yoshioka K, Aoki Y, Mori S, Yoshikawa H. Establishment and characterization of a murine osteosarcoma (LM8) with high metastatic potential to the lung. Int J Cancer. 1998;76:418–22.
5. Egeblad M, Werb Z. New functions for the matrix metalloproteinases in cancer progression. Nat Rev Cancer. 2002;3:161–74.
6. Yui Y, Itoh K, Yoshioka K, Naka N, Watanabe M, Hiraumi Y, Matsubara H, Watanabe K, Sano K, Nakahata T, Adachi S. Mesenchymal mode of migration participates in pulmonary metastasis of mouse osteosarcoma LM8. Clin Exp Metastasis. 2010;27:619–30.
7. McCarthy M. Antiangiogenesis drug promising for metastatic colorectal cancer. Lancet. 2003;361:1959.
8. Steeg PS, Anderson RL, Bar-Eli M, Chambers AF, Eccles SA, Hunter K, Itoh K, Kang Y, Matrisian LM, Sleeman JP, Theodorescu D, Thompson EW, Welch DR. Preclinical drug development must consider the impact on metastasis. Clin Cancer Res. 2009;15:4529–30.
9. Tanaka T, Yui Y, Naka N, Wakamatsu T, Yoshioka K, Araki N, Yoshikawa H, Itoh K. Dynamic analysis of lung metastasis by mouse osteosarcoma LM8-VEGF is a candidate for anti-metastasis therapy. Clin Exp Metastasis. 2013;30:369–79.
10. Joyama S, Naka N, Tsukamoto Y, Yoshikawa H, Itoh K. Dendritic cell immunotherapy for lung metastasis from murine osteosarcoma. Clin Orthop Relat Res. 2006;453:318–27.
11. Mouw JK, Yui Y, Damiano L, Bainer RO, Lakins NL, Acerbi I, Ou G, Wijekoon AC, Levental KR, Gilbert PM, Hwang ES, Chen YY, Weaver VM. Tissue mechanics modulate microRNA-dependent PTEN expression to regulate malignant progression. Nat Med. 2014;20:360–7.

Immunotherapy for Osteosarcoma

3

Tomohide Tsukahara and Takuro Wada

Abstract

Osteosarcoma is a highly malignant neoplasm occurring in young persons. The prognosis of nonresponders to chemotherapy is still poor and new treatment modalities are required. We have been working on the development and clinical application of immunotherapy for osteosarcoma since 1998. In this chapter, we describe our studies and discussed the future directions of immunotherapy for osteosarcoma.

Keywords

Tumor-associated antigen • Peptide vaccination • PBF • HLA-A24 • HLA-A2

3.1 Introduction

Osteosarcoma is a highly malignant neoplasm occurring primarily in young persons. The survival rate of patients was under 20 % before 1970. The introduction of chemotherapy raised the 5-year survival rate to 60–70 % in the 1970s [1]. Around the same time, pioneering adjuvant immunotherapy trials using autologous tumor vaccines for patients with osteosarcoma were conducted and surprisingly showed clinical benefits [2]. However, immunotherapy did not draw much attention because of the strong effects of chemotherapy. In the 2000s, the survival rate of patients with osteosarcoma has reached a plateau, and the limitations of chemotherapy have led to the spotlight focusing on immunotherapy again. In this chapter,

T. Tsukahara (✉)
Sapporo Medical University School of Medicine, South-1, West-17, Chuo-ku, Sapporo 060-8556, Japan
e-mail: tukahara@sapmed.ac.jp

T. Wada
Saiseikai Otaru Hospital, 10-1, Chikko, Otaru 047-9997, Japan

T. Ueda, A. Kawai (eds.), *Osteosarcoma*, DOI 10.1007/978-4-431-55696-1_3

we describe and discuss our studies conducted for the development of peptide-based immunotherapy for osteosarcoma from basic experiments to clinical trials and the perspectives for the future.

3.2 Development of Immunotherapy for Osteosarcoma

3.2.1 Establishment of Osteosarcoma Cell Line OS2000 Showing Humoral and Cellular Immunogenicity

First, we established the new osteosarcoma cell line OS2000 from a biopsy specimen of osteosarcoma of the right distal femur of a 16-year-old female who underwent surgical resection of both eyes due to retinoblastoma because of the lack of the tumor suppressor gene Rb at infancy. Establishing the cell line took more than 3 years [3]. OS2000 cells showed in vivo tumorigenicity in nude mice and expressed osteocalcin mRNA when treated with $1,25(OH)_2D_3$. These findings suggested that the characteristics of OS2000 were compatible with osteosarcoma. Using OS2000 and autologous sera, we performed serological identification using a recombinant expression cloning (SEREX) method to identify tumor-associated antigens recognized by the humoral immune system. As a result, we cloned cDNA coding smooth muscle myosin light chain and HLA-Cw*01:02 identical to the wild type. However, we could not detect any reactivity against these molecules in the sera of other patients with osteosarcoma.

Therefore, we next performed mixed lymphocyte-tumor cell culture using irradiated OS2000 cells as the antigenic stimulator and autologous peripheral blood mononuclear cells as the responder. The responder, TcOS2000, showed specific cytotoxicity against OS2000 cells. After limiting dilution of TcOS2000, we obtained three CTL clones specifically recognizing autologous OS2000 cells. Among them, we selected CTL clone TcOS cl-303 on the basis of the high cytotoxic ability. OS2000 expressed HLA-A*24:02, B*55:02, and Cw*01:02. TcOS cl-303 could recognize OS2000 and allogeneic osteosarcoma cell lines in the context of HLA-B*55:02.

These results suggested that human osteosarcoma could naturally prime humoral and cellular immunity. Moreover, the autologous pair of TcOS cl-303 and OS2000 could be useful as a probe to identify the antigenic peptide naturally presented by HLA-B*55:02 on osteosarcoma cells.

3.2.2 Identification of the Osteosarcoma Antigen, Papillomavirus Binding Factor (PBF)

Using the autologous pair of OS2000 and CTL clone TcOS cl-303, we performed cDNA library expression cloning. First, we constructed a cDNA library containing more than 100,000 clones from OS2000 mRNA. Next, we transiently transfected pools of library cDNA (80–120 clones per pool) into 293EBNA cells stably expressing exogenous HLA-B*55:02, followed by coculture of TcOS cl-303. The cytotoxicity of TcOS cl-303 was measured by LDH release assay, detecting LDH released from dead cells in the supernatant. After screening approximately 1000 pools of library cDNA, we selected the cDNA pool 1B9. The cDNA pool was divided into single clones (approximately 400 clones) and screened again. Four cDNA clones were recognized by TcOS cl-303 and encoded the identical cDNA sequence. We designated the antigenic cDNA clone 1B9.1H4. cDNA clone 1B9.1H4 contained the 3′ part of the open reading frame of papillomavirus binding factor (PBF). No mutations and no frameshift were identified. TcOS cl-303 could recognize the full length of PBF cDNA as well as the cDNA clone 1B9.1H4. Next, to identify CTL epitope of TcOS cl-303, we performed epitope mapping using truncated variants of PBF mRNA. We made more than 90 truncated variants. The C-terminus part of PBF was antigenic, and arginine at position 510 of 512 was the C-terminus amino acid of the CTL epitope. Subsequently, we synthesized peptides with various lengths and screened the response of TcOS cl-303 against 293EBNA cells expressing HLA-B*55:02 pulsed with each peptide. Finally, we identified a 12-mer peptide (CTACRWKKACQR) as the epitope of TcOS cl-303 and simultaneously proved that PBF was the osteosarcoma antigen recognized by the autologous CTL clone [4].

3.2.3 Expression and Function of the Osteosarcoma Antigen PBF

mRNA of PBF was expressed in various sarcoma tissues, including osteosarcoma (79 %), Ewing's sarcoma (92 %), and synovial sarcoma (90 %). In addition, mRNA of PBF was expressed in epithelial cancer tissues such as lung cancer (90 %), gastric cancer (56 %), colon cancer (14 %), and breast cancer (80 %). On the other hand, mRNA of PBF was expressed in some normal organs, including the pancreas, ovary, and spleen. However, immunohistochemistry using an anti-PBF polyclonal antibody revealed that PBF protein was detected in tumors but not in normal organs expressing PBF mRNA [4]. As shown in Table 3.1, PBF protein was expressed in osteosarcoma (92 %), Ewing's sarcoma (90 %), and synovial sarcoma (100 %). Moreover, PBF expression was significantly correlated with poor prognoses for patients with osteosarcoma and Ewing's sarcoma [5]. These results suggested that PBF might be a good candidate molecule to target in an immunotherapeutic approach using antigenic peptide vaccination.

PBF is a transcription factor containing a Zn finger domain. It was first reported to regulate transcriptional activity in the human papillomavirus type 8 genome DNA [6]. However, osteosarcoma is not related to papillomavirus infection. Therefore, we hypothesized that PBF might regulate cell survival or apoptosis in osteosarcoma cells. To characterize the function of PBF, we performed yeast two-hybrid screening using a cDNA library of OS2000 and PBF as the bait to isolate the binding partners of PBF. As a result, we obtained cDNA clone 93 encoding Scythe/BAT3 (currently designated BAG6) as the associated molecule of PBF [7]. Scythe/BAT3 was reported to be an essential factor for cell proliferation [8] and inhibitor of

Table 3.1 Expression of PBF protein in bone and soft tissue sarcoma

	PBF status*			
	Number	Negative	Low	High
Bone tumors				
Osteosarcoma				
Primary lesion	83	7	27	49
Lung metastatic lesion	8	1	2	5
Chondrosarcoma	5	2	0	3
Malignant fibrous histiocytoma	2	1	0	1
Soft tissue tumors				
Malignant fibrous histiocytoma	15	2	7	6
Liposarcoma	5	1	0	4
Rhabdomyosarcoma	3	0	0	3
Clear-cell sarcoma	3	0	1	2
Ewing's sarcoma	2	0	0	2
Synovial sarcoma	2	0	1	1
Leiomyosarcoma	2	0	1	1
Alveolar soft-part sarcoma	2	0	0	2
MPNST	1	0	0	1
Total	133	14	39	80

MPNST malignant peripheral nerve sheath tumor

*Expression of PBF was graded according to the number of tumor cells stained positively with the anti-PBF antibody; negative (<5 % positive cells), low (5–50 % positive cells), or high (>50 % positive cells)

apoptosis [9]. Surprisingly, overexpression of PBF could induce apoptosis in 293EBNA cells and OS2000 cells. However, coexpression of Scythe/BAT3 could inhibit cell death induced by PBF. Moreover, PBF and Scythe/BAT3 colocalized in the nuclei of osteosarcoma cells but in the cytoplasm of normal tissues. These results suggested that colocalization of PBF and BAG6 in nuclei might be important for the survival of osteosarcoma cells. Recently, PBF was reported to be associated with innate immunity [10] and adipogenesis [11]. The function of PBF is variable and other characteristics might be revealed in the future.

3.2.4 Expression Status of HLA Class I in Osteosarcoma

For peptide-based immunotherapy for osteosarcoma, expression of target molecules in tumor cells is required. However, the expression of HLA class I molecules is also important to present antigenic peptides toward T-cell receptors of CTLs recognizing tumor cells. To assess this issue, we analyzed the expression status of HLA class I molecules on formalin-fixed paraffin-embedded sections of primary osteosarcoma tissues by immunohistochemistry using the pan-HLA class I monoclonal antibody EMR8-5 [12]. HLA class I molecules were detected as high grade (positive cells >50 %) in 48 %, low grade (5 $\leq$ positive cells $\leq$50 %) in 32 %, and negative (positive cells <5 %) in 20 % of primary lesions of osteosarcoma. Surprisingly, the overall survival and event-free survival of the patients with HLA class I-positive osteosarcoma were significantly better than those with HLA class I-negative osteosarcoma [13]. These findings suggested that osteosarcoma might be an immunogenic tumor surveyed by the human cellular immune system. In addition, peptide-based immunotherapy might be able to elicit the response of CTLs naturally reacting with tumor cells.

3.2.5 Identification of CTL Epitopes Presented by HLA-A24 and HLA-A2

As described above, we identified the antigenic peptide encoded by PBF in the context of HLA-B*55:02. However, this epitope is not adequate to clinically immunize patients with osteosarcoma because the frequency of the allele is too low (less than 2 %) in Japanese. Therefore, we identified the CTL epitopes of PBF in the context of HLA-A*24:02 and HLA-A*02:01. At first, ten candidate peptides each for HLA-A*24:02 and HLA-A*02:01 were selected using the peptide motif prediction system BIMAS. Using in vitro peptide binding assay, we selected peptides PBF A24.2 (AYRPVSRNI) and PBF A2.2 (ALPSFQIPV) as candidates to assess their immunogenicity. Next, we synthesized MHC/peptide tetramers (HLA-A*24:02/PBF A24.2 and HLA-A*02:01/PBF A2.2) and assessed the frequency of tetramer-positive cells in peripheral mononuclear cells of patients with osteosarcoma. We found that the frequencies of tetramer-positive cells ranged from 5×10^{-7} to 7×10^{-6} and from 2×10^{-7} to 5×10^{-6} in HLA-A*24:02-positive and HLA-A*02:01-positive patients, respectively [14]. These frequencies were compatible with that of anti-MAGE-3 peptide CTL in preimmunized HLA-A1 patients with melanoma ($<1.3 \times 10^{-6}$) [15]. Moreover, tetramer-positive cells could recognize allogeneic osteosarcoma cell lines in the context of HLA-A*24:02 or HLA-A*02:01. Therefore, peptides PBF A24.2 and PBF A2.2 were used for studies of clinical vaccination.

3.2.6 Clinical PBF-Derived Peptide Vaccination Study in HLA-A24-Positive and HLA-A2-Positive Patients with Osteosarcoma

Under approval by the IRB, we started a clinical phase I peptide vaccination trial in 2008. To date, five HLA-A24-positive patients and five HLA-A2-positive patients with osteosarcoma have been enrolled in the study. Three had shown stable disease (SD) and the other seven had progressive disease (PD). One HLA-A2-positive patient with metastatic lesions in the bilateral lungs and subcutaneous region of the right lower back vaccinated with peptide PBF A2.2 survived for 31 months without any other therapeutic intervention. The patient received the peptide PBF A2.2 vaccination under three protocols: Protocol 1 (six subcutaneous vaccinations with 1 mg of peptide PBF A2.2 mixed with incomplete Freund's adjuvant [IFA] at

14-day intervals), Protocol 2 (vaccination with 10 mg of the peptide mixed with IFA), and Protocol 3 (vaccination with 1 mg of the peptide mixed with IFA and subcutaneous injection of interferon-α on the same day and 3 days after the vaccination). Although Protocol 1 and Protocol 2 were successfully completed, Protocol 3 was discontinued after the 1st vaccination because of leukopenia that might have been a side effect of interferon-α. Vaccine peptide-specific immunological responses were observed by ELISpot assay [16] in Protocols 1, 2, and 3 (Fig. 3.1a). Protocol 2 showed the best immunological response. High-dose vaccination of the peptide seemed to be more important than combination with interferon-α. Although clinical responses were evaluated as PD due to the appearance of new metastatic lesions in the lung at the end of Protocol 1, a subcutaneous metastatic lesion showed marginal calcification (Fig. 3.1b, c). Such marginal calcification was occasionally observed after chemotherapy and considered to be a partial response. For Protocol 2 and Protocol 3, clinical responses were evaluated as SD. Considering the good immunological responses and the clinical observation of marginal calcification of the subcutaneous lesion, we investigated a resected specimen of the subcutaneous metastatic lesion after Protocol 1 (Fig. 3.1d). Microscopically viable tumor cells were observed. However, immunohistochemistry reveled CD8+ T-cell infiltration into the metastatic tumor, which was not observed in the primary biopsy specimen before the vaccination therapy. Obviously, a natural nonspecific response could not be denied. Nevertheless, we believe that the tumor-infiltrating lymphocytes were elicited by the peptide vaccination and contributed to killing the tumor for a long time. The clinical phase I trial is still continuing in our institute. After the trial, we are planning a vaccination trial for HLA-A24 patients with sarcoma with high risk for metastasis, including osteosarcoma, synovial sarcoma, and Ewing's sarcoma in the adjuvant setting using a peptide cocktail. In addition to peptide PBF, an inhibitor of apoptosis protein-derived peptide survivin 2B [16] is also used.

3.3 Future Perspectives of Immunotherapy for Osteosarcoma

Recently, monoclonal antibodies against immune checkpoint molecules (ipilimumab for CTLA-4 and nivolumab for PD-1) showed dramatic clinical responses in patients with melanoma [17, 18]. However, the response might be limited to some cancers having the characteristics of natural immunogenicity. In melanoma, many mutated antigens are recognized by tumor-infiltrating lymphocytes [19, 20]. In addition, melanoma antigens could be presented to and efficiently prime specific CTLs by Langerhans cells existing abundantly in the skin around the tumor. Indeed, ipilimumab did not show any clinical benefit for patients with synovial sarcoma [21]. However, we found that chromosomal translocation SYT-SSX-derived peptide vaccination could induce an immune response and provide clinical benefits including long SD (>20 months) [22]. On the other hand, adoptive cell transfer using engineered T lymphocytes expressing TCR directed to cancer-testis antigen NY-ESO-1 showed a clinical response in synovial

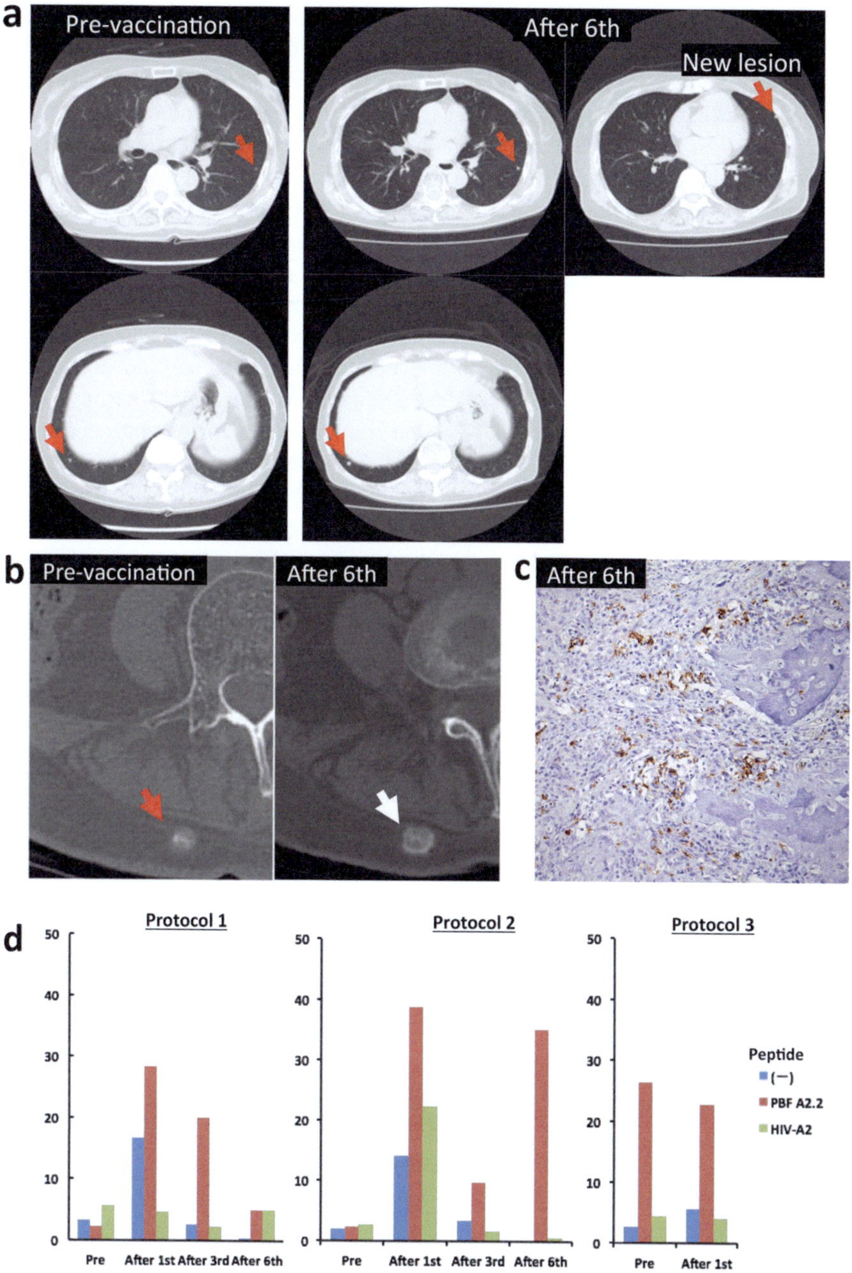

Fig. 3.1 Immunological and clinical responses against PBF peptide vaccination. (**a**) ELISpot assay. PBMC obtained from peripheral blood samples of the patient was in vitro stimulated with the peptide PBF A2.2 and used as responders for ELISpot assay. T2 cells pulsed with indicated peptides were used as stimulators. (**b**, **c**) Computed tomography of the bilateral lungs (**b**) and right lower back (**c**) before and after vaccination in Protocol 1. Metastatic lesions were indicated in *red arrows*. Marginal calcification appeared after 6th vaccination was indicated in a *white arrow*. (**d**) Immunohistochemistry of the resected subcutaneous lesion. Tumor-infiltrating CD8-positive lymphocytes were demonstrated. Original magnification was ×100

sarcoma [23]. These findings suggest that synovial sarcoma cells are sensitive to CTL and also support the idea that specific antigenic stimulation is still required for the effectiveness of immune checkpoint antibodies, especially for sarcomas.

Since the first report of human CTL-defined tumor-associated antigen MAGE [24], many tumor-associated antigens and peptides have been reported in various tumors [25]. However, we believe that many other antigens that are more suitable for immunotherapy remain undiscovered. Suitable criteria for tumor-associated antigens in the next generation are (i) overexpression in tumor cells, (ii) regulation of proliferation, and (iii) undetectable expression in normal organs except for the testis lacking expression of HLA class I molecules. Recently, Rosenberg et al. wrote that "an ideal source of antigens to target using genetically modified lymphocytes are shared mutations that are unique to each cancer type and are not found on normal tissues" [26, 27]. Adoptive transfer therapy using lymphocytes expressing exogenous TCR or a chimeric antigenic receptor combined with lymphodepletion chemotherapy showed dramatic clinical responses [28, 29]; however, excessively boosted antigen-specific T-cell immunity also destroyed normal organs expressing the same or a mimicking tumor-associated antigen and caused serious adverse effects [30, 31]. Therefore, it is imperative to identify ideal tumor-associated antigens with ultrafine specificity. Since 2006 we have focused on cancer stemlike cells/cancer-initiating cells of bone and soft tissue sarcomas, "sarcoma stem cells (SSCs)," because SSCs might be rich sources of novel tumor-associated antigens conferring on SSCs higher tumorigenicity, proliferation ability, and mobility capacity. In addition, such SSC antigens might make it possible for the immune system to distinguish highly malignant tumor cells from normal cells. We identified SSCs in bone MFH cell line MFH2003 [32] using side population analysis based on the higher drug efflux ability of SSCs more than non-SSCs [33]. Subsequently, we established a CTL clone recognizing SSCs in the context of HLA class I, aiming to identify an autologous CTL-defined SSC antigen [34]. Next, we identified SSCs in epithelioid sarcoma using the ALDEFLUOR assay based on the higher aldehyde dehydrogenase activity in SSCs and found that CD109 was highly expressed in SSCs compared to non-SSCs [35]. CD109 is also expressed in normal organs, including platelets, lung epithelium, and hematopoietic stem cells [36]. However, the glycosylation pattern of CD109 might be different in epithelioid sarcoma and normal cells. Therefore, we are trying to isolate monoclonal antibodies against CD109 with tumor-specific glycosylation. Moreover, we are currently isolating SSCs from a newly established osteosarcoma cell line based on sphere-formation ability and trying to identify SSC antigens.

On the other hand, sometimes it is very hard to activate CTLs recognizing antigenic peptides presented by HLA class I using peptide vaccination. To overcome this obstacle, we attempted to generate artificial monoclonal antibodies reacting with the HLA/peptide complex. We constructed a single-chain variable fragment (scFv) phage display library and isolated the scFv clone reacting with the HLA-A*02:01/peptide PBF A2.2 complex with high affinity ($K_D = 1.53 \times 10^{-9}$ M) [37]. Now we are trying to isolate more specific antibodies reacting with various tumor-associated antigens in the context of HLA class I with the aim of the development and clinical application of novel therapeutic antibodies.

References

1. Ferrari S, Palmerini E. Adjuvant and neoadjuvant combination chemotherapy for osteogenic sarcoma. Curr Opin Oncol. 2007;19:341–6.
2. Southam CM, Marcove RC, Levin AG, Buchsbaum HJ, Mike V. Proceedings: clinical trial of autogenous tumor vaccine for treatment of osteogenic sarcoma. Proc Natl Cancer Conf. 1972;7:91–100.
3. Nabeta Y, Kawaguchi S, Sahara H, Ikeda H, Hirohashi Y, Goroku T, Sato Y, Tsukahara T, Torigoe T, Wada T, Kaya M, Hiraga H, Isu K, Yamawaki S, Ishii S, Yamashita T, Sato N. Recognition by cellular and humoral autologous immunity in a human osteosarcoma cell line. J Orthop Sci. 2003;8:554–9.
4. Tsukahara T, Nabeta Y, Kawaguchi S, Ikeda H, Sato Y, Shimozawa K, Ida K, Asanuma H, Hirohashi Y, Torigoe T, Hiraga H, Nagoya S, Wada T, Yamashita T, Sato N. Identification of human autologous cytotoxic T-lymphocyte-defined osteosarcoma gene that encodes a transcriptional regulator, papillomavirus binding factor. Cancer Res. 2004;64:5442–8.
5. Yabe H, Tsukahara T, Kawaguchi S, Wada T, Sato N, Morioka H, Yabe H. Overexpression of papillomavirus binding factor in Ewing's sarcoma family of tumors conferring poor prognosis. Oncol Rep. 2008;19:129–34.
6. Boeckle S, Pfister H, Steger G. A new cellular factor recognizes E2 binding sites of papillomaviruses which mediate transcriptional repression by E2. Virology. 2002;293:103–17.
7. Tsukahara T, Kimura S, Ichimiya S, Torigoe T, Kawaguchi S, Wada T, Yamashita T, Sato N. Scythe/BAT3 regulates apoptotic cell death induced by papillomavirus binding factor in human osteosarcoma. Cancer Sci. 2009;100:47–53.
8. Desmots F, Russell HR, Lee Y, Boyd K, McKinnon PJ. The reaper-binding protein scythe modulates apoptosis and proliferation during mammalian development. Mol Cell Biol. 2005;25:10329–37.
9. Minami R, Shimada M, Yokosawa H, Kawahara H. Scythe regulates apoptosis through modulating ubiquitin-mediated proteolysis of the Xenopus elongation factor XEF1AO. Biochem J. 2007;405:495–501.
10. Jordanovski D, Herwartz C, Pawlowski A, Taute S, Frommolt P, Steger G. The hypoxia-inducible transcription factor ZNF395 is controlled by IkB kinase-signaling and activates genes involved in the innate immune response and cancer. PLoS One. 2013;8:e74911.
11. Hasegawa R, Tomaru Y, de Hoon M, Suzuki H, Hayashizaki Y, Shin JW. Identification of ZNF395 as a novel modulator of adipogenesis. Exp Cell Res. 2013;319:68–76.
12. Torigoe T, Asanuma H, Nakazawa E, Tamura Y, Hirohashi Y, Yamamoto E, Kanaseki T, Hasegawa T, Sato N. Establishment of a monoclonal anti-pan HLA class I antibody suitable for immunostaining of formalin-fixed tissue: unusually high frequency of down-regulation in breast cancer tissues. Pathol Int. 2012;62:303–8.
13. Tsukahara T, Kawaguchi S, Torigoe T, Asanuma H, Nakazawa E, Shimozawa K, Nabeta Y, Kimura S, Kaya M, Nagoya S, Wada T, Yamashita T, Sato N. Prognostic significance of HLA class I expression in osteosarcoma defined by anti-pan HLA class I monoclonal antibody, EMR8-5. Cancer Sci. 2006;97:1374–80.
14. Tsukahara T, Kawaguchi S, Torigoe T, Murase M, Wada T, Kaya M, Nagoya S, Yamashita T, Sato N. HLA-A*0201-restricted CTL epitope of a novel osteosarcoma antigen, papillomavirus binding factor. J Transl Med. 2009;7:44.
15. Coulie PG, Karanikas V, Colau D, Lurquin C, Landry C, Marchand M, Dorval T, Brichard V, Boon T. A monoclonal cytolytic T-lymphocyte response observed in a melanoma patient vaccinated with a tumor-specific antigenic peptide encoded by gene MAGE-3. Proc Natl Acad Sci U S A. 2001;98:10290–5.
16. Kameshima H, Tsuruma T, Kutomi G, Shima H, Iwayama Y, Kimura Y, Imamura M, Torigoe T, Takahashi A, Hirohashi Y, Tamura Y, Tsukahara T, Kanaseki T, Sato N, Hirata K. Immunotherapeutic benefit of alpha-interferon (IFNalpha) in survivin2B-derived peptide vaccination for advanced pancreatic cancer patients. Cancer Sci. 2013;104:124–9.

17. Hodi FS, O'Day SJ, McDermott DF, Weber RW, Sosman JA, Haanen JB, Gonzalez R, Robert C, Schadendorf D, Hassel JC, Akerley W, van den Eertwegh AJ, Lutzky J, Lorigan P, Vaubel JM, Linette GP, Hogg D, Ottensmeier CH, Lebbe C, Peschel C, Quirt I, Clark JI, Wolchok JD, Weber JS, Tian J, Yellin MJ, Nichol GM, Hoos A, Urba WJ. Improved survival with ipilimumab in patients with metastatic melanoma. N Engl J Med. 2010;363:711–23.
18. Wolchok JD, Kluger H, Callahan MK, Postow MA, Rizvi NA, Lesokhin AM, Segal NH, Ariyan CE, Gordon RA, Reed K, Burke MM, Caldwell A, Kronenberg SA, Agunwamba BU, Zhang X, Lowy I, Inzunza HD, Feely W, Horak CE, Hong Q, Korman AJ, Wigginton JM, Gupta A, Sznol M. Nivolumab plus ipilimumab in advanced melanoma. N Engl J Med. 2013;369:122–33.
19. Robbins PF, El-Gamil M, Li YF, Kawakami Y, Loftus D, Appella E, Rosenberg SA. A mutated beta-catenin gene encodes a melanoma-specific antigen recognized by tumor infiltrating lymphocytes. J Exp Med. 1996;183:1185–92.
20. Robbins PF, Lu YC, El-Gamil M, Li YF, Gross C, Gartner J, Lin JC, Teer JK, Cliften P, Tycksen E, Samuels Y, Rosenberg SA. Mining exomic sequencing data to identify mutated antigens recognized by adoptively transferred tumor-reactive T cells. Nat Med. 2013;19:747–52.
21. Maki RG, Jungbluth AA, Gnjatic S, Schwartz GK, D'Adamo DR, Keohan ML, Wagner MJ, Scheu K, Chiu R, Ritter E, Kachel J, Lowy I, Old LJ, Ritter G. A pilot study of anti-CTLA4 antibody ipilimumab in patients with synovial sarcoma. Sarcoma. 2013;2013:168145.
22. Kawaguchi S, Tsukahara T, Ida K, Kimura S, Murase M, Kano M, Emori M, Nagoya S, Kaya M, Torigoe T, Ueda E, Takahashi A, Ishii T, Tatezaki S, Toguchida J, Tsuchiya H, Osanai T, Sugita T, Sugiura H, Ieguchi M, Ihara K, Hamada K, Kakizaki H, Morii T, Yasuda T, Tanizawa T, Ogose A, Yabe H, Yamashita T, Sato N, Wada T. SYT-SSX breakpoint peptide vaccines in patients with synovial sarcoma: a study from the Japanese Musculoskeletal Oncology Group. Cancer Sci. 2012;103:1625–30.
23. Robbins PF, Morgan RA, Feldman SA, Yang JC, Sherry RM, Dudley ME, Wunderlich JR, Nahvi AV, Helman LJ, Mackall CL, Kammula US, Hughes MS, Restifo NP, Raffeld M, Lee CC, Levy CL, Li YF, El-Gamil M, Schwarz SL, Laurencot C, Rosenberg SA. Tumor regression in patients with metastatic synovial cell sarcoma and melanoma using genetically engineered lymphocytes reactive with NY-ESO-1. J Clin Oncol. 2011;29:917–24.
24. Van der Bruggen P, Traversari C, Chomez P, Lurquin C, De Plaen E, Van den Eynde B, Knuth A, Boon T. A gene encoding an antigen recognized by cytolytic T lymphocytes on a human melanoma. Science. 1991;254:1643–7.
25. Van Der Bruggen P, Stroobant V, Van Pel A, Van den Eynde B. Peptide database: T cell-defined tumor antigens. Cancer Immun. 2013;13:15.
26. Rosenberg SA. Finding suitable targets is the major obstacle to cancer gene therapy. Cancer Gene Ther. 2014;21:45–7.
27. Tran E, Turcotte S, Gros A, Robbins PF, Lu YC, Dudley ME, Wunderlich JR, Somerville RP, Hogan K, Hinrichs CS, Parkhurst MR, Yang JC, Rosenberg SA. Cancer immunotherapy based on mutation-specific CD4+ T cells in a patient with epithelial cancer. Science. 2014;344:641–5.
28. Rosenberg SA, Restifo NP, Yang JC, Morgan RA, Dudley ME. Adoptive cell transfer: a clinical path to effective cancer immunotherapy. Nat Rev Cancer. 2008;8:299–308.
29. Porter DL, Levine BL, Kalos M, Bagg A, June CH. Chimeric antigen receptor-modified T cells in chronic lymphoid leukemia. N Engl J Med. 2011;365:725–33.
30. Morgan RA, Yang JC, Kitano M, Dudley ME, Laurencot CM, Rosenberg SA. Case report of a serious adverse event following the administration of T cells transduced with a chimeric antigen receptor recognizing ERBB2. Mol Ther. 2010;18:843–51.
31. Morgan RA, Chinnasamy N, Abate-Daga D, Gros A, Robbins PF, Zheng Z, Dudley ME, Feldman SA, Yang JC, Sherry RM, Phan GQ, Hughes MS, Kammula US, Miller AD, Hessman CJ, Stewart AA, Restifo NP, Quezado MM, Alimchandani M, Rosenberg AZ, Nath A,

Wang T, Bielekova B, Wuest SC, Akula N, McMahon FJ, Wilde S, Mosetter B, Schendel DJ, Laurencot CM, Rosenberg SA. Cancer regression and neurological toxicity following anti-MAGE-A3 TCR gene therapy. J Immunother. 2013;36:133–51.
32. Tsukahara T, Kawaguchi S, Ida K, Kimura S, Tamura Y, Ikeda T, Torigoe T, Nagoya S, Wada T, Sato N, Yamashita T. HLA-restricted specific tumor cytolysis by autologous T-lymphocytes infiltrating metastatic bone malignant fibrous histiocytoma of lymph node. J Orthop Res. 2006;24:94–101.
33. Murase M, Kano M, Tsukahara T, Takahashi A, Torigoe T, Kawaguchi S, Kimura S, Wada T, Uchihashi Y, Kondo T, Yamashita T, Sato N. Side population cells have the characteristics of cancer stem-like cells/cancer-initiating cells in bone sarcomas. Br J Cancer. 2009;101:1425–32.
34. Kano M, Tsukahara T, Emori M, Murase M, Torigoe T, Kawaguchi S, Wada T, Yamashita T, Sato N. Autologous CTL response against cancer stem-like cells/cancer-initiating cells of bone malignant fibrous histiocytoma. Cancer Sci. 2011;102:1443–7.
35. Emori M, Tsukahara T, Murase M, Kano M, Murata K, Takahashi A, Kubo T, Asanuma H, Yasuda K, Kochin V, Kaya M, Nagoya S, Nishio J, Iwasaki H, Sonoda T, Hasegawa T, Torigoe T, Wada T, Yamashita T, Sato N. High expression of CD109 antigen regulates the phenotype of cancer stem-like cells/cancer-initiating cells in the novel epithelioid sarcoma cell line ESX and is related to poor prognosis of soft tissue sarcoma. PLoS One. 2013;8:e84187.
36. Hwang SM, Kim MJ, Chang HE, Hong YJ, Kim TS, Song EY, Park KU, Song J, Han KS. Human platelet antigen genotyping and expression of CD109 (human platelet antigen 15) mRNA in various human cell types. Biomed Res Int. 2013;2013:946403.
37. Tsukahara T, Emori M, Murata K, Hirano T, Muroi N, Kyono M, Toji S, Watanabe K, Torigoe T, Kochin V, Asanuma H, Matsumiya H, Yamashita K, Himi T, Ichimiya S, Wada T, Yamashita T, Hasegawa T, Sato N. Specific targeting of a naturally presented osteosarcoma antigen PBF peptide using an artificial monoclonal antibody. J Biol Chem. 2014;289:22035.

Part II

Clinical Features

Outcome of Treatment for Osteosarcoma of the Extremities Over the Last 20 Years: Report from 11 Referral Centers in Japan

4

Koichi Ogura, Hiroaki Hiraga, Takeshi Ishii, Toshifumi Ozaki, Yoshihiro Nishida, Hideo Morioka, Toru Hiruma, Takafumi Ueda, Nobuhito Araki, Norifumi Naka, Hirotaka Kawano, and Akira Kawai

K. Ogura
Department of Musculoskeletal Oncology, National Cancer Center Hospital, 5-1-1 Tsukiji, Chuo-ku, Tokyo 104-0045, Japan

Department of Orthopaedic Surgery, The University of Tokyo Hospital, Tokyo, Japan

H. Hiraga
Department of Orthopaedic Surgery, Hokkaido Cancer Center, Hokkaido, Japan

T. Ishii
Department of Orthopaedic Surgery, Chiba Cancer Center, Chiba, Japan

T. Ozaki
Department of Orthopaedic Surgery, Okayama University, Okayama, Japan

Y. Nishida
Department of Orthopaedic Surgery, Nagoya University, Aichi, Japan

H. Morioka
Department of Orthopaedic Surgery, Keio University, Tokyo, Japan

T. Hiruma
Department of Orthopaedic Surgery, Kanagawa Cancer Center, Kanagawa, Japan

T. Ueda
Department of Orthopaedic Surgery, Osaka National Hospital, Osaka, Japan

N. Araki
Department of Orthopaedic Surgery, Osaka Medical Center for Cancer and Cardiovascular Diseases, Osaka, Japan

N. Naka
Department of Orthopaedic Surgery, Osaka University, Osaka, Japan

H. Kawano
Department of Orthopaedic Surgery, The University of Tokyo Hospital, Tokyo, Japan

A. Kawai (✉)
Department of Musculoskeletal Oncology, National Cancer Center Hospital, 5-1-1 Tsukiji, Chuo-ku, Tokyo 104-0045, Japan
e-mail: akawai@ncc.go.jp

T. Ueda, A. Kawai (eds.), *Osteosarcoma*, DOI 10.1007/978-4-431-55696-1_4

Abstract

The survival of patients with osteosarcoma has improved dramatically due to the introduction of effective systemic chemotherapy. The key standard drugs for osteosarcoma chemotherapy are methotrexate, doxorubicin, and cisplatin, and multi-institutional trials based on these drugs have been conducted in Japan since the 1990s. However, there have been no nationwide data on treatment outcome, especially with regard to survival and prognostic factors. In this chapter, therefore, we present data from a large nationwide cohort of patients with osteosarcoma treated at 11 referral centers in Japan during the period 1990–2010 with special reference to survival and relevant prognostic factors. The 3-, 5-, and 10-year metastasis-free survival and overall survival rates for the 529 patients were 70 %, 64 %, and 62 % and 88 %, 83 %, and 77 %, respectively. The prognosis for patients with osteosarcoma in Japan was comparable to, or slightly better than, those reported in other countries. International collaboration should also be conducted in Asian countries including Japan to improve the outcome further and find the optimal treatment for osteosarcoma.

Keywords

Osteosarcoma • Prognosis • Prognostic factor • Japan

4.1 Background

Osteosarcoma is the most common sarcoma of bone, characterized by production of immature osteoid by the tumor cells. The long-term survival of osteosarcoma patients has improved dramatically since the 1970s following the introduction of effective systemic chemotherapy [1–4]. The key drugs employed in standard chemotherapy for osteosarcoma have been high-dose methotrexate, doxorubicin, and cisplatin (MAP) [5]. Ifosfamide has also been reported to be active against osteosarcoma [6]. A more favorable outcome with 5-year survival rates of 60–80 % has been reported for patients with nonmetastatic osteosarcoma receiving intensive multidrug chemotherapy with these key drugs and aggressive surgery for local control [5, 7–12].

In Japan, a multi-institutional phase II study of neoadjuvant chemotherapy for osteosarcoma (the NECO study) [13] was conducted between 1993 and 2004, and currently the randomized trial JCOG 0905 study [14], started in 2010, is now in progress. In these trials, patients with nonmetastatic osteosarcoma received the MAP regimen, or MAP plus ifosfamide, and neoadjuvant chemotherapy using these key drugs and surgery has been the standard treatment in Japan since the 1990s.

In this chapter, we present nationwide data pertaining to survival and associated prognostic factors of patients with nonmetastatic osteosarcoma of the extremities since the treatment became standardized in the 1990s.

Table 4.1 Descriptive characteristics of the study population

Characteristic	No. of patients	%
Entire population	529	100
Age, years; mean [SD]	20.0 [12.9]	
≤12	134	25.3
13–19	227	42.9
20–39	121	22.9
40–	47	8.9
Sex		
Male	326	61.6
Female	203	38.4
Tumor size, cm: mean [SD]	9.6 [4.1]	
≤8	237	44.8
>8	292	55.2
Tumor site		
Distal extremity[a]	42	7.9
Distal femur	251	47.4
Proximal tibia/fibula	151	28.5
Proximal humerus	47	8.9
Proximal femur	38	7.2
Pathologic fracture		
No	489	92.4
Yes	40	7.6
Histologic response (tumor necrotic rate, %)		
Grade 1 (<50)	133	25.1
Grade 2 (50–89)	161	30.4
Grade 3 (90–99)	169	31.9
Grade 4 (100)	66	12.5
Type of surgery		
Limb salvage	420	79.4
Amputation	71	13.4
Unknown	38	7.2
Surgical margin		
Negative	193	36.5
Positive	1	0.2
Unknown	335	63.3

SD standard deviation

[a]The distal extremity was defined as any location distal to the knee or elbow joint with the exception of the proximal tibia/fibula (i.e., the radius, ulna, distal tibia, or hand and foot)

4.2 Eligibility and Data Extraction

The inclusion criteria for patients were (1) a histological diagnosis of high-grade osteosarcoma of the extremity, (2) no distant metastasis at presentation, (3) scheduled for neoadjuvant chemotherapy and surgery, and (4) a follow-up period of more than 3 years for survivors. During the whole period 1990–2010, we identified 529 eligible patients who met the inclusion criteria and for whom sufficient data were available.

The following data were extracted from 11 major referral centers in Japan (National Cancer Center Hospital ($N=104$), Hokkaido Cancer Center ($N=74$), Chiba Cancer Center ($N=61$), Okayama University ($N=50$), Nagoya University ($N=48$), Keio University ($N=42$), Kanagawa Cancer Center Hospital ($N=37$), Osaka Medical Center for Cancer and Cardiovascular Diseases ($N=36$), the University of Tokyo Hospital ($N=29$), Osaka National Hospital ($N=27$), and Osaka University ($N=21$)): patient age at diagnosis, sex, primary tumor site, maximal tumor size, presence or absence of pathologic fracture before surgery (i.e., at diagnosis and during preoperative chemotherapy), type of surgery (limb salvage surgery or amputation), surgical margin (positive or negative), and histologic response to preoperative chemotherapy. The demographic data for the 529 patients are shown in Table 4.1. The mean follow-up period was 94 months (range, 12–291 months).

4.3 Survival and Prognostic Factors

Distant metastasis and tumor-related death occurred in 194 patients and 106 patients, respectively. The data for metastasis-free survival (MFS) and overall survival (OAS) estimated using the Kaplan-Meier method are shown Fig. 4.1a, b.

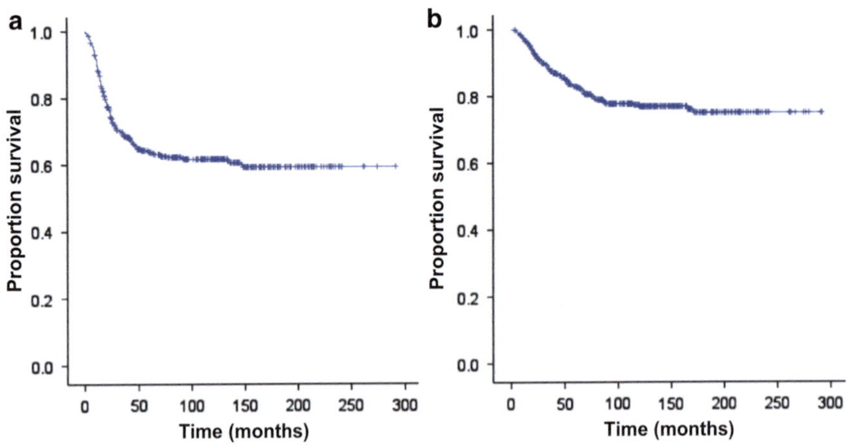

Fig. 4.1 Kaplan-Meier plots for the patients overall (MFS (**a**) and OAS (**b**))

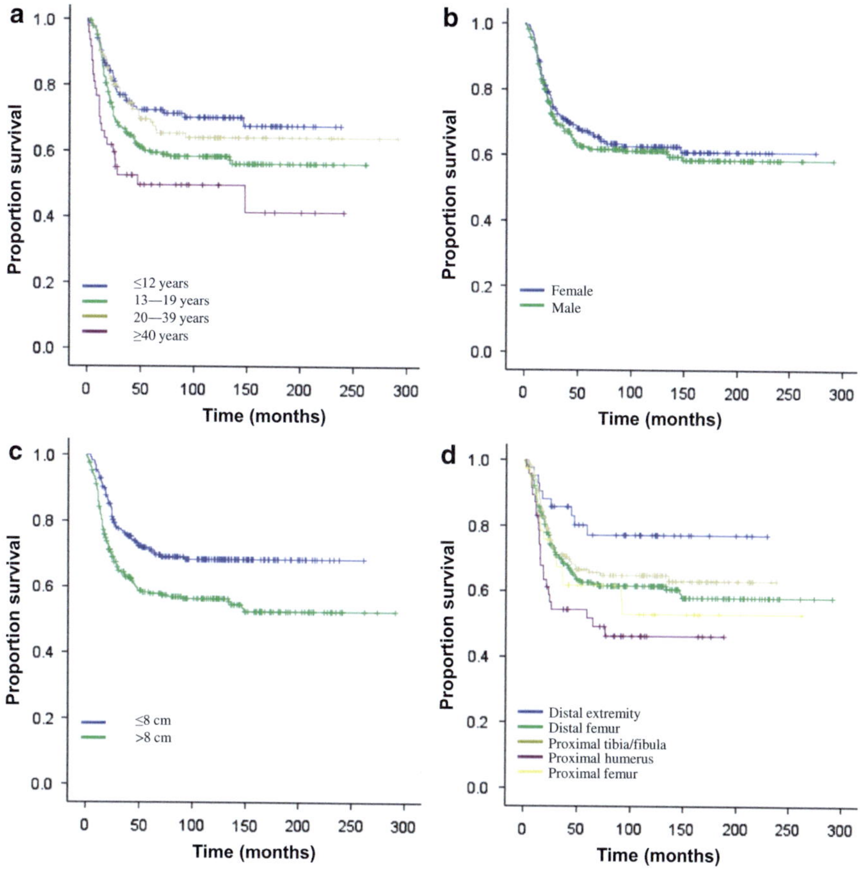

Fig. 4.2 (continued)

The 3-, 5-, and 10-year MFS rates and OAS rates for the 529 patients were 70 %, 64 %, and 62 % and 88 %, 83 %, and 77 %, respectively. The univariate associations of the various factors with the MFS and OAS rates determined using Kaplan-Meier plots are shown in Figs. 4.2a–g and 4.3a–g, respectively.

Table 4.2 shows the univariate and multivariate Cox proportional hazard models for MFS and OAS. Multivariate analyses demonstrated significant associations between distant metastasis and a patient age of 13–19 years (hazard ratio [HR], 1.56; 95 % confidence interval [CI], 1.07–2.29; $P = 0.022$) or ≥40 years (HR, 2.13; 95 % CI, 1.26–3.59; $P = 0.005$), tumor size >8 cm (HR, 1.58; 95 % CI, 1.17–2.14; $P = 0.003$), tumor location in the proximal humerus (HR, 2.86; 95 % CI, 1.32–6.19; $P = 0.008$), presence of pathologic fracture (HR, 1.75; 95 % CI, 1.10–2.78; $P = 0.018$), and tumor necrotic rate (50–89 % (HR, 0.66; 95 % CI, 0.47–0.94; $P = 0.021$), 90–99 % (HR, 0.53; 95 % CI, 0.36–0.77; $P = 0.001$), and 100 % (HR,

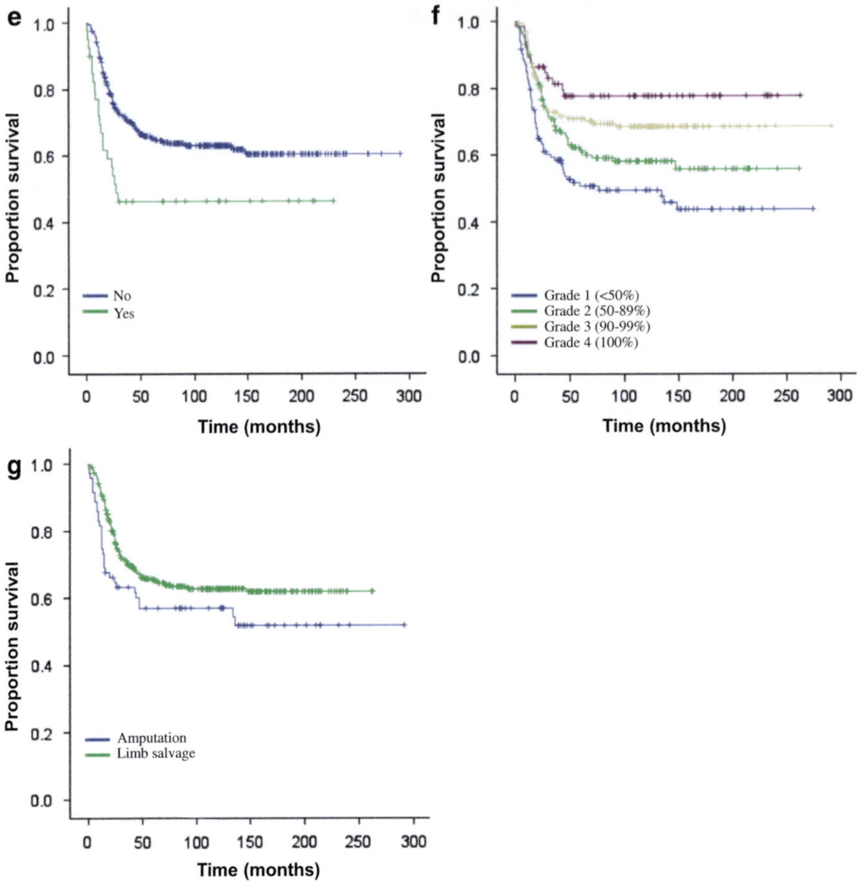

Fig. 4.2 Kaplan-Meier survival plots stratified by predictor variables on MFS: (**a**) age (≤12, 13–19, 20–39, ≥40 year), (**b**) sex, (**c**) tumor size (≤8 cm, >8 cm), (**d**) tumor site (distal extremity, distal femur, proximal tibia/fibula, proximal humerus, proximal femur), (**e**) pathologic fracture, (**f**) histologic response to preoperative chemotherapy, and (**g**) type of surgery (limb salvage, amputation)

0.36; 95 % CI, 0.20–0.65; *P* = 0.001)). Moreover, multivariate analyses demonstrated significant associations between tumor-related death and a patient age of 13–19 years (HR, 1.76; 95 % CI, 1.00–3.08; *P* = 0.048) or ≥40 years (HR, 3.91; 95 % CI, 1.96–7.78; *P* < 0.001), tumor size >8 cm (HR, 1.61; 95 % CI, 1.06–2.46; *P* = 0.026), tumor site (distal femur (HR, 8.48; 95 % CI, 1.17–61.68; *P* = 0.035), proximal tibia/fibula (HR, 10.94; 95 % CI, 1.49–80.32; *P* = 0.019), proximal humerus (HR, 9.42; 95 % CI, 1.20–73.89; *P* = 0.033), and proximal femur (HR, 14.07; 95 % CI, 1.83–108.16; *P* = 0.011)), presence of pathologic fracture (HR, 2.72; 95 % CI, 1.56–4.74; *P* < 0.001), and tumor necrotic rate (50–89 % (HR,

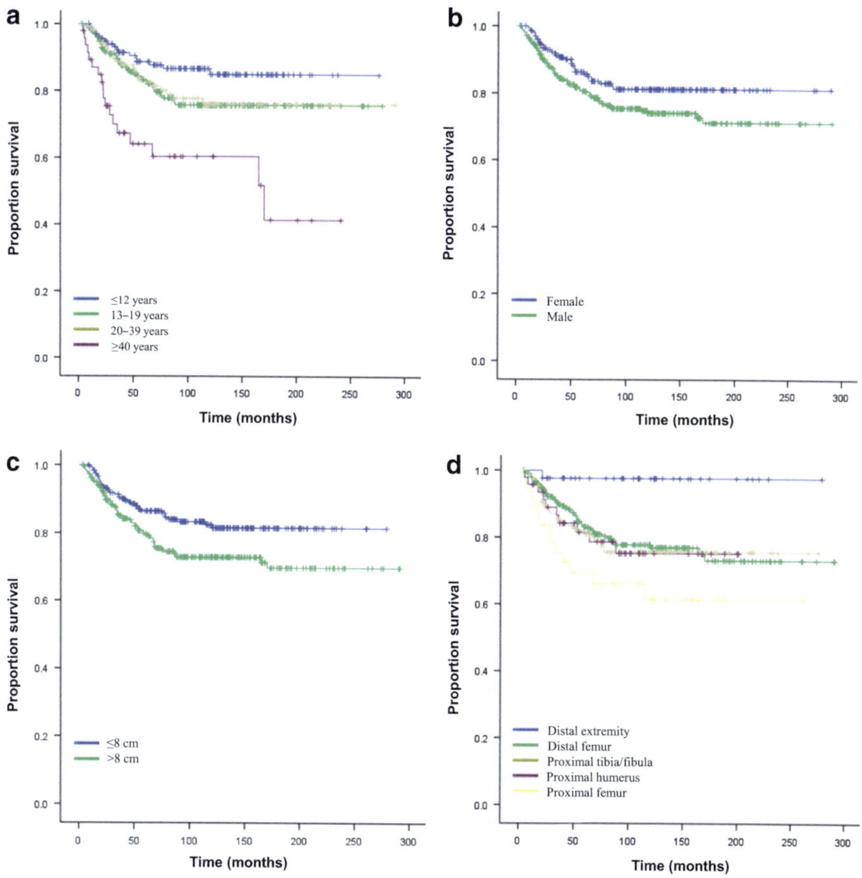

Fig. 4.3 (continued)

0.56; 95 % CI, 0.35–0.90; $P = 0.015$), 90–99 % (HR, 0.48; 95 % CI, 0.29–0.79; $P = 0.004$), and 100 % (HR, 0.30; 95 % CI, 0.13–0.68; $P = 0.004$)).

4.4 Comparison with Previous Reports

Table 4.3 gives a summary of previous reports of large series published after 2000 in relation to survival and prognostic factors for osteosarcoma [11, 15–19]. The survival rate in the present series (5-year MFS 64 %, OAS 83 %) is comparable to, or slightly better than, those in previous reports. Tumor size, tumor location, and histologic response to preoperative chemotherapy were prognostic factors common to all these reports, whereas age, sex, and pathologic fracture were not consistent

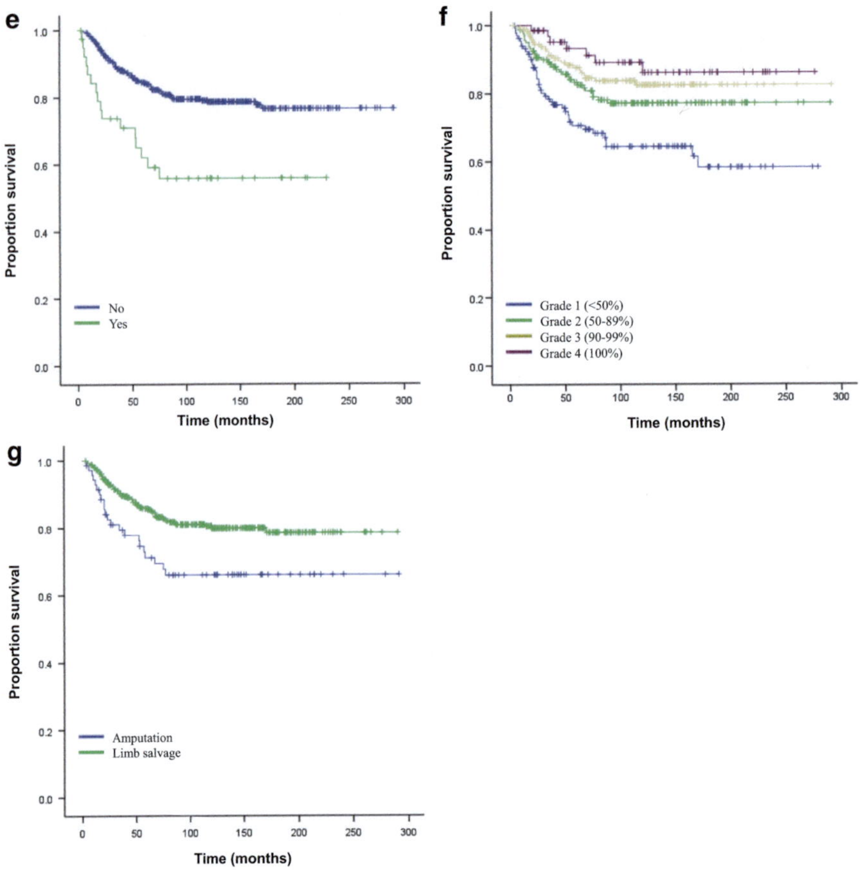

Fig. 4.3 Kaplan-Meier survival plots stratified by predictor variables on OAS: (**a**) age ($\leq$12, 13–19, 20–39, $\geq$40 year), (**b**) sex, (**c**) tumor size ($\leq$8 cm, >8 cm), (**d**) tumor site (distal extremity, distal femur, proximal tibia/fibula, proximal humerus, proximal femur), (**e**) pathologic fracture, (**f**) histologic response to preoperative chemotherapy, and (**g**) type of surgery (limb salvage, amputation)

[11, 15–19]. Among these inconsistent factors, we have shown that age and pathologic fracture both had a significant impact on survival.

4.5 Future Direction

On the basis of a nationwide patient cohort treated between 1990 and 2010 in Japan, we have identified survival rate (MFS and OAS) and prognostic factors related to the survival of patients with nonmetastatic osteosarcoma of the extremity receiving

Table 4.2 Cox proportional hazards models for MFS and OAS

	MFS				OAS			
	Univariate analysis		Multivariate analysis		Univariate analysis		Multivariate analysis	
	Hazard ratio (95 % CI)	*P* value	Hazard ratio (95 % CI)	*P* value	Hazard ratio (95 % CI)	*P* value	Hazard ratio (95 % CI)	*P* value
Age (year)								
≤12	Reference		Reference		Reference		Reference	
13–19	1.51 (1.04–2.21)	0.032	1.56 (1.07–2.29)	0.022	1.71 (0.98–2.97)	0.059	1.76 (1.00–3.08)	0.048
20–39	1.17 (0.75–1.82)	0.496	1.18 (0.75–1.86)	0.470	1.64 (0.88–3.04)	0.121	1.81 (0.96–3.42)	0.067
40–	2.41 (1.45–4.02)	0.001	2.13 (1.26–3.59)	0.005	4.31 (2.22–8.38)	<0.001	3.91 (1.96–7.78)	<0.001
Sex								
Male	Reference	0.505	Reference		Reference		Reference	
Female	0.91 (0.68–1.21)	0.506	0.92 (0.69–1.24)	0.591	0.82 (0.66–1.00)	0.055	0.68 (0.45–1.04)	0.074
Tumor size								
≤8 cm	Reference		Reference		Reference		Reference	
>8 cm	1.66 (1.24–2.22)	0.001	1.58 (1.17–2.14)	0.003	1.66 (1.11–2.47)	0.013	1.61 (1.06–2.46)	0.026
Tumor site								
Distal extremity	Reference		Reference		Reference		Reference	
Distal femur	1.99 (1.00–3.94)	0.049	1.81 (0.91–3.61)	0.091	9.30 (1.29–67.39)	0.027	8.48 (1.17–61.68)	0.035
Proximal tibia/fibula	1.75 (0.86–3.55)	0.123	1.73 (0.85–3.54)	0.131	10.25 (1.40–74.92)	0.022	10.94 (1.49–80.32)	0.019
Proximal humerus	3.16 (1.47–6.79)	0.003	2.86 (1.32–6.19)	0.008	10.41 (1.33–81.31)	0.026	9.42 (1.20–73.89)	0.033
Proximal femur	2.32 (1.03–5.26)	0.043	1.92 (0.84–4.37)	0.122	18.00 (2.35–137.59)	0.005	14.07 (1.83–108.16)	0.011
Pathologic fracture								

(continued)

Table 4.2 (continued)

	MFS				OAS			
	Univariate analysis		Multivariate analysis		Univariate analysis		Multivariate analysis	
	Hazard ratio (95 % CI)	*P* value	Hazard ratio (95 % CI)	*P* value	Hazard ratio (95 % CI)	*P* value	Hazard ratio (95 % CI)	*P* value
No	Reference		Reference		Reference		Reference	
Yes	1.95 (1.24–3.07)	0.004	1.75 (1.10–2.78)	0.018	2.60 (1.53–4.42)	<0.001	2.72 (1.56–4.74)	<0.001
Histologic response (tumor necrotic rate, %)								
Grade 1 (<50)	Reference		Reference		Reference		Reference	
Grade 2 (50–89)	0.69 (0.49–0.97)	0.032	0.66 (0.47–0.94)	0.021	0.55 (0.35–0.87)	0.010	0.56 (0.35–0.90)	0.015
Grade 3 (90–99)	0.50 (0.35–0.72)	<0.001	0.53 (0.36–0.77)	0.001	0.40 (0.24–0.66)	<0.001	0.48 (0.29–0.79)	0.004
Grade 4 (100)	0.34 (0.19–0.61)	<0.001	0.36 (0.20–0.65)	0.001	0.27 (0.12–0.60)	0.001	0.30 (0.13–0.68)	0.004

CI confidence interval

Table 4.3 Summary of previous reports regarding survival and prognostic factors

Report	Journal	Institution	*N*	Survival	Prognostic factors
Bielack [11]	J Clin Oncol, 2002	Cooperative Osteosarcoma Study Group	1702	5-year OAS, 65 %	OAS: macroscopic residual tumor, response to chemotherapy (necrotic rate), metastases at diagnosis, tumor location, tumor size
				5-year EFS, 52 %	
Grimer [16]	JBJS Br, 2002	European Osteosarcoma Intergroup Study	202	5-year OAS, 57 %	OAS: tumor size and volume, tumor location, ALP, response to chemotherapy (necrotic rate), type of surgery, local recurrence
				5-year EFS, 63 %	
Smeland [19]	Eur J Cancer, 2003	Scandinavian Sarcoma Group Osteosarcoma	113	5-year OAS, 74 %	EFS: tumor volume, 24-h serum methotrexate level, sex
				5-year EFS, 63 %	
Bacci [15]	Cancer, 2006	Istituto Ortopedico Rizzoli	789	5-year OAS, 66 %	EFS: age, ALP, protocol of chemotherapy, surgical margin, response to chemotherapy (necrotic rate)
				5-year EFS, 60 %	
Kim [18]	Ann Oncol, 2009	Korea Cancer Center Hospital	365	5-year MFS, 60 %	MFS: age, tumor size, tumor location, response to chemotherapy (necrotic rate)
Janeway [17]	Cancer, 2012	Children's Oncology Group	1054	5-year OAS, 69 %	OAS: age, tumor site, metastases at diagnosis
				5-year EFS, 56 %	EFS: age, tumor site, metastases at diagnosis
Present study		Japanese 11 referral centers	529	5-year OAS, 69 %	OAS and MFS: age, tumor size, tumor site, pathologic fracture, response to chemotherapy (necrotic rate)
				5-year EFS, 56 %	

intensive multidrug chemotherapy and surgery. Over the two decades covered by the study, treatment outcome in Japan was comparable to, or slightly better than, those in previous reports. However, despite the recent improvement in survival, a substantial number of patients still develop metastases or suffer tumor-related death. With regard to studies abroad, the EURAMOS-1 study, an open-label phase III randomized controlled trial, is currently in progress through collaboration among four osteosarcoma study groups in the USA and Europe [20, 21]. International collaboration should also be conducted in Asian countries including Japan to improve the outcome of osteosarcoma and find an optimal treatment for it.

Acknowledgments The authors would like to acknowledge Tsukasa Yonemoto, Shintaro Iwata, Hiroto Kamoda, and Yoko Hagiwara (Chiba Cancer Center); Tomohiro Fujiwara (Okayama University); Eiji Kozawa (Nagoya University); Shigeki Kakunaga (Osaka National Hospital); and Yusuke Shinoda and Yusuke Tsuda (The University of Tokyo Hospital) for data collection and kind assistance.

References

1. Rosen G, Marcove RC, Huvos AG, Caparros BI, Lane JM, Nirenberg A, et al. Primary osteogenic sarcoma: eight-year experience with adjuvant chemotherapy. J Cancer Res Clin Oncol. 1983;106(Suppl):55–67.
2. Eilber F, Giuliano A, Eckardt J, Patterson K, Moseley S, Goodnight J. Adjuvant chemotherapy for osteosarcoma: a randomized prospective trial. J Clin Oncol. 1987;5(1):21–6.
3. Link MP, Goorin AM, Miser AW, Green AA, Pratt CB, Belasco JB, et al. The effect of adjuvant chemotherapy on relapse-free survival in patients with osteosarcoma of the extremity. N Engl J Med. 1986;314(25):1600–6. doi:10.1056/NEJM198606193142502.
4. Link MP, Goorin AM, Horowitz M, Meyer WH, Belasco J, Baker A, et al. Adjuvant chemotherapy of high-grade osteosarcoma of the extremity. Updated results of the multi-institutional osteosarcoma study. Clin Orthop Relat Res. 1991;270:8–14.
5. Meyers PA, Schwartz CL, Krailo M, Kleinerman ES, Betcher D, Bernstein ML, et al. Osteosarcoma: a randomized, prospective trial of the addition of ifosfamide and/or muramyl tripeptide to cisplatin, doxorubicin, and high-dose methotrexate. J Clin Oncol. 2005;23(9):2004–11. doi:10.1200/JCO.2005.06.031.
6. Harris MB, Cantor AB, Goorin AM, Shochat SJ, Ayala AG, Ferguson WS, et al. Treatment of osteosarcoma with ifosfamide: comparison of response in pediatric patients with recurrent disease versus patients previously untreated: a Pediatric Oncology Group study. Med Pediatr Oncol. 1995;24(2):87–92.
7. Goorin AM, Schwartzentruber DJ, Devidas M, Gebhardt MC, Ayala AG, Harris MB, et al. Presurgical chemotherapy compared with immediate surgery and adjuvant chemotherapy for nonmetastatic osteosarcoma: Pediatric Oncology Group Study POG-8651. J Clin Oncol. 2003;21(8):1574–80. doi:10.1200/JCO.2003.08.165.
8. Bacci G, Bertoni F, Longhi A, Ferrari S, Forni C, Biagini R, et al. Neoadjuvant chemotherapy for high-grade central osteosarcoma of the extremity. Histologic response to preoperative chemotherapy correlates with histologic subtype of the tumor. Cancer. 2003;97(12):3068–75. doi:10.1002/cncr.11456.
9. Patel SJ, Lynch Jr JW, Johnson T, Carroll RR, Schumacher C, Spanier S, et al. Dose-intense ifosfamide/doxorubicin/cisplatin based chemotherapy for osteosarcoma in adults. Am J Clin Oncol. 2002;25(5):489–95.
10. Wilkins RM, Cullen JW, Odom L, Jamroz BA, Cullen PM, Fink K, et al. Superior survival in treatment of primary nonmetastatic pediatric osteosarcoma of the extremity. Ann Surg Oncol. 2003;10(5):498–507.
11. Bielack SS, Kempf-Bielack B, Delling G, Exner GU, Flege S, Helmke K, et al. Prognostic factors in high-grade osteosarcoma of the extremities or trunk: an analysis of 1,702 patients treated on neoadjuvant cooperative osteosarcoma study group protocols. J Clin Oncol. 2002;20(3):776–90.

12. Crews KR, Liu T, Rodriguez-Galindo C, Tan M, Meyer WH, Panetta JC, et al. High-dose methotrexate pharmacokinetics and outcome of children and young adults with osteosarcoma. Cancer. 2004;100(8):1724–33. doi:10.1002/cncr.20152.
13. Iwamoto Y, Tanaka K, Isu K, Kawai A, Tatezaki S, Ishii T, et al. Multiinstitutional phase II study of neoadjuvant chemotherapy for osteosarcoma (NECO study) in Japan: NECO-93J and NECO-95J. J Orthop Sci. 2009;14(4):397–404. doi:10.1007/s00776-009-1347-6.
14. Iwamoto Y, Tanaka K. The activity of the Bone and Soft Tissue Tumor Study Group of the Japan Clinical Oncology Group. Jpn J Clin Oncol. 2012;42(6):467–70. doi:hys059 [pii] 10.1093/jjco/hys059 [doi].
15. Bacci G, Longhi A, Versari M, Mercuri M, Briccoli A, Picci P. Prognostic factors for osteosarcoma of the extremity treated with neoadjuvant chemotherapy: 15-year experience in 789 patients treated at a single institution. Cancer. 2006;106(5):1154–61. doi:10.1002/cncr.21724 [doi].
16. Grimer RJ, Taminiau AM, Cannon SR. Surgical outcomes in osteosarcoma. J Bone Joint Surg (Br). 2002;84(3):395–400.
17. Janeway KA, Barkauskas DA, Krailo MD, Meyers PA, Schwartz CL, Ebb DH, et al. Outcome for adolescent and young adult patients with osteosarcoma: a report from the Children's Oncology Group. Cancer. 2012;118(18):4597–605. doi:10.1002/cncr.27414 [doi].
18. Kim MS, Lee SY, Lee TR, Cho WH, Song WS, Koh JS, et al. Prognostic nomogram for predicting the 5-year probability of developing metastasis after neo-adjuvant chemotherapy and definitive surgery for AJCC stage II extremity osteosarcoma. Ann Oncol. 2009;20(5):955–60. doi:mdn723 [pii] 10.1093/annonc/mdn723 [doi].
19. Smeland S, Muller C, Alvegard TA, Wiklund T, Wiebe T, Bjork O, et al. Scandinavian Sarcoma Group Osteosarcoma Study SSG VIII: prognostic factors for outcome and the role of replacement salvage chemotherapy for poor histological responders. Eur J Cancer. 2003;39(4):488–94.
20. Bielack SS, Smeland S, Whelan JS, Marina N, Jovic G, Hook JM et al. Methotrexate, doxorubicin, and cisplatin (MAP) plus maintenance pegylated interferon alpha-2b versus MAP alone in patients with resectable high-grade osteosarcoma and good histologic response to preoperative MAP: first results of the EURAMOS-1 good response randomized controlled trial. J Clin Oncol. 2015;33(20):2279–87. doi:JCO.2014.60.0734 [pii] 10.1200/JCO.2014.60.0734 [doi].
21. Whelan JS, Bielack SS, Marina N, Smeland S, Jovic G, Hook JM et al. EURAMOS-1, an international randomised study for osteosarcoma: results from pre-randomisation treatment. Ann Oncol. 2015;26(2):407–14. doi:mdu526 [pii] 10.1093/annonc/mdu526 [doi].

5 Osteosarcoma in the Elderly: Clinical Features and Outcome

Yoshihiro Nishida

Abstract

Osteosarcoma developing in elderly persons has several characteristic features. A predilection for the axial skeleton, particularly the pelvis, has been noted. Secondary osteosarcoma due to preexisting conditions such as irradiated bone, Paget's disease, fibrous dysplasia, and bone infarct is occasionally observed in the elderly. Because osteosarcoma is relatively rare in the aged persons, diagnostic delay is common, with this exerting a possibly adverse effect on prognosis. Treatment-related factors also may affect the prognosis of elderly patients with osteosarcoma. Difficulty in achieving wide resection is reported because axial bones are affected in a high proportion of elderly osteosarcoma patients. Tolerability and completion rate of chemotherapy are lower in the elderly as compared with younger patients. In this chapter, tumor-related features and treatment-related characteristics are described in elderly patients with osteosarcoma.

Keywords

Secondary osteosarcoma • Elderly • Surgical treatment • Axial skeleton

5.1 Introduction

Osteosarcoma is known to have a double peak of incidence. Most osteosarcomas occur in adolescents during the growth spurt, with a second peak in the seventh and eighth decades [1]. Elderly patients with osteosarcoma have several particular problems including etiology, diagnostic difficulty, unusual site of predilection,

Y. Nishida (✉)
Department of Orhtopaedic Surgery, Nagoya University Graduate School and School of Medicine, 65 Tsurumai-cho, Showa-ku, Nagoya, Aichi 466-8550, Japan
e-mail: ynishida@med.nagoya-u.ac.jp

T. Ueda, A. Kawai (eds.), *Osteosarcoma*, DOI 10.1007/978-4-431-55696-1_5

advanced stage at diagnosis, and feasibility of multidisciplinary treatment in the same manner as that for younger patients with osteosarcoma.

In most developed world countries, the age of 65 years is accepted as the definition of "elderly" person. The United Nations has accepted that age over 60 years may be usually indicated as old age (http://www.who.int/healthinfo/survey/ageingdefnolder/en/ (Accessed July 26, 2014.)). In the context of osteosarcoma treatment, the peak age of onset is between 10 and 20 years, and most clinical therapeutic trials for patients with osteosarcoma have excluded those over the age of 40 years. For this reason physicians involved in the treatment of osteosarcoma have tended to variously define "elderly" as over 40, over 50, or over 60 years.

In this chapter, barriers to adequate diagnosis and therapeutic approach and the prognosis and prognostic factors of the present status are outlined for elderly patients with osteosarcoma, based on the findings of previous reports. Additionally, perspectives of novel therapeutic possibility are provided for this group.

5.2 Secondary Osteosarcoma

Osteosarcomas arising in adolescents are commonly de novo neoplasms, although in elderly patients they occasionally occur in the setting of a preexisting condition such as irradiated bone, Paget's disease, and bone infarct [2–6] (Table 5.1).

In secondary osteosarcoma, previous studies indicated that the prognosis of elderly patients is dependent on the presence of preexisting conditions. Generally, osteosarcomas arising from a preexisting condition have a dismal prognosis, particularly from Paget's disease of bone [2, 7]. However, little progress has been made in the treatment of Paget's sarcoma in the last 60 years [8]. The proportion of Paget's disease in secondary osteosarcoma as a preexisting condition has been differently reported even from Western countries (Table 5.1). Because osteosarcoma arising from Paget's disease has been reported to be uncommon in Japan [9], two subsequent studies from Japan have reconfirmed the unlikelihood of this disease as an underlying pathological condition in this country. The significance of Paget's disease of bone as a preexisting condition of osteosarcoma thus differs markedly among countries.

The carcinogenic effect of radiation is one of the crucial concerns in the treatment of patients with primary malignancy. Prior radiation of bone is a well-

Table 5.1 Secondary osteosarcoma in the elderly patients

Study	Age	Total number (secondary/%)	Number of Paget's disease of bone
Huvos [5]	60<	117 (66/56 %)	58 (50 %)
Grimer [11]	40<	481 (83[a]/17 %)	42 (8.7 %)
Longhi [16]	65<	43 (14/33 %)	13 (30 %)
Okada [13]	50<	64 (14/22 %)	0 (0 %)
Nishida [14]	60<	95 (12/13 %)	0 (0 %)

[a]Paget's disease and radiation-induced osteosarcoma described in the study

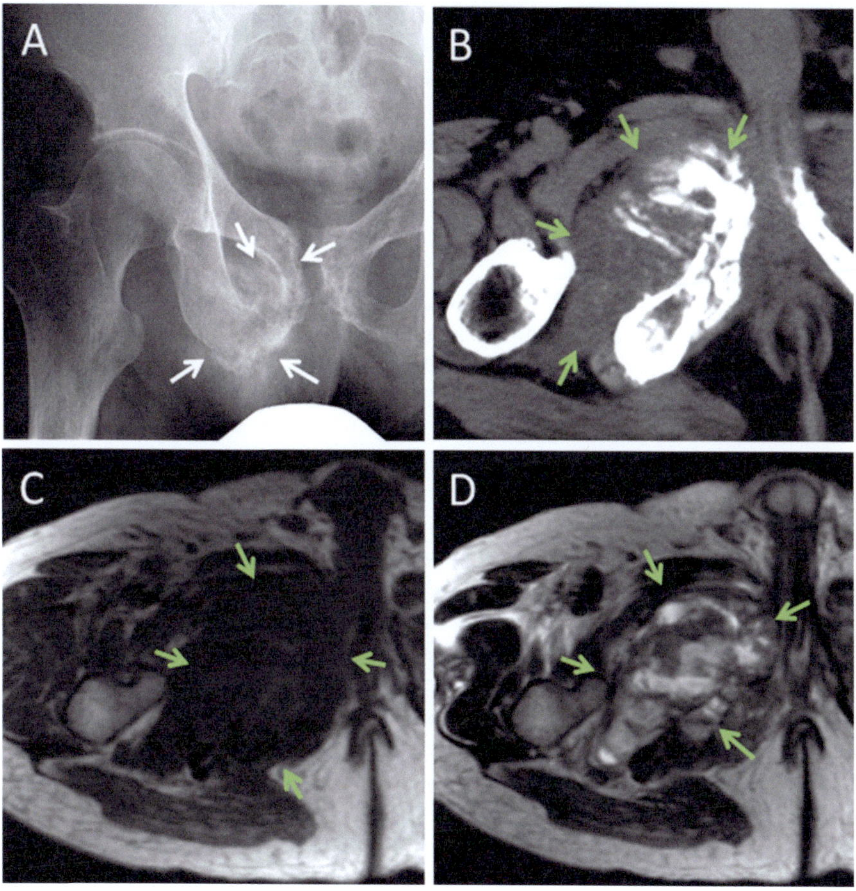

Fig. 5.1 70-year-old male. He received 60 Gy of radiotherapy for the treatment of his prostate cancer 7 years before. He developed radiation-induced osteosarcoma in his right pubic bone (*white arrows*) (**a**). Axial sections of CT image (**b**) and MR images of T1 weighted (**c**) and T2 weighted (**d**) show extraosseously invading tumor (*green arrows*)

known risk factor for the development of secondary osteosarcoma [2, 6, 10]. The median latency period between radiotherapy for the primary cancer and the development of postradiation sarcoma ranges from 8 to 16 years. Grimer et al. reported that the time lag between radiotherapy and subsequent development of osteosarcoma ranged from 6 to 23 years [11]. Historically, radiotherapy was less used for patients with cancer in Japan than those in Western countries. However, comparing the past few decades, radiotherapy has recently assumed more prominent roles in the treatment of cancer. Thus it is likely that the number of secondary osteosarcomas, particularly radiation-induced osteosarcoma (Fig. 5.1), will increase in the near future. Grimer et al. reported that analyses of 41 patients with radiation-induced osteosarcoma confirmed that cure can be achieved even in the older (over 40 years) group of patients if treated aggressively with multidisciplinary treatment including surgery and chemotherapy [11], which is consistent with other previous studies [2, 6]. Contrary results have also been reported. Lewis et al. reported that despite multi-agent chemotherapy, postradiation osteosarcoma continues to have a poor prognosis. Possible contributing factors may include the advanced age and worsened performance status of this patient population [12].

5.3 Delay in Diagnosis

Malignancies of bone are commonly metastases from other primary malignancies in elderly patients, possibly resulting in the misdiagnosis and/or delay in diagnosis of osteosarcoma. Okada et al. reported that the duration between development of symptoms and referral to a specialist ranged from 1 to 276 months (mean 18 months). Clinical and radiological misdiagnoses at the initial presentation were observed in 15 (23 %) of the 64 cases. The length of time in the delay of the diagnosis ranged from 3 to 12 months (average, 6 months) [13]. Nishida et al. reported that although the median duration from the initial presentation at any clinic to the definitive diagnosis of osteosarcoma at specialist centers was 2 months, the mean duration from presentation was 5.2 months. There were 23 cases in which it took more than 5 months between presentation and the making of the correct diagnosis. In many cases, the lesion was considered to be a bone metastasis from carcinoma at another site [14]. A possible reason for such a misdiagnosis is that rare periosteal reactions in osteosarcoma in elderly patients (Fig. 5.2) were previously reported [15], occasionally leading to the radiological diagnosis of metastatic disease of bone.

The results of these Japanese studies agree with those of another report in which the median time interval from onset of symptoms to diagnosis was 4 months [16]. In the younger population, the median time interval has been reported to be 10 weeks [17].

A major concern is the association between delay in diagnosis and patient prognosis. A previous report indicated that misdiagnosis is associated with a poor prognosis in elderly patients with osteosarcoma. The 10-year survival rate of patients with inadequate diagnoses was much lower than that of patients with adequate diagnoses, although the difference was not statistically significant [13]. In contrast, another study demonstrated that a prolonged latency period before the correct diagnosis was made was not an individual prognostic factor [14].

5.4 Site of Predilection

The knee region is affected in approximately 62 % of adolescents with osteosarcoma [18]. Several reports have shown a predilection for axial localization in elderly persons with osteosarcoma (Table 5.2), including Longhi's report in which 4 (9.3 %) of 43 patients were noted to have had a primary tumor in the

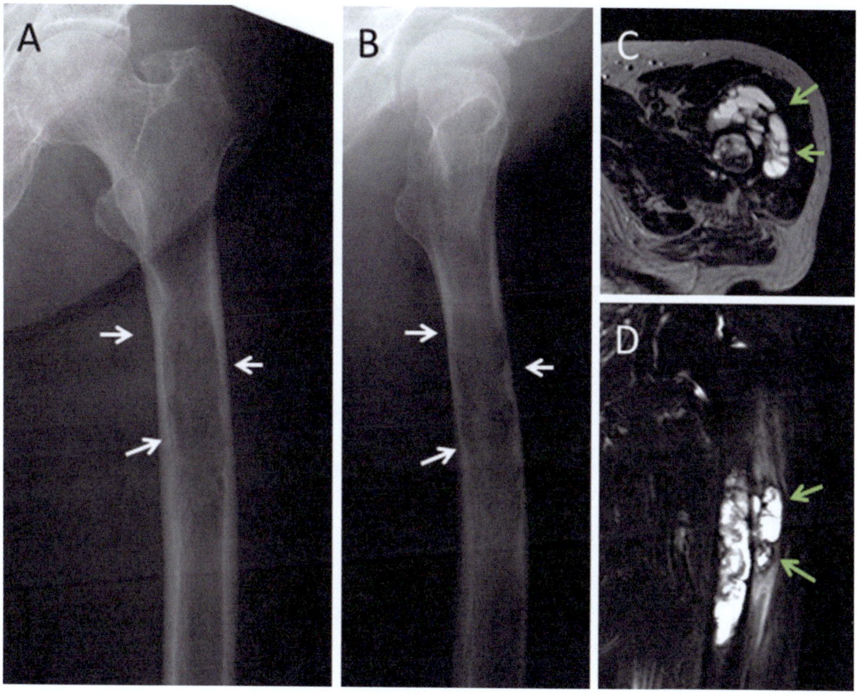

Fig. 5.2 78-year-old female. Primary osteosarcoma developed in her left shaft of femur. X-ray indicated permeative osteolytic lesion without obvious periosteal reaction (*white arrows*) (**a** and **b**). T2-weighted axial image (**c**) and STIR coronal image (**d**) demonstrated the extraosseously invading tumorous lesion (*green arrows*)

Table 5.2 Site of osteosarcoma in elderly patients

Study	Age	Number of patients	Axial bone, number (%)
Huvos[a] [5]	60<	117	32 (27 %)
Carsi [19]	40<	47	18 (38 %)
Grimer [11]	40<	481	100 (21 %)
Okada [13]	50<	64	24 (38 %)
Longhi [16]	65<	43	10 (23 %)
Manoso[b] [21]	40<	58	11 (19 %)
Nishida [14]	60<	95	31 (33 %)
Iwata[b] [20]	40<	86	42 (49 %)

[a]Site of craniofacial bone is included
[b]Secondary osteosarcoma is not included. Site of craniofacial bone is included

knee area and 10 (23 %) a tumor in the axial skeleton [16]. Grimer's study based on 481 cases over 40 years revealed that 21 % of cases had tumor in the axial bones [11]. Other series including primary and secondary osteosarcoma reported higher rates (27–38 %) of axial skeleton as the site of involvement in elderly patients

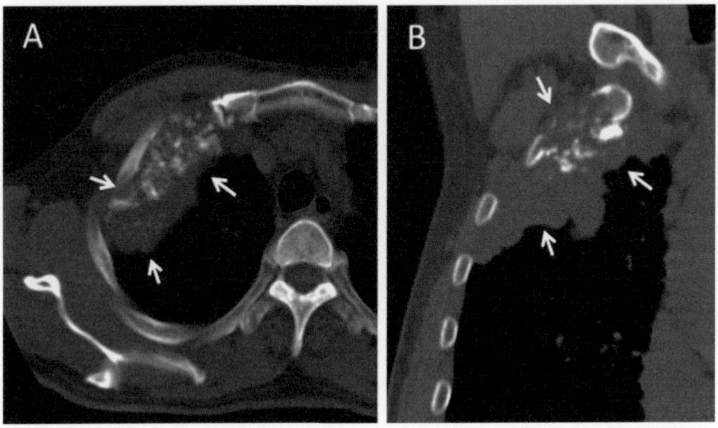

Fig. 5.3 64-year-old male. Primary osteosarcoma occurred in his right first rib, an atypical site. CT axial (**a**) and coronal (**b**) images show extraosseously expanding lesion (*white arrows*)

[5, 13, 14, 19]. Secondary osteosarcoma due to conditions such as postradiation sarcoma and Paget's sarcoma often occurs in the pelvis [2, 7, 8], contributing to a higher tumor incidence in axial bone. However, Manoso et al. and Iwata et al.'s studies focusing on primary osteosarcoma in the elderly [20, 21] also demonstrated the predilection of primary osteosarcoma for axial bones (19 % and 49 %, respectively). Taking these results together, it may be that primary osteosarcoma in elderly patients is also more likely to involve axial bone (Fig. 5.3).

5.5 Stage at Diagnosis

The Cooperative Osteosarcoma Study Group (COSS) had a uniform treatment protocol for two decades. The registration was not limited to the young patients with localized limb tumors, but included all patients with osteosarcoma. The results of this study [22] reflecting the long-term outcome of a wide spectrum of patients with high-grade osteosarcoma after the introduction of multi-agent chemotherapy may be representative of the whole osteosarcoma cohort, thereby facilitating comparison with those of elderly patients with osteosarcoma. In this study, of 1702 patients, 1491 (87.6 %) presented with localized disease, and 211 (12.4 %) had distant metastases.

Regarding the cohort of elderly patients with primary and secondary osteosarcoma, Longhi et al. reported the results of 43 osteosarcoma patients over 65 years of whom 13 had metastatic disease (30.2 %) and 30 (69.8 %) localized disease [16]. Nishida et al. reported that 12 (13 %) of 91 patients had distant metastases at diagnosis [14]. According to the results of Okada et al. who analyzed patients over 50 years, 11 % had lung metastasis at the initial presentation [13]. In the cohort of elderly patients with only primary osteosarcoma, Grimer et al. described that

48 (18 %) of 270 patients with high-grade primary osteosarcoma over 40 years had distant metastasis at diagnosis [11]. Manoso et al. noted a lower proportion of the cases with distant metastasis at diagnosis (5 %) in their cases over 40 years. Iwata et al. reported that 28 % of patients with primary osteosarcoma over 40 years had distant metastasis at diagnosis [20]. In this way the reported proportion of distant metastasis at diagnosis in the cohort of elderly patients has been reported to range from 5 to 30 %. Stage at diagnosis, particularly with distant metastasis, is slightly higher compared with the all-age cohort (12.4 %) [22]. It is likely that the feasibility of chemotherapy and/or surgical treatment and response to chemotherapy may be more important for elderly patients with osteosarcoma.

5.6 Treatment Modality

5.6.1 Surgery

As discussed later, "operability" has been reported as a significant good prognostic factor for elderly patients with osteosarcoma in several studies [14, 16, 20]. However, as was described above, the axial skeleton, in particular the pelvis, is significantly more often affected in elderly patients with osteosarcoma, which makes definitive surgery more difficult to achieve. A previous report, reflecting the whole osteosarcoma cohort based on 1702 cases, indicated that 113 (6.6 %) of 1702 cases retained macroscopic residual tumor at the primary tumor site [22]. Among the 113 patients with macroscopic residual tumor, 84 had not been surgically treated, while 29 had residual tumor after definitive surgery.

In their cohort of elderly patients over 40 years, Carsi et al. reported that 42 (89 %) of 47 cases were operable [19]. According to Grimer's study of a cohort over 40 years, of 238 cases with high-grade nonmetastatic extremity primary osteosarcoma, 212 (92 %) underwent amputation or limb salvage surgery, while of elderly patients with pelvic osteosarcoma, 37 (51 %) of 72 cases underwent surgery [11]. Iwata et al. investigated elderly patients with primary osteosarcoma over 40 years, of whom 63 (73 %) of 86 received surgical treatment [20]. Nishida et al. noted that 81 (85 %) of 95 cases received surgical treatment in an analysis of patients over 60 years [14]. Of the cohort of aged over 65 years, 74.4 % underwent surgery [16]. Together, the predilection of osteosarcoma in the elderly for axial bone may be the main factor precluding the achievement of complete resection of primary tumors.

Another concern arises in terms of limb salvage surgery when osteosarcoma arises in an extremity. In contrast to an incidence of limb salvage in the younger population of approximately 90 % [23], in Longhi's study of patients over 65 years it was limited to only 18 patients (56 %) [16]. In Nishida et al.'s investigation of patients over 60 years, 22 (27 %) of the 81 patients underwent amputation and 59 (73 %) limb salvage surgery [14]. As described in Grimer's study, the proportion having limb salvage was higher in the under 60-year age group (64 %) compared with those over 60 years (49 %) [11], indicating that the rate of limb salvage as a definitive surgery may decrease with increasing age. However, as described later in this chapter, considering that the feasibility of definitive surgery has been a significant prognostic factor in several reports [14, 16, 20] with multivariate analysis, operable cases should be treated aggressively to improve the prognosis.

5.6.2 Chemotherapy

Chemotherapy has made a major contribution to improving patient prognosis for children, adolescents, and young adults with osteosarcoma [24, 25]. However, such efficacy was not confirmed in a study of relatively elderly patients [5]. In addition, because elderly patients may not tolerate aggressive multi-agent chemotherapy, patients over 40 years who develop osteosarcoma are commonly excluded from clinical trials of treatment for it.

Chemotherapeutic agents used for elderly patients with osteosarcoma have been basically the same as those used for young patients, namely, cisplatin, doxorubicin, ifosfamide, and methotrexate (Table 5.3). Several reports have described the tolerability of chemotherapy for elderly patients with osteosarcoma. Grimer et al. noted that chemotherapy was used in 154 patients, with only 29 % of patients over 60 years receiving it in contrast to 80 % of those under 60 years. No patient over 60 years was recorded to have completed the full planned course of chemotherapy, whereas 73 % of those under 60 years did so. There were four treatment-related deaths associated with the use of chemotherapy [11]. Nishida et al. reported that the mean age of patients administered chemotherapy was 67 ± 4.6 years, while that of those not administered it was 71 ± 6.6 years ($P = 0.0007$). No deaths in their series were caused by chemotherapy. Twelve of 51 cases with chemotherapy could tolerate similar doses and regimens to those used for young patients [14]. Manoso et al. reported that among 40 patients who received chemotherapy, six were unable to complete the full course of chemotherapy because of toxicity. An additional

Table 5.3 Chemotherapeutic agents used in previous studies

Study	Age	Agents	Benefit for prognosis
Grimer [11]	40<	Cisplatin, doxorubicin, ifosfamide, methotrexate	Yes
Carsi [19]	40<	Cisplatin, doxorubicin, mitomycin C, ifosfamide, cyclophosphamide, etoposide, high-dose methotrexate	No
Okada [13]	50<	Cisplatin, doxorubicin, ifosfamide, methotrexate	No
Manoso [21]	40<	Cisplatin, doxorubicin, ifosfamide, methotrexate, etoposide, vincristine, bleomycin, cyclophosphamide, dactinomycin	Yes
Bacci [26]	41–60	Cisplatin, doxorubicin, ifosfamide	Yes
Longhi [16]	65<	Ifosfamide, anthracycline	No
Nishida [14]	60<	Cisplatin, doxorubicin, ifosfamide, methotrexate	No
Iwata [20]	40<	Cisplatin, doxorubicin, ifosfamide, methotrexate	No

seven patients required a reduction in dosage during treatment. No deaths were caused by chemotherapy [21]. Longhi et al. reported that in patients over 65 years, none received methotrexate due to its high nephrotoxicity. All patients received ifosfamide and an anthracycline. All drugs were delivered at doses reduced by 20 % as compared with standard protocols and for a reduced number of cycles. Twenty-nine (67 %) of 43 patients did not receive chemotherapy, of whom 10 were excluded because of impaired cardiac or renal function. The physician decided not to conduct chemotherapy due to the patient's age in 15 cases [16].

A most important point of interest to physicians is whether chemotherapy can improve the prognosis of elderly patients with osteosarcoma. Grimer et al., in a review of 481 patients older than age 40 years in the EMSOS study, found that chemotherapy significantly improved survival. Patients treated with chemotherapy had a 5-year OS of 51 % compared with 39 % in those patients undergoing surgery alone [11]. Manoso et al. reported the results of the Memorial Sloan Kettering experience in which multimodality treatment with surgery and chemotherapy statistically improved survival ($P = 0.02$) compared with surgery alone in patients with high-grade osteosarcoma. The chemotherapy group had a median survival of 113 months versus the surgery-only group with a median survival of 5 months. The subset analysis of patients older than 60 years with high-grade disease showed that the chemotherapy significantly increased the overall survival ($P < 0.0008$). The median survival with chemotherapy was 68 months as compared to 5 months without chemotherapy. However, the two groups had only seven patients each [21]. Bacci et al. reported the results of the Rizzoli experience in which the 5-year overall survival rate was 70 % in patients aged 41–60 years with chemotherapy, which is similar to that of 296 patients under 40 years treated with a more aggressive protocol of chemotherapy (5-year overall survival, 71 %) [26].

In contrast to these beneficial effects of chemotherapy, Okada et al. reported that in a group of 22 patients receiving preoperative chemotherapy, 82 % of cases showed a poor response rate. They were unable to show any beneficial impact of chemotherapy on prognosis [13]. Carsi et al. showed that 35.7 % of their patients received chemotherapy, but found no difference in survival [19]. Lewis et al. reported that current chemotherapy regimens fail to impact survival in postradiation osteosarcoma [12]. Nishida et al. reported that chemotherapy had no impact on patient survival in those aged over 60 years [14]. Iwata et al. reported that in patients without metastasis at diagnosis who subsequently underwent definitive surgery, chemotherapy had no significant impact on survival (with chemotherapy, 63.4 %; without chemotherapy, 65.2 %), despite the absence of any significant differences in the tumor site, stage, or surgical margin between the groups [20].

No definitive conclusion was drawn from previous reports due to the heterogeneity of the cohort studies, chemotherapeutic regimens, and their indications. Prospective, multi-institutional, well-directed clinical trials will be needed to help clarify the role of chemotherapy for elderly patients with osteosarcoma.

5.7 Prognosis and Prognostic Factors

The prognosis of elderly patients with osteosarcoma has been shown to be worse than that of younger patients. Of the cohort of elderly patients with both primary and secondary osteosarcoma, Huvos et al. indicated a 5-year overall survival of only 8 % in the whole cohort, being however, 37 % in primary osteosarcoma and 7.5 % in secondary osteosarcoma [5]. Longhi et al. showed that in patients over 65 years, overall survival was 22 % at 5 years and 45 % when patients with distant metastasis at diagnosis were excluded [16]. Okada et al. revealed the overall survival at 5 years to be 55.5 % in patients over 50 years. Nishida et al. reported an overall survival rate of 46.7 % at 5 years in patients over 60 years including those with low-grade malignancy. Patients with high-grade malignancy showed 42.8 % survival at 5 years and patients with extremity location 51.9 % [14].

Regarding a cohort limited to primary osteosarcoma, Grimer et al. reported an overall survival rate of 46 % at 5 years in high-grade and conventional osteosarcoma without metastasis at diagnosis [11]. Carsi et al. showed the overall survival at 5 years to be 42 % in their cohort over 40 years (distant metastasis at diagnosis: 17 %) [19]. Iwata et al. described the 5-year overall survival to be 38.8 % in their cohort aged over 40 years. Prognosis was poor compared with results from other studies, but their cohort included 24 patients (28 %) with AJCC stage IV [20]. Manoso analyzed 58 patients with primary osteosarcoma over 40 years including 3 with initial distant metastasis and revealed that overall survival was 58 % at 5 years and 44 % at 10 years. Focusing on high-grade tumors, overall survival was 53 % at 5 years and 41 % at 10 years [21]. Bacci et al. reported that patients with nonmetastatic extremity osteosarcoma aged 41–60 years showed a 5-year overall survival of 70 % [26].

The results of whole-aged cohort including distant metastasis at diagnosis showed overall survival rates at 5 years and 10 years to be 65.3 % and 59.8 %, respectively [22]. Compared to this survival rate, outcome in the elderly patients including initial distant metastasis was lower (8–58 %) at 5 years as shown above.

Prognostic factors in the elderly patients with osteosarcoma have been variously reported (Table 5.4). In general, inoperable cases, distant metastasis at diagnosis, large size, and older age were reported as poor prognostic factors. Of interest, site of upper limb (or proximal humerus) was shown to be a poor prognostic factor in two studies [11, 27].

5.8 Perspective

Osteosarcoma in the elderly had some characteristic features including unusual site of predilection, high proportion of secondary osteosarcomas as compared to adolescents, delay in diagnosis, higher proportion of amputation in extremity location, and poor tolerability of chemotherapy. Of the tumor-related variables, none can be modified, whereas diagnosis and treatment-related factors may be improved and/or newly innovated in the near future.

Table 5.4 Prognostic factors for overall survival in elderly patients with osteosarcoma (multivariate)

Study	Age	Significant factors
Carsi [19]	40<	Metachronous metastasis
Grimer [11]	40<	Age >60, upper limb
Longhi [16]	65<	M1, large size, inoperability
Okada [13]	50<	Axial bone, M1, large size
Manoso [21]	40<	Age >60, large size, M1, positive margin, high ALP, recurrence
Nishida [14]	60<	Inoperability
Song [27]	40–60	Large size, proximal humerus, poor histologic response
Iwata [20]	40<	M1, inoperability

Grimer's study: high-grade nonmetastatic extremity osteosarcoma M1: distant metastasis at diagnosis
Song's study: prognostic factors of metastasis-free survival

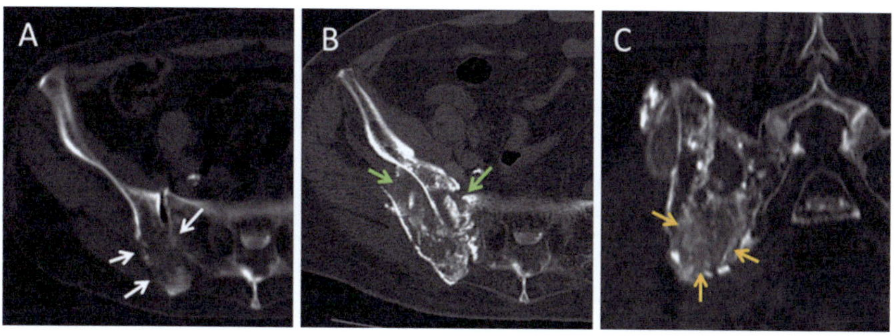

Fig. 5.4 83-year-old female. Primary osteosarcoma occurred in her right ilium adjacent to sacrum (*white arrows*) (**a**). She received carbon ion radiotherapy of 70.4 GyE. Six years after carbon ion radiotherapy, axial section of CT image indicates postradiation fractures (*green arrows*) (**b**). Coronal section of CT shows the osteogenic response in the irradiated field (*orange arrows*) (**c**). She could walk with T-cane at the latest follow-up

Raising awareness regarding the occurrence of osteosarcoma in the elderly population is important for its early diagnosis, particularly in developed countries in which society is experiencing unprecedented aging. Prospective, well-organized, multi-institutional studies should be planned for elderly osteosarcoma patients and should help to clarify the indications of chemotherapy in greater detail. Targeted therapy will be introduced into the area of osteosarcoma in the future. Although osteosarcoma is a group of heterogeneous tumors, pazopanib is now being used for patients with soft tissue sarcomas, which are also composed of heterogeneous tumors.

A novel therapeutic tool is particle radiotherapy. The efficacy of heavy ion radiotherapy has already been reported in patients with primary malignant bone tumors including osteosarcoma [28, 29]. Given that osteosarcoma in the elderly often arises in the axial skeleton where wide resection is difficult to achieve and surgical treatment-related morbidity is a concern, charged particle radiation therapy including carbon ion radiotherapy and proton therapy are promising tools for elderly patients with osteosarcoma (Fig. 5.4). Accumulated data will be needed to more precisely elucidate their fascinating details and clarify issues such as efficacy and indications.

References

1. Dorfman HD, Czerniak B. Osteosarcoma. In: Dorfman HD, Czemiak B, editors. Bone tumors. St. Louis: Mosby; 1998. p. 128–252.
2. Bielack SS, et al. Combined modality treatment for osteosarcoma occurring as a second malignant disease. Cooperative German-Austrian-Swiss Osteosarcoma Study Group. J Clin Oncol. 1999;17(4):1164.
3. Dahlin DC, Coventry MB. Osteogenic sarcoma. A study of six hundred cases. J Bone Joint Surg Am. 1967;49(1):101–10.
4. Duffaud F, et al. Osteosarcomas of flat bones in adolescents and adults. Cancer. 2000;88 (2):324–32.
5. Huvos AG. Osteogenic sarcoma of bones and soft tissues in older persons. A clinicopathologic analysis of 117 patients older than 60 years. Cancer. 1986;57(7):1442–9.
6. Huvos AG, et al. Postradiation osteogenic sarcoma of bone and soft tissues. A clinicopathologic study of 66 patients. Cancer. 1985;55(6):1244–55.
7. Shaylor PJ, et al. Paget's osteosarcoma – no cure in sight. Sarcoma. 1999;3(3–4):191–2.
8. Mankin HJ, Hornicek FJ. Paget's sarcoma: a historical and outcome review. Clin Orthop Relat Res. 2005;438:97–102.
9. Naka T, et al. Osteosarcoma versus malignant fibrous histiocytoma of bone in patients older than 40 years. A clinicopathologic and immunohistochemical analysis with special reference to malignant fibrous histiocytoma-like osteosarcoma. Cancer. 1995;76(6):972–84.
10. Mindell ER, Shah NK, Webster JH. Postradiation sarcoma of bone and soft tissues. Orthop Clin North Am. 1977;8(4):821–34.
11. Grimer RJ, et al. Osteosarcoma over the age of forty. Eur J Cancer. 2003;39(2):157–63.
12. Lewis VO, et al. Outcome of postradiation osteosarcoma does not correlate with chemotherapy response. Clin Orthop Relat Res. 2006;450:60–6.
13. Okada K, et al. Second primary osteosarcoma with rosette-like structure in a patient with retinoblastoma. Virchows Arch. 2004;445(4):421–4.
14. Nishida Y, et al. Osteosarcoma in the elderly over 60 years: a multicenter study by the Japanese Musculoskeletal Oncology Group. J Surg Oncol. 2009;100(1):48–54.
15. de Santos LA, et al. Osteogenic sarcoma after the age of 50: a radiographic evaluation. AJR Am J Roentgenol. 1978;131(3):481–4.
16. Longhi A, et al. Osteosarcoma in patients older than 65 years. J Clin Oncol. 2008;26 (33):5368–73.
17. Bacci G, et al. Delay in diagnosis of high-grade osteosarcoma of the extremities. Has it any effect on the stage of disease? Tumori. 2000;86(3):204–6.
18. Campanacci M. Bone tumors. Philadelphia: Lippincott-Verlag; 1999. p. 1418–68.
19. Carsi B, Rock MG. Primary osteosarcoma in adults older than 40 years. Clin Orthop Relat Res. 2002;397:53–61.
20. Iwata S, et al. Prognostic factors in elderly osteosarcoma patients: a multi-institutional retrospective study of 86 cases. Ann Surg Oncol. 2014;21(1):263–8.
21. Manoso MW, et al. De novo osteogenic sarcoma in patients older than forty: benefit of multimodality therapy. Clin Orthop Relat Res. 2005;438:110–5.
22. Bielack SS, et al. Prognostic factors in high-grade osteosarcoma of the extremities or trunk: an analysis of 1,702 patients treated on neoadjuvant cooperative osteosarcoma study group protocols. J Clin Oncol. 2002;20(3):776–90.

23. Ferrari S, et al. Neoadjuvant chemotherapy with high-dose Ifosfamide, high-dose methotrexate, cisplatin, and doxorubicin for patients with localized osteosarcoma of the extremity: a joint study by the Italian and Scandinavian Sarcoma Groups. J Clin Oncol. 2005;23(34):8845–52.
24. Meyers PA, et al. Chemotherapy for nonmetastatic osteogenic sarcoma: the Memorial Sloan-Kettering experience. J Clin Oncol. 1992;10(1):5–15.
25. Rosen G, et al. Preoperative chemotherapy for osteogenic sarcoma: selection of postoperative adjuvant chemotherapy based on the response of the primary tumor to preoperative chemotherapy. Cancer. 1982;49(6):1221–30.
26. Bacci G, et al. Neoadjuvant chemotherapy for osteosarcoma of the extremities in patients aged 41–60 years: outcome in 34 cases treated with adriamycin, cisplatinum and ifosfamide between 1984 and 1999. Acta Orthop. 2007;78(3):377–84.
27. Song WS, et al. Prognosis of extremity osteosarcoma in patients aged 40–60 years: a cohort/case controlled study at a single institute. Eur J Surg Oncol. 2010;36(5):483–8.
28. Imai R, et al. Cervical spine osteosarcoma treated with carbon-ion radiotherapy. Lancet Oncol. 2006;7(12):1034–5.
29. Kamada T, et al. Efficacy and safety of carbon ion radiotherapy in bone and soft tissue sarcomas. J Clin Oncol. 2002;20(22):4466–71.

Prognostic Factors for Osteosarcoma Patients

6

Mitsunori Kaya

Abstract
It is necessary to clarify the prognostic factor for the patients with osteosarcoma to improve their clinical results. Many research works have been published in several fields including clinical, molecular, and genetic aspect and immunology.

Keywords
Osteosarcoma • Prognostic factor • Research

6.1 Background

Osteosarcoma is the most commonly diagnosed primary malignant bone tumor, with similar global incidence rate across childhood and adolescence. Patients with localized disease have a 5-year survival period of 80 %; however, the prognosis is poor in those with metastatic osteosarcoma. From the standpoint that clarification of the prognostic factors is critical for the further improvement of the prognosis for the patients with osteosarcoma, many research works have been published even from the Japanese institutes. The objective of the current review is to introduce the research works about the prognostic factors of osteosarcoma (Table 6.1).

M. Kaya (✉)
Department of Orthopaedic Surgery, Sapporo Medical University, School of Medicine, S-1 W-16, Chuo-ku, Sapporo 060-8543, Japan
e-mail: kayamitsunori@yahoo.co.jp

T. Ueda, A. Kawai (eds.), *Osteosarcoma*, DOI 10.1007/978-4-431-55696-1_6

Table 6.1 Summary of prognostic factors for patients with osteosarcoma

Factors	
Clinical factors	
Metastatic disease at presentation	Patients who have metastases at the time of presentation indicative of a poor prognosis
Tumor necrosis after chemotherapy	Good response to chemotherapy (>90 % tumor necrosis) is suggestive of a good survival
Tumor location	Truncal tumors appears to be indicative of a poor prognosis
Tumor suppressor genes	
Rb gene	Loss of heterozygosity at the Rb locus is a predictor of poor outcome
Oncogene	
ErbB2	Overexpression was correlated with decreased event-free survival
	Increased levels of ErbB2 was associated with good survival
Angiogenesis	
VEGF	Patients with high serum VEGF had poor survival
Immunology	
PBF	PBF-positive osteosarcoma conferred poorer prognosis
Cyclooxygenase inhibitor	
COX-2	Patients with strong COX-2 expression had a poor prognosis

6.2 Clinical Prognostic Factors

The single most predictive factor in osteosarcoma is the presence or absence of detectable metastatic disease at presentation. As mentioned, the survival rate for patients who have metastases at the time of presentation is between 10 and 20 % [1, 2]. Those who present with bone or skip metastases fare even worse [3, 4]. The degree of tumor necrosis after neoadjuvant chemotherapy is also an important prognostic factor. Patients who have tumors with a good response to chemotherapy (>90 % tumor necrosis) have a considerably better long-term survival rate than those who have tumors with a poor response (<90 % tumor necrosis) [5–7]. The response to chemotherapy is commonly assessed by histological analysis, although it is difficult to evaluate the chemotherapeutic effects before tumor excision. Miwa et al. evaluated the impact of various radiological examinations on overall survival and event-free survival. They concluded that 99mTc-MIBI scintigraphy and combined radiological score (CRS) could be considered as significant predictor of overall survival and event-free survival [8]. Large tumor size has been implicated as a negative prognostic indicator in several studies; however, inconsistent methods of determining size in these studies make it difficult to ascertain its true influence. Other poor prognostic variable was patient's age at diagnosis. The prognosis of elderly patients was generally considered to be worse compared to those of the young patients. Iwata et al. conducted the multi-institutional retrospective study to investigate clinical features and prognostic factors in patients older than 40 years with osteosarcoma. They demonstrated the distinct clinical features, such as the high incidence of truncal tumors or metastasis at diagnosis, in patients older than 40 years with osteosarcoma. Additionally, prognostic factor analyses revealed that tumor site, metastasis at diagnosis, definitive surgery, and surgical margins were significant prognostic factors, whereas chemotherapy did not influence survival [9]. A tumor located in the pelvis, proximal part of the femur, or proximal part of the humerus also appears to be indicative of a poor prognosis [10].

6.3 Molecular and Genetic Considerations

6.3.1 Tumor Suppressor Genes

A tumor suppressor gene is any gene that by its loss of function contributes to the pathogenesis or progression of a tumor. This can occur at the level of the gene or at the level of the protein for which it codes. Often, tumor suppressors function as cell-cycle regulators. The hallmark of a putative suppressor gene is loss of the genetic material coding for a protein that is important in the regulation of the cell cycle or its proliferation. The known tumor suppressor gene p53 and the retinoblastoma (Rb) gene are the most frequently mutated in osteosarcoma (mutated in 25–80 %) and are localized to chromosome arm 17p and 13q, respectively [11].

The retinoblastoma (Rb) gene was the first characterized tumor suppressor gene. It acts as a negative transcriptional regulator of genes involved in the cell-cycle progression from G1 to S phase. Loss of this function allows cells to progress through the cell cycle unchecked. Allele loss of the Rb gene has been reported in approximately 50–60 % of osteosarcomas [11]. A recent study has demonstrated that loss of heterozygosity at the Rb locus on chromosome arm 13q is a predictor of poor outcome in patients with osteosarcoma [12].

6.3.2 Oncogenes

The effect of oncogenes on tumorigenesis is different from that of tumor suppressors in that mutation of a normal proto-oncogene to an oncogene confers a gain of function, as opposed to a loss, driving the cell toward a malignant phenotype.

Her2/erbB-2 is a cellular proto-oncogene that encodes the human epidermal growth factor receptor 2 (Her2). Overexpression of this oncogene induces malignant transformation of rodent fibroblasts and has been implicated in decreased survival of patients with breast carcinoma. Recently, two studies have shown overexpression in approximately 40 % of the osteosarcomas and a correlation with decreased event-free survival and histological response to neoadjuvant chemotherapy [13, 14]. With the development of additional prospective studies, the presence of the Her2/erbB-2 receptor eventually may emerge as a significant prognostic indicator. In contrast, Akatsuka et al. demonstrated that the presence of increased levels of ErbB2 in tumor cells was associated with a significantly increased probability of event-free and overall survival in patients with high-grade osteosarcoma without metastatic disease at presentation and treated with surgery and chemotherapy [15].

The MDM2 gene codes for a p53 binding protein and is located on chromosome arm 12q13, a region that is often amplified in a variety of sarcomas. It has the ability to inhibit the transcriptional activity of p53, providing an alternative pathway of p53 inactivation. MDM2 has been found to be amplified in approximately 4–7 % of osteosarcomas. It is marginally associated with locally recurrent and metastatic disease but cannot be used currently as a prognostic marker [16].

6.4 Angiogenesis

One of the most interesting topics in cancer therapy is that of anti-angiogenesis. Very little work on sarcomas has been done in this field. Anti-angiogenic agents have been shown to inhibit tumor growth and cause tumor regression in mouse models [17]. There are currently many anti-angiogenic agents being tested in Phase I and II clinical trials of their effects on human cancers. Two of the targets of these trials are vascular endothelial growth factor and its receptors. Kaya et al. recently demonstrated expression of vascular endothelial growth factor in 17 (63 %) of 27 osteosarcomas [18]. They also correlated this expression with a high prevalence of pulmonary metastasis, suggesting that expression of vascular endothelial growth factor may play a role in the metastatic cascade of osteosarcoma [18]. Kaya et al. also evaluated the prognostic significance of the serum levels of vascular endothelial growth factor (VEGF) in predicting the survival of patients with osteosarcoma prospectively. Patients with a serum VEGF >1000 pg/ml had significantly worse survival than those with a level <1000 pg/ml ($p=0.002$). They concluded that serum VEGF level might be useful in predicting the prognosis for survival in patients with osteosarcoma [19]. It may also become a treatment target, and anti-angiogenic therapy using antivascular endothelial growth factor antibody and a vascular endothelial growth factor receptor inhibitor is expecting to offer a potentially useful strategy for lung metastasis from osteosarcoma. This was supported by the experimental research work by Tanaka et al. They demonstrated that disruption of the vascular barrier and transendothelial migration of syngeneic mouse spontaneous highly metastatic osteosarcoma cell line LM8 is dependent, at least one part, on VEGF [20]. They also demonstrated that daily oral administration of pazopanib reduced the rate and size of pulmonary metastasis in vivo [20].

6.5 Immunology

Currently, there is a growing realization that active immunotherapy serves as the fourth therapeutic modality for malignant tumors following surgery, chemotherapy, and radiotherapy. To establish the immunotherapy for osteosarcoma, the identification of tumor-associated antigens recognized by cytotoxic T cells (CTLs) was performed. Tsukahara et al. identified papillomavirus binding factor (PBF) as a cytotoxic T lymphocytes (CTL)-defined osteosarcoma antigen in the context of HLA-B55 [21]. They also analyzed the prognostic impact of PBF expression in 78 patients with osteosarcoma who had completed the standard treatment protocols and demonstrated that PBF-positive osteosarcoma conferred significantly poorer prognosis than those with negative expression of PBF [22]. These findings suggested prognostic significance and immunodominancy of PBF in patients with osteosarcoma. PBF is the candidate target for immunotherapy in patients with osteosarcoma, and subsequent clinical trials of peptide-based immunotherapy for osteosarcoma have just started.

6.6 Cyclooxygenase Inhibitor

Cyclooxygenase (COX) is an enzyme implicated in the conversion of arachidonic acid into prostaglandin. There are two isoforms of COX, designated COX-1 and COX-2. COX-2 is an inducible enzyme associated with inflammatory disease and cancer. Various reports have indicated that COX is overexpressed in many types of malignant tumors such as colorectal [23], prostate [24], breast [25], and lung [26]. Urakawa et al. found that patients with strong COX-2 expression had a poor prognosis with regard to metastasis, and all patients with increased COX-2 expression in lung metastases died of the disease. They concluded that COX-2 could be one of the key enzymes directly or indirectly involved in the process of metastasis in osteosarcoma [27].

References

1. Bacci G, Mercuri M, Briccoli A, Ferrari S, Bertoni F, Donati D, Monti C, Zanoni A, Forni C, Manfrini M. Osteogenic sarcoma of the extremity with detectable lung metastases at presentation. Results of treatment of 23 patients with chemotherapy followed by simultaneous resection of primary and metastatic lesions. Cancer. 1997;79:245–54.
2. Meyers PA, Heller G, Healey JH, Huvos A, Appelwhite A, Sun M, LaQuaglia M. Osteogenic sarcoma with clinically detectable metastasis at initial presentation. J Clin Oncol. 1993;11:449–53.
3. Wuisman P, Enneking WF. Prognosis for patients who have osteosarcoma with skip metastasis. J Bone Joint Surg Am. 1990;72:60–8.
4. Ward WG, Mikaelian K, Dorey F, Mirra JM, Sassoon A, Holmes EC, Eilbert FR, Eckardt JJ. Pulmonary metastases of stage IIB extremity osteosarcoma and subsequent pulmonary metastases. J Clin Oncol. 1994;12:1849–58.
5. Provisor AJ, Ettinger LJ, Nachman JB, Krailo MD, Makley JT, Yunis EJ, Huvos AG, Betcher DL, Baum ES, Kisker CT, Miser JS. Treatment of nonmetastatic osteosarcoma of the extremity with preoperative and postoperative chemotherapy: a report from the Children's Cancer Group. J Clin Oncol. 1997;15:76–84.
6. Glasser DB, Lane JM, Huvos AG, Marcove RC, Rosen G. Survival, prognosis, and therapeutic response in osteogenic sarcoma. The Memorial Hospital experience. Cancer. 1992;69:698–708.

7. Davis AM, Bell RS, Goodwin PJ. Prognostic factors in osteosarcoma: a critical review. J Clin Oncol. 1994;12:423–31.
8. Miwa S, Takeuchi A, Shirai T, Taki J, Yamamoto N, Nishida H, Hayashi K, Tanzawa Y, Kimura H, Igarashi K, Ooi A, Tsuchiya H. Prognostic value of radiological response to chemotherapy in patients with osteosarcoma. PLoS One. 2013;8(7):e70015.
9. Iwata S, Ishii T, Kawai A, Hiruma T, Yonemoto T, Kamoda H, Asano N, Takeyama M. Prognostic factors in elderly osteosarcoma patients: a multi-institutional retrospective study of 86 cases. Ann Surg Oncol. 2014;21(1):263–8.
10. Shin KH, Rougraff BT, Simon MA. Oncologic outcomes of primary bone sarcomas of the pelvis. Clin Orthop. 1994;304:207–17.
11. Yamaguchi T, Toguchida J, Yamamuro T, Kotoura Y, Takada N, Kawaguchi N, Kaneko Y, Nakamura Y, Sasaki MS, Ishizaki K. Allelotype analysis in osteosarcomas: frequent allele loss on 3q, 13q, 17p, and 18q. Cancer Res. 1992;52:2419–23.
12. Feugeas O, Guriec N, Babin-Boilletot A, Marcellin L, Simon P, Babin S, Thyss A, Hofman A, Terrier P, Kalifa C, Brunat-Mentigny M, Patricot LM, Oberling F. Loss of heterozygosity of the RB gene is a poor prognostic factor in patients with osteosarcoma. J Clin Oncol. 1996;14:467–72.
13. Gorlick R, Huvos AG, Heller G, Aledo A, Beardsley GP, Healey JH, Meyers PA. Expression of HER2/erbB-2 correlates with survival in osteosarcoma. J Clin Oncol. 1999;17:2781–8.
14. Onda M, Matsuda S, Higaki S, Iijima T, Fukushima J, Yokokura A, Kojima T, Horiuchi H, Kurokawa T, Yamamoto T. ErbB-2 expression is correlated with poor prognosis for patients with osteosarcoma. Cancer. 1996;77:71–8.
15. Akatsuka T, Wada T, Kokai Y, Kawaguchi S, Isu K, Yamashiro K, Yamashita T, Sawada N, Yamawaki S, Ishii S. ErbB2 expression is correlated with increased survival of patients with osteosarcoma. Cancer. 2002;94:1397–404.
16. Lonardo F, Ueda T, Huvos AG, Healey J, Ladanyi M. p53 and MDM2 alterations in osteosarcomas: correlation with clinicopathologic features and proliferative rate. Cancer. 1997;79:1541–7.
17. Bergers G, Javaherian K, Lo KM, Folkman J, Hanahan D. Effects of angiogenesis inhibitors on multistage carcinogenesis in mice. Science. 1999;284:808–12.
18. Kaya M, Wada T, Akatsuka T, Kawaguchi S, Nagoya S, Shindoh M, Higashino F, Mezawa F, Okada F, Ishii S. Vascular endothelial growth factor expression in untreated osteosarcoma is predictive of pulmonary metastasis and poor prognosis. Clin Cancer Res. 2000;6:572–7.
19. Kaya M, Wada T, Nagoya S, Sasaki M, Matsumura T, Yamashita T. The level of vascular endothelial growth factor as a predictor of a poor prognosis in osteosarcoma. J Bone Joint Surg Br. 2009 Jun;91(6):784–8.
20. Tanaka T, Yui Y, Wakamatsu T, Yoshioka K, Araki N, Yoshikawa H, Itoh K. Dynamic analysis of lung metastasis by mouse osteosarcoma LM8: VEGF is a candidate for anti-metastasis therapy. Clin Exp Metastasis. 2013;30(4):369-79.
21. Tsukahara T, Nabeta Y, Kawaguchi S, Ikeda H, Satp Y, Shimozawa K, Ida K, Asanuma H, Hirohashi Y, Torigoe T, Hiraga H, Nagoya S, Wada T, Yamashita T, Sat N. Identification of human autologous cytotoxic T-lymphocyte-defined osteosarcoma gene that encodes a transcriptional regulator, papillomavirus binding factor. Cancer Res. 2004;64(15):5442–8.
22. Tsukahara T, Kawaguchi S, Torigoe T, Kimura S, Murase M, Ichimiya S, Wada T, Kaya M, Nagoya S, Ishii T, Tatezaki S, Yamashita T, Sato N. Prognostic impact and immunogenicity of a novel osteosarcoma antigen, papillomavirus binding factor, in patients with osteosarcoma. Cancer Sci. 2008;99(2):368–75. Clin Exp Metastasis 2013;30:369–379.
23. Eberhart CE, Coffey RJ, Radhika A, Giardiello FM, Ferrenbach S, Dubois RN. Up-regulation of cyclooxygenase-2 gene-expression in human colorectal adenomas and adenocarcinomas. Gastroenterology. 1994;107:1183–8.
24. Gupta S, Srivastava M, Ahmad N, Bostwick DG, Mukhtar H. Over-expression of cyclooxygenase-2 in human prostate adenocarcinoma. Prostate. 2000;42:73–8.

25. Hwang D, Scollard D, Byrne J, Levine E. Expression of cyclooxygenase-1 and cyclooxygenase-2 in human breast cancer. J Natl Cancer Inst. 1998;90:455–60.
26. Watkins DN, Lenzo JC, Segal A, Garlepp MJ, Thompson PJ. Expression and localization of cyclo-oxygenase isoforms in non-small cell lung cancer. Eur Respir J. 1999;14:412–8.
27. Urakawa H, Nishida Y, Naruse T, Nakashima H, Ishiguro N. Cyclooxygenase-2-overexpression predicts poor survival in patients with high-grade extremity osteosarcoma: a pilot. Study Clin Orthop Relat Res. 2009;467(11):2932–8.

Part III

Chemotherapy

Neoadjuvant Chemotherapy Developed in Japan

7

Hiroaki Hiraga

Abstract

Adjuvant chemotherapy is a standard treatment for osteosarcoma, which was verified by two randomized controlled trials (RCTs). Preoperative chemotherapy and limb-preserving procedure have been developed in the USA since around 1970 and in Japan since around 1980. In addition, histologic evaluation concerned with the rate of necrosis of excised tumors after preoperative chemotherapy has been tried, and it has been reported that patients with higher rate of necrosis result in better survival. Neoadjuvant chemotherapy for osteosarcoma (NECO) study tried to improve survival of the patients with lower rate of necrosis, called as "poor responders," by the changes or addition of chemotherapeutic agents on the basis of the histologic evaluation in Japan, and the study found the possibility to rescue poor responders. Such strategies, however, have not been verified by RCT yet. Now additional effects of ifosfamide (IFO) to postoperative chemotherapy for poor responders after preoperative chemotherapy and surgery are just tested by two RCTs.

Keywords

Osteosarcoma • Adjuvant chemotherapy • Multi-institutional study

H. Hiraga (✉)
Department of Orthopaedic Surgery, Hokkaido Cancer Center, Kikusui 4-2-3-54, Shiroishi-ku, Sapporo 003-0804, Japan
e-mail: hhiraga@sap-cc.go.jp

T. Ueda, A. Kawai (eds.), *Osteosarcoma*, DOI 10.1007/978-4-431-55696-1_7

7.1 Adjuvant Chemotherapy for Osteosarcoma

7.1.1 Establishment of Adjuvant Chemotherapy

Surgical resection is always required, as it is difficult to achieve a curative effect for high-grade malignant primary osteosarcoma through the use of only chemotherapy or radiotherapy. However, even in cases with no distant metastases on initial examination, pulmonary metastases may occur 1–2 years postoperatively, requiring amputation or disarticulation; thereby, this results in a poor prognosis with a 2-year relapse-free survival (RFS) rate of 15–20 %, as pulmonary micrometastasis may have already occurred by the time of surgery.

On the other hand, reports from the early 1970s indicated that doxorubicin (ADM), cisplatin (CDDP), high-dose methotrexate (HD-MTX), and cyclophosphamide (CPA) were effective chemotherapeutic agents in patients with progressive disease with distant metastases [1]. It is a natural way of thinking that the use of these drugs at an early postoperative stage may result in suppression against radiographically undetectable micrometastases and prolonged RFS and overall survival (OS). Some single-arm adjuvant chemotherapy trials performed in the 1970s reported favorable outcomes when compared with historical controls [2–4]. At the same time that chemotherapy was being adopted for osteosarcoma, however, there were significant changes in other aspects of the management of this disease. CT became a routine for the evaluation of pulmonary metastasis at the time of diagnosis and was demonstrated to be significantly more sensitive than plain radiography or conventional tomography. Because good outcomes might be achieved from selection of patients without lung metastases by CT, but not from adjuvant chemotherapy, it remains unclear whether the prognosis of patients without metastases improves by means of adjuvant chemotherapy or not. For this reason, the first RCT was conducted at the Mayo Clinic (Rochester, MN, USA) to elucidate the effectiveness of adjuvant chemotherapy with HD-MTX [5]. Subjects were 38 patients with osteosarcoma of the extremities, including the pectoral and pelvic girdles. First, the tumor was resected (37 underwent amputation and one had limb-preserving surgery), and subjects were then randomly assigned to either a surgery-only group ($n = 18$) or an adjuvant chemotherapy group ($n = 20$) treated with vincristine (VCR) + HD-MTX. The 5-year OS and RFS rates were 52 % and 42 %, respectively. There were no significant differences between groups. The RFS rate of the surgery-only group was the highest of all reports to date. However, the effectiveness of this adjuvant chemotherapy regimen was inconclusive because the patient cohort was relatively small; thus, a larger-scale study is required to verify the results. For this reason, the Multi-Institutional Osteosarcoma Study (MIOS), a phase III clinical trial, was initiated in June 1982 to assess the role of adjuvant chemotherapy for the treatment of osteosarcoma of the extremities after amputation of the affected limb [6]. The five drugs used were MTX, ADM, bleomycin (BLM), CPA, and actinomycin D (ACT-D). Informed consent for randomized allocation was obtained from 36 patients who were allocated to two groups of 18 subjects each: a surgery-only group and a postoperative adjuvant chemotherapy group.

Furthermore, they also analyzed 18 subjects who were nonrandomly allocated to the surgery-only group and 59 who were nonrandomly allocated to the postoperative adjuvant chemotherapy group. The 5-year RFS and OS rates of the postoperative adjuvant chemotherapy group were significantly greater than those of the surgery-only group (61 % and 71 % vs. 17 % and 50 %, respectively). The clinical courses were similar among subjects who were and were not randomly assigned to a treatment group. Eilber et al. also demonstrated similar outcomes [7]; thus, these two RCTs experimentally confirmed the efficacy of surgical resection followed by postoperative adjuvant chemotherapy, which has since been adopted as the standard treatment for osteosarcoma.

7.1.2 Introduction of Preoperative Adjuvant Chemotherapy

From the first half of 1970 when adjuvant chemotherapy was first introduced, Rosen et al. introduced neoadjuvant chemotherapy already in order to gain time for a custom-made artificial joint used for limb preservation [8]. Thereafter, modular-type artificial joints were developed, and the initial significance of preoperative chemotherapy began to decrease. The POG-8651 trial in the US was designed to demonstrate the superiority of preoperative and postoperative chemotherapy over postoperative chemotherapy only [9]. Although there were no significant differences in the 5-year event-free survival and OS rates between the pre-/postoperative chemotherapy group and the postoperative chemotherapy-only group (61 % and 76 % vs. 69 % and 79 %, respectively), the former group showed a lower point estimate. Accordingly, the superiority of preoperative chemotherapy was not verified. The rate of limb preservation in both groups in this study was approximately 50 %, and the outcomes of limb preservation modalities were also similar. For this reason, the authors were unable to identify a superior treatment strategy. The duration of the POG-8651 trial, which enrolled 100 subjects, was 8 years, but we believe that this trial did not have a major impact on the establishment of standard treatment for osteosarcoma that followed because: (1) the rate of limb preservation in the two groups was too low; (2) the impression gained through experience was that the primary lesion shrank due to preoperative chemotherapy; thus, it was possible to perform more efficient and safe surgery; and (3) performing preoperative chemotherapy allowed the adoption of the treatment strategy of changing postoperative treatment based on the histologic necrosis rate. For these reasons, although efficacy was not verified, preoperative chemotherapy was still administered. In addition, regarding the future direction, the results of ongoing clinical trials and the protocols of future clinical trials will need to be carefully scrutinized.

7.1.3 Histologic Necrosis Rate Following Preoperative Chemotherapy

By calculating the histologic necrosis rate of resected specimens obtained after the introduction of preoperative chemotherapy, we established that tumors with a high necrosis rate have a good prognosis and that tumors with a low necrosis rate have a poor prognosis. Differences in prognosis based on the histologic necrosis rates in the trials conducted to date are summarized in Table 7.1. Therefore, we believe that therapeutic effects will improve in patients who experienced limited preoperative therapeutic effects after administration of additional drugs that were not used in the preoperative regimen. Rosen added CDDP to the T-10 regimen in patients with a low histologic necrosis rate (poor responders) [10]. The results of this study indicated that there was no significant difference between the prognosis of these patients and those with a high histologic necrosis rate (good responders). They concluded that salvage by means of CDDP was possible. This conclusion was later refuted by Meyer PA, who conducted a long-term observational study [11]. The strategy of changing the postoperative chemotherapy regimen based on the histologic necrosis rate has been a main clinical question in treatment for osteosarcoma.

7.2 Development of Adjuvant Chemotherapy in Japan

7.2.1 The Dawn of a New Era in Osteosarcoma Treatment

In Japan, the development of treatments for osteosarcoma has been supported by the orthopedic surgeons with passion of the institutes engaged in multi-institutional studies. In addition, the bone tumor registry, which was started by Professor Amako

Table 7.1 Results of adjuvant chemotherapy for nonmetastatic osteosarcoma with respect to histological response

Protocol	Histological response	EFS		OS	
POG-8651	Viable tumor <10 % ($n = 26$)	5 years	73 % ± 8 %	5 years	77 % ± 9 %
	Viable tumor ≧10 % ($n = 16$)		44 % ± 15		80 % ± 12 %
CCG-782	Viable tumor <5 %	8 years	81 %	8 years	87 %
	Viable tumor ≧5 %		46 %		52 %
IOR/OS-2	Good responder ($n = 115$)	5 years	71.3 %		
	Poor responder ($n = 47$)		57.4 %		
IOR/OS-3a	Good responder ($n = 53$)	7 years	60 %	7 years	66 %
	Poor responder		45 %		55 %
COSS-80	Good responder ($n = 31$)	4 years	84 %		
	Poor responder ($n = 27$)		52 %		
COSS-82	Good responder ($n = 48$)	4 years	77 %		
	Poor responder ($n = 62$)		44 %		

(Kyushu University) in 1954, facilitated early advancements in the development of treatments for bone tumors. The bone tumor registry expanded to Japanese bone tumor registry after the decision at the annual meeting of the Japanese Orthopaedic Association in 1957. It has been managed in National Cancer Center since 1964 and paper registration forms have been substituted by digital media since 2006.

In 1960, osteosarcoma treatment was limited to amputation or disarticulation, and the survival rate of patients without metastases was 3–15 % [12]. Thereafter, in 1964, Miki et al. reported a treatment regimen of regional perfusion of anticancer drugs [13]. Subsequently, in 1966, Akahosi et al. and Masuda et al. reported the efficacy of continuous intra-arterial infusion [14]. For prevention of pulmonary metastases, Ohno et al. reported a method of continuous infusion of anticancer drugs into the bronchial artery [15]. As such, the primary methods of preoperative arterial infusion and regional perfusion were adopted. In 1971, Tateishi et al. reported a 5-year OS rate of 31.7 % in 64 patients who received regional perfusion therapy comprising 5-fluorouracil (5-FU), mitomycin C (MMC), and nitromin between 1960 and 1970 [16]. In addition, Akaboshi et al. reported a 5-year OS rate of 31.4 % in patients receiving intra-arterial infusion of 5-FU and MMC [17].

7.2.2 Introduction of Preoperative Adjuvant Chemotherapy by Multi-institutional Studies

Thereafter, several multi-institutional studies of adjuvant therapy for treatment of osteosarcoma were started in 1975. First, the Japanese Orthopedic Oncology Group (JOOG) conducted a multicenter study of postoperative adjuvant chemotherapy with ADM [18]. During this study, osteosarcoma patients without metastasis and who underwent amputation or disarticulation during the period between 1973 and 1980 received ADM at 0.6–0.8 mg/kg for 3 days by intravenous infusion beginning on postoperative week 1 and received multiple doses until a total dose of 600 mg (500 mg/m^2) was reached. However, in 1976, many investigators began to introduce combined therapy with ADM + HD-MTX, and the final report in 1988 was structured as a comparative study between ADM as monotherapy and combined therapy with ADM + HD-MTX. In addition, during this period, the decision of whether to administer preoperative therapy via intra-arterial infusion or regional perfusion therapy varied among studies. Among the accumulated cases, 59 were excluded, and 117 were included for analysis. The 5-year OS and DFS rates of all cases were 50.2 % and 39.4 %, respectively, whereas the 5-year OS and RFS rates of the 80 subjects in the ADM-only group were 44.4 % and 35.6 % compared with the rates of 63.1 % and 47.8 % in the combined treatment group, respectively, indicating more favorable outcomes, although these differences were not significant. When restricted to the 65 subjects who received a total ADM dose of $\geq$500 mg, the 5-year OSR was significantly greater in combined treatment group than in the 48 subjects in the ADM-only group (76.5 % vs. 52.1 %, respectively).

They concluded that combined ADM and HD-MTX treatment was more appropriate as adjuvant chemotherapy for osteosarcoma. Furthermore, another analysis of the cases who developed pulmonary metastases after initial treatment was based on the 23 subjects who underwent resection of metastatic lesions compared with 43 who did not. The 5-year OS rate was significantly greater in the resection group than in the nonresection group (43.5 % vs. 2.6 %, respectively), suggesting that resection of pulmonary metastases was the more effective method to prolong survival.

In addition, a study conducted by the Ministry of Health and Welfare (MHW) during approximately the same period (1973–1981) reported the 5-year OS and DFS rates of 52.6 % and 37.0 %, respectively, in 1983 [19]. The 5-year OS and DFS rates in the ADM-only group were 32.7 % and 26.1 % compared with the rates of 59.5 % and 41.4 % in the MTX combination therapy group, respectively, again showing more favorable outcomes for combination therapy. Because these two multi-institutional studies included many of the same institutions, there is a high likelihood that patients were duplicated. However, even if this is the case, the efficacy of combination therapy was confirmed by both multicenter studies.

7.2.3 Introduction of Preoperative Adjuvant Chemotherapy

Preoperative adjuvant chemotherapy was first introduced in 1980. Between 1980 and 1981, the MTX osteosarcoma research group registered 35 patients who received VCR and HD-MTX preoperatively and VCR, HD-MTX, ADM, and CPM postoperatively and reported the 3-year OS and DFS rates of 58.2 % and 40 %, respectively [20]. The histological response to preoperative chemotherapy was determined, and although there was no statistically significant difference, the survival time tended to be longer in those with a favorable histological response.

In addition, during this period, CDDP and ifosfamide (IFO) were introduced as novel drugs to treat osteosarcoma in Japan. In 1984, CDDP was introduced into the market for the treatment of cancers of the testes, bladder, renal pelvis and ureters, prostate, and ovaries. In 1989, the therapeutic effects of CDDP monotherapy for primary and metastatic lesions in patients with osteosarcoma were reported [21]. Although the evaluation methods differed from those used today, this treatment was successful in 3 of 18 subjects. Ten years later, in December 1999, CDDP was approved for use for the additional indication of osteosarcoma. In addition, from July 1978 to September 1980, joint studies of IFO to treat malignant bone and soft tissue tumor reported effective outcomes in 12 of 22 subjects with osteosarcoma [22]. Although the use of IFO was covered by the national insurance program for this and other indications in 1985, hematuria and bladder dysfunction were observed as characteristic adverse drug reactions of IFO; thus, wide-scale use was delayed until the 1994 commercialization of mesna, a detoxifying agent that inhibits hemorrhagic cystitis induced by IFO.

Limb-preserving surgery became popular in the 1980s. From 1980 to 1985, 250 cases of osteosarcoma were accumulated retrospectively from 22 Japanese institutions and were reported in 1992 as the 10-year intergroup study [23]. All subjects who underwent limb-preserving surgery received adjuvant chemotherapy consisting mainly of MTX, ADM, and CDDP. This study reported that subjects who underwent amputation or disarticulation also usually received the same adjuvant chemotherapy regimen, but the details were not mentioned. The 5-year OS rate was 58 % in all 250 subjects, 70 % in the 107 subjects (42.8 %) who underwent limb-preserving surgery, and 49 % in the 143 subjects (57.2 %) who underwent amputation or disarticulation, indicating significantly better outcomes after limb-preserving surgery. Analysis of the resection margin was also performed, and resection with wide margin and marginal margin partially and resection with wide margin fully had the same outcome. The outcomes after limb-preserving surgery were favorable; thus, it was concluded that the optimal strategy was to perform limb-preserving surgery to achieve more favorable long-term limb function. It was also concluded that this strategy required more aggressive localized chemotherapy and radiotherapy to get higher rate of tumor necrosis and development of reconstructive surgery, involving joint replacement and bone grafts.

7.2.4 Changes in Postoperative Chemotherapy Based on the Histologic Necrosis Rate

Outcomes of the T-10 and T-12 protocols reported by Rosen in the US during the mid-1980s had a major impact on strategies for osteosarcoma [10]. In both protocols, the postoperative treatment was changed based on the histologic necrosis rate of the tumor after resection, with preoperative treatment composed mainly of HD-MTX. Fundamentally, groups that achieved good results continued to receive HD-MTX treatment, and those with insufficient results received treatment with CDDP and ADM. Of 87 subjects who received treatment according to the T-10 protocol, DFS was reported in 67 subjects (77 %) and OS was reported in 71 subjects (81.6 %) after a follow-up period of 3–6 years. Of 51 subjects treated according to the T-12 protocol, DFS was reported in 38 subjects (75 %) and OS was reported in 39 (76 %) after a median short-term follow-up period of 2 years. Based on these results, Rosen concluded that it was possible to avoid administering drugs that could cause further adverse reactions to patients who had favorable results after preoperative treatment and to complete treatment early. As mentioned above, these results were later refuted by Meyers after long-term follow-up observations, but at that time, the outcome was very impressive, and several studies to verify this result were conducted in other countries.

A study to verify the efficacy of T-12 protocol was also conducted as a multi-institutional study including six institutes in Japan between 1987 and 1990 [24]. The T-12 protocol was based on preoperative administration of six courses of HD-MTX and two courses of BCD (bleomycin, cyclophosphamide, and dactinomycin), and postoperative chemotherapy was based on the histological response. Good responders received treatment with four courses of ADM and HD-MTX, and poor responders received six courses of ADM + CDDP + BCD

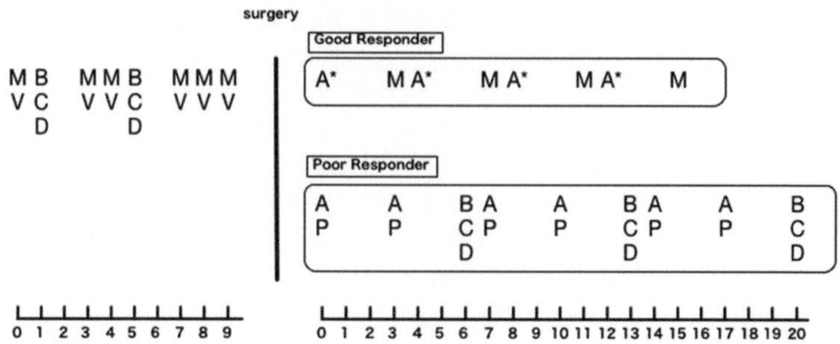

Fig. 7.1 The schema of T-12 protocol used by Japanese multi-institutional study. M, high-dose MTX 8–12 g/m^2; V, vincristine 1.5 mg/m^2; BCD, bleomycin 15 mg/m^2, cyclophosphamide 600 mg/m^2, dactinomycin 0.6 mg/m2; A, ADM 30 mg/m^2 × 2 days; A*, ADM 30 mg/m^2 × 3 days; P, CDDP 120 mg/m^2

(Fig. 7.1). The 5-year OS and DFS rates of 37 registered subjects over a mean follow-up period of 60.3 months were 68.7 % and 48.3 %, respectively. The 5-year OS and DFS rates were 85.6 % and 64.7 % in the 17 subjects who were good responders to preoperative chemotherapy and 55.0 % and 35.0 % in the 20 subjects who were poor responders, respectively. Compared with good responders, poor responders exhibited a significant decrease in overall and disease-free survival. This study showed the fact that changes of drugs in poor responders was not effective, which may arise because the tumor was originally multidrug resistant or the tumor size increased due to the ineffectiveness of preoperative drug administration.

This study above mentioned reported that changes in the postoperative chemotherapy regimen used to treat poor responders resulted in unfavorable outcomes. Thereafter, the bone tumor research group was awarded a grant from the MHLW Japanese Foundation for Cancer Research to conduct a multi-institutional phase II study of neoadjuvant chemotherapy for osteosarcoma (NECO)-93J and NECO-95J protocols with the following characteristics [25] (Fig. 7.2):

1. Use of three key drugs for osteosarcoma, i.e., ADM, HD-MTX, and CDDP (MAP therapy), preoperatively and an increase in the treatment intensity.
2. Introduction of IFO preoperatively if there is exacerbation during preoperative treatment.
3. Determination of the histological response of the resected tumor in patients who showed no exacerbation during preoperative treatment. If the results were favorable, MAP therapy was continued. If not, IFO was then introduced.

During the NECO-93J trial, which was conducted first, only 44 % of subjects were able to complete the treatment schedule, primarily because of hemotoxicity. In particular, a total of eight courses of IFO which composed of 16 g/m^2/course was added to postoperative MAP therapy in subjects who responded poorly to preoperative treatment during phase V of the trial and to the postoperative treatment schedule in subjects who experienced preoperative exacerbation during phase

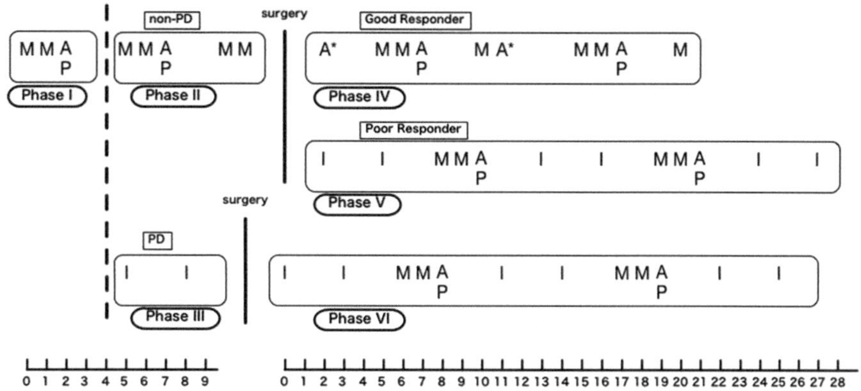

Fig. 7.2 The schema of NECO-95J protocol. M, high-dose MTX 8–12 g/m^2; A, ADM 30 mg/m^2 × 2 days; A*, ADM 30 mg/m^2 × 3 days; P, CDDP 120 mg/m^2; I, IFO total 16 g/m^2/7 days (4 g/m^2 on the first day followed by 2 g/m^2/day × 6 days)

VI. However, during these phases, the treatment completion rate was approximately halved; therefore, in the NECO-95J trial, a total course of IFO during phases V and VI was shortened to six courses. Between October 1993 and May 2001, 50 subjects were enrolled in the NECO-93J trial and 63 in the NECO-95J trial. From a total of 113 subjects, the 5-year RFS and OS rates after a median observation period of 75.6 months (range, 11–140 months) were 65.5 % and 77.9 %, respectively. When the histological response was determined in those who underwent surgery, 46 were considered as good responders and 63 as poor responders; thus, approximately 40 % were good responders. The 5-year OSR was 78.7 % among 47 subjects who experienced no exacerbation during preoperative treatment and were determined to be good responders postoperatively. In the other hand, the 5-year OSR was 89.5 % among 38 subjects who experienced no exacerbation during preoperative treatment and were determined to be poor responders postoperatively; there was no significant difference in these two groups. In addition, the 5-year OS rate was 68.2 % among the 22 subjects who progressed from phase III to VI after being diagnosed with exacerbation during preoperative treatment, and although this rate was somewhat low, there was no statistically significant difference. These results implied that the addition of IFO to the treatment regimen of subjects who responded poorly to MAP therapy may improve prognosis. During the NECO study, the IFO dosage was usually high compared with the total doses in protocols used in other countries, which ranged from 34 to 60 g/m^2; the dose was 128 g/m^2 in the NECO-93J trial and 96 g/m^2 in the NECO-95J trial during phase V and 160 g/m^2 in the NECO-93J trial and 128 g/m^2 when subjects progressed from phase III to VI in the NECO-95J trial. Although the increase of IFO dose makes the treatment period prolonged and may raise concerns regarding male infertility, increases in renal dysfunction, such as Fanconi's syndrome, or the onset of secondary cancers, this treatment was expected to contribute to prolonged survival.

The increased effectiveness clinically observed through the addition of IFO remained inconclusive for 20 years. In the USA, 793 subjects were enrolled in the 4-year INT-0133 trial conducted by the Children's Oncology Group (COG), which began in 1993 (Fig. 7.3). At the start of the treatment, subjects were randomly allocated to four groups to receive MAP therapy, MAP therapy + IFO, MAP therapy + mifamurtide, or MAP therapy + IFO + mifamurtide, and the two groups undergoing therapy involving IFO received this drug at a total preoperative and postoperative dose of 45 mg/m^2. In 2008, the final results, which included a follow-up observation period, showed no significant differences in the 6-year DFS and OS of the MAP therapy groups (MAP and MAP + mifamurtide groups) compared with those of the MAP + IFO groups (MAP + IFO and MAP + IFO + mifamurtide groups; 63 % and 73 % vs. 64 % and 75 %, respectively), which indicated that there were no additional benefits from the addition of IFO [26]. In this final report, changes were made to the subject population as compared with the population in the initial report, and the statistical methods were difficult to interpret; thus, it was difficult to determine whether a consensus in terms of a conclusion was reached between research groups from different countries. Nonetheless, at the very least, some groups in the USA have already abandoned the idea that the addition of IFO offers further benefits.

The aim of the NECO study was to determine whether the outcome of poor responders only, as opposed to all patients, was improved by the addition of IFO. Similar studies were conducted in Germany by the Cooperative Osteosarcoma Study Group (COSS) and in Italy. The Italian group reported that outcomes improved when IFO or IFO + VP-16 was administered to poor responders after MAP therapy. Currently, two RCTs are ongoing to verify if there are any additional benefits for the treatment outcome from the addition of IFO to the regimens of poor responders.

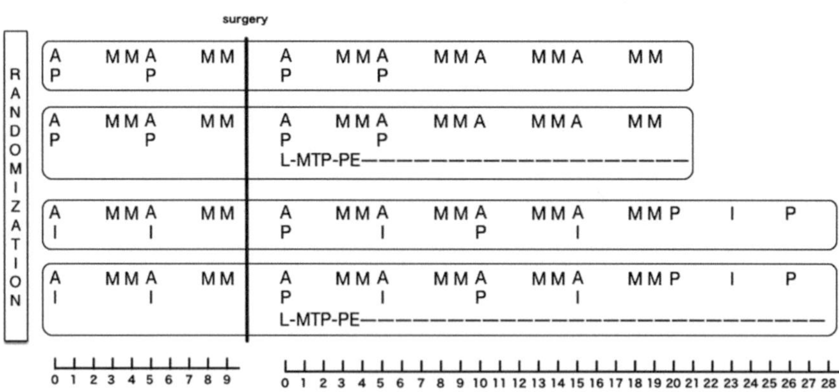

Fig. 7.3 The schema of INT-0133. M, high-dose MTX 12 g/m^2 (max 20 g/m^2); A, ADM 75 mg/m^2/72-h civ; P, CDDP 120 mg/m^2/4 h; I, IFO 1.8 g/m2 × 5 days; L-MTP-PE, liposomal muramyl tripeptide phosphatidylethanolamine 2 mg/m^2 (escalation to 4 mg by 1 mg)

The European and American Osteosarcoma Study Group (EURAMOS) was founded in 2001 and is composed of four clinical research groups, namely, COSS; COG; the European Osteosarcoma Intergroup (EOI), which focuses on the UK; and the Scandinavian Sarcoma Group (SSG) (http://www.ctu.mrc.ac.uk/euramos/default.asp). In the EURAMOS-1 trial, good responders were randomized to receive either MAP therapy or MAP therapy + interferon α, while poor responders were randomized to receive either MAP therapy or MAP therapy + IFO +VP-16 (Fig. 7.4). The total dose of IFO was greater than that used in the INT-0133 trial, which was 60 g/m^2. Because the additional effects were 10 % greater than those of experimental treatment in both the good and poor responder groups, initial enrollment of 1,400 subjects for a 4-year study was scheduled to begin in 2005. However, the end of the registration was delayed, and approximately 6.5 years later, 2260 subjects were enrolled. In 2013, the results of good responders were reported by the American Society of Clinical Oncology, and the 3-year DFS rates of the MAP and MAP + interferon groups were 74 % and 77 %, respectively. The additional effects of interferon α were not confirmed (HR = 0.77; 95% CI = 0.50–1.19) [27]. The results of poor responders were also reported by the Connective Tissue Oncology Society in October 2014; no evidence of an advantage of MAP + IFO + VP-16 for this group was shown in terms of EFS-hazard ratio 1.01 (95 % CI 0.80–1.26) nor in survival-hazard ratio 0.99 (95 % CI 0.74–1.32) [28].

In Japan, enrollment for the JCOG0905 RCT, conducted by the Japan Clinical Oncology Group (JCOG) bone and soft tissue tumor research group, was started in

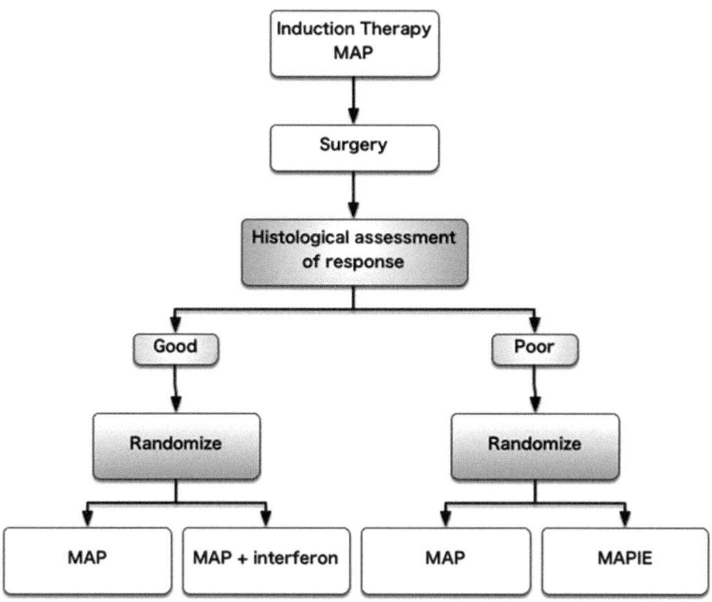

Fig. 7.4 The schema of EURAMOS-1. MAP, high-dose MTX, ADM, and CDDP; MAPIE, high-dose MTX, ADM, CDDP, IFO, VP-16

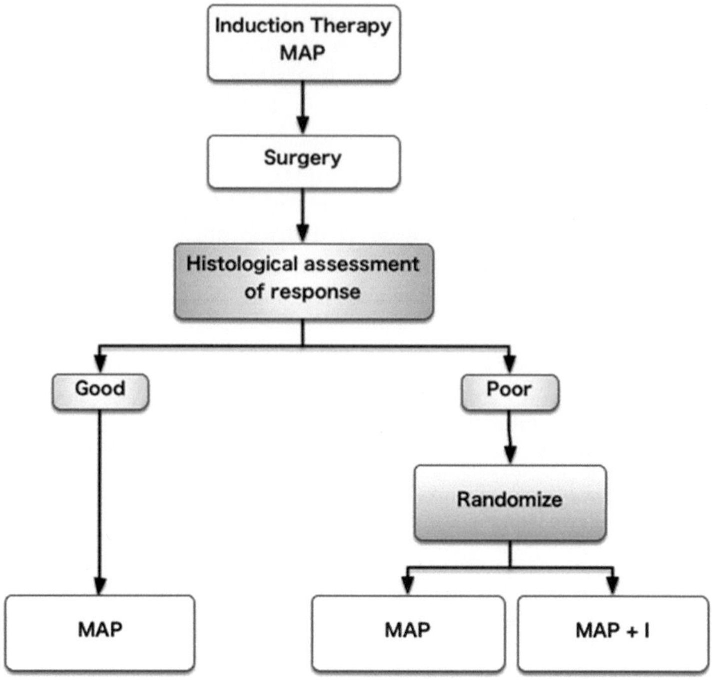

Fig. 7.5 The schema of JCOG0905. MAP, high-dose MTX, ADM, and CDDP; MAP + I, high-dose MTX, ADM, CDDP, IFO

February 2012 (https://upload.umin.ac.jp/cgi-open-bin/ctr/ctr.cgi?function=brows&action=brows&type=summary&recptno=R000003846&language=J) (Fig. 7.5). This study is the first osteosarcoma phase III study conducted in Japan. In the JCOG0905 trial, poor responders were randomly allocated to receive either standard chemotherapy with MAP or experimental treatment with MAP therapy + IFO as postoperative chemotherapy. The experimental treatment regimen was approximately the same as that used in the NECO-95J trial with a total dose of 90 g/m^2. We believe that the results from the EURAMOS-1 and JCOG0905 trials will provide conclusive results regarding the effectiveness of changes in postoperative chemotherapy regimens for poor responders, which had long remained inconclusive.

References

1. Cores EP, Holland JF, Wang JJ, Sinks LF. Doxorubicin in disseminated osteosarcoma. JAMA. 1972;221(10):1132–8.
2. Sutow WW, Sullivan MP, Fernbach DJ, Cangir A, George SL. Adjuvant chemotherapy in primary treatment of osteogenic sarcoma. A Southwest Oncology Group study. Cancer. 1975;36(5):1598–602.

3. Jaffe N, Frei E, Traggis D, Bishop Y. Adjuvant methotrexate and citrovorum-factor treatment of osteogenic sarcoma. N Engl J Med. 1974;291(19):994–7.
4. Cortes EP, Holland JF, Wang JJ, Sinks LF, Blom J, Senn H, et al. Amputation and adriamycin in primary osteosarcoma. N Engl J Med. 1974;291(19):998–1000.
5. Edmonson JH, Green SJ, Ivins JC, Gilchrist GS, Creagan ET, Pritchard DJ, et al. A controlled pilot study of high-dose methotrexate as postsurgical adjuvant treatment for primary osteosarcoma. J Clin Oncol. 1984;2(3):152–6.
6. Link MP, Goorin AM, Horowitz M, Meyer WH, Belasco J, Baker A, et al. Adjuvant chemotherapy of high-grade osteosarcoma of the extremity. Updated results of the Multi-Institutional Osteosarcoma Study. Clin Orthop Relat Res. 1991;270:8–14.
7. Eilber F, Giuliano A, Eckardt J, Patterson K, Moseley S, Goodnight J. Adjuvant chemotherapy for osteosarcoma: a randomized prospective trial. J Clin Oncol. 1987;5(1):21–6.
8. Rosen G, Murphy ML, Huvos AG, Gutierrez M, Marcove RC. Chemotherapy, en bloc resection, and prosthetic bone replacement in the treatment of osteogenic sarcoma. Cancer. 1976;37(1):1–11.
9. Goorin AM. Presurgical chemotherapy compared with immediate surgery and adjuvant chemotherapy for nonmetastatic osteosarcoma: Pediatric Oncology Group Study POG-8651. J Clin Oncol. 2003;21(8):1574–80.
10. Rosen G, Nirenberg A. Neoadjuvant chemotherapy for osteogenic sarcoma: a five year follow-up (T-10) and preliminary report of new studies (T-12). Prog Clin Biol Res. 1985;201:39–51.
11. Meyers PA, Heller G, Healey J, Huvos A, Lane J, Marcove R, et al. Chemotherapy for nonmetastatic osteogenic sarcoma: the memorial Sloan-Kettering experience. J Clin Oncol. 1992;10(1):5–15.
12. Furuse K, Maeyama I, Morimoto K, Orito T. Adjuvant chemotherapy for osteosarcoma in Japan – past, present and future. Gan To Kagaku Ryoho. 1984;11(9):1746–56.
13. Miki I, Azuma H, Tateishi A. Seiganzai kyokusho kanryuhou niyoru shishiakuseishuyou no chiryou. Seikeigeka. 1964;15:87–97 (in Japanese).
14. Akahoshi Y. Chronometric Infusor hiraku kotsushuyou no chiryou heno ouyou. Rinshou Seikeigeka. 1966;1:315–9 (in Japanese).
15. Ohno T, Osuwari K. Kotsugensei nikusyu no haitenni yobou wo mokutekitoseru seiganzai no kikanshidoumyaku chunyu. Seikeigeka. 1966;1:724–31 (in Japanese).
16. Tateishi A. kyokusho kanryuhou niyoru kotsunikushu no chiryou seiseki. Nichiganchi. 1971;6:632–8 (in Japanese).
17. Akahoshi Y, Takeuchi S. Kotsunikushuni taisuru kagaku ryohou – Tokuni jutsuzen kyokusho domyakunai touyohou to shujutsu no heiyou nitsuite. Rinshou Seikeigeka. 1976;11:790–7 (in Japanese).
18. Maeyama I, Furuse K, Yamawaki S, Abe M, Tateishi A, Takeyama S, et al. Evaluation of adjuvant chemotherapy of osteosarcoma with special reference to adriamycin (final report). Gan To Kagaku Ryoho. 1988;15(12):3245–51.
19. Furuse K, Maeyama I, Inada O, et al. Adjuvant chemotherapy for bone and soft tissue sarcomas in Japan. In: Ogawa M, Muggia FM, Rozencweig M, editors. Adriamycin its expanding role in cancer treatment (Proceedings of the international symposium on Adriamycin, Japna, 1983). Amsterdam: Excerpta Medica; 1984. p. 307–18.
20. Fukuma H, Yamawaki S, Sasaki T, et al. High-dose methotrexate with citrovorum factor rescue for bone and soft tissue sarcoma. In: Kimura K, Wang YM, editors. Methotrexate in cancer therapy, progress in cancer research and therapy, vol. 33. New York: Raven Press; 1986. p. 239–47.
21. Fukuma H, Beppu Y, Chuman H, Yagi T, Yamawaki S, Isu K, et al. Cis-dichlorodiammineplatinum in osteosarcoma. Osteosarcoma Cooperative Study Group report. Gan To Kagaku Ryoho. 1989;16(4 Pt 1):811–7.
22. Akahoshi Y, Takeuchi S, Ishii S, Yamawaki S, Inoue S, Takada N, Toriyama S, Abe M, Tateishi A, Nomura S, Sugiura I, Ogihara Y, Ishida T, Maeyama I, Kitagawa T. Clinical

experience with ifosfamide in malignant bone and soft-tissue tumors. Gan To Kagaku Ryoho. 1981;8(3):395–405.
23. Tsuchiya H, Tomita K. Prognosis of osteosarcoma treated by limb-salvage surgery: the ten-year intergroup study in Japan. Jpn J Clin Oncol. 1992;22(5):347–53.
24. Isu K, Yamawaki S, Fukuma H, Kawaguchi T, Tatezaki S-I, Furuse K, Usui M. Results of a group study of T-12 protocol as neo-adjuvant chemotherapy for osteosarcoma. The 68th Annual Meeting of the Japanese Orthopaedic Association, proceeding, S394.
25. Iwamoto Y, Tanaka K, Isu K, Kawai A, Tatezaki S-I, Ishii T, et al. Multiinstitutional phase II study of neoadjuvant chemotherapy for osteosarcoma (NECO study) in Japan: NECO-93J and NECO-95J. J Orthop Sci. 2009;14(4):397–404.
26. Meyers PA, Schwartz CL, Krailo MD, Healey JH, Bernstein ML, Betcher D, et al. Osteosarcoma: the addition of muramyl tripeptide to chemotherapy improves overall survival – a report from the Children's Oncology Group. J Clin Oncol. 2008;26(4):633–8.
27. Bielack SS, Smeland S, Whelan J, Marina N, Hook J, Jovic G, Krailo MD, Butterfass-Bahloul T, Kühne T, Eriksson M, Teot LA, Gelderblom H, Kager L, Hall KS, Gorlick RG, Randall RL, Hogendoorn PCW, Calaminus G, Sydes MR, Bernstein ML, Klinikum Stuttgart, Olgahospital, Cooperative Osteosarcoma Study Group (COSS), Stuttgart, Germany; Oslo University Hospital, The Norwegian Radium Hospital, Scandinavian Sarcoma Group, Oslo, Norway; University College London Hospitals NHS Foundation Trust, London, United Kingdom; Stanford University, School of Medicine, Palo Alto, CA; MRC Clinical Trials Unit, London, United Kingdom; Children's Oncology Group, Arcadia, CA; Center for Clinical Trials, University of Muenster, Muenster, Germany; University Children's Hospital Basel, Basel, Switzerland; Skane University Hospital and Lund University, Lund, Sweden; Children's Hospital Boston, Boston, MA; Department of Clinical Oncology, Leiden University Medical Center, Leiden, Netherlands; St Anna's Children's Hospital, Vienna, Austria; The Children's Hospital, Bronx, NY; Huntsman Cancer Institute, University of Utah, Salt Lake City, UT; Department of Pathology, Leiden University Medical Center, Leiden, Netherlands; University Hospital of Muenster, Muenster, Germany; IWK Health Center, Dalhousie University, Halifax, NS, Canada. MAP plus maintenance pegylated interferon α-2b (MAPIfn) versus MAP alone in patients with resectable high-grade osteosarcoma and good histologic response to preoperative MAP: First results of the EURAMOS-1 "good response" randomization. J Clin Oncol. 2013;31 (suppl; abstr LBA10504).
28. Marina N, Smeland S, Bielack SS, Bernstein M, Jovic G, Hook JM, Krailo MD, Butterfass-Bahloul T, Kühne T, Eriksson M, Teot L, Gelderblom H, Kager L, Hall KS, Gorlick R, Randall RL, Hogendoorn PW, Calaminus G, Sydes MR, Whelan JS. MAPIE vs MAP as postoperative chemotherapy in patients with a poor response to preoperative chemotherapy for newly-diagnosed osteosarcoma: results from EURAMOS-1 (Paper 032). 2014, Presented at Connective Tissue Oncology Society (CTOS) 2014.

Neoadjuvant Chemotherapy: Osaka University Osteosarcoma (OOS) Regimen

8

Shigeki Kakunaga, Takafumi Ueda, Norifumi Naka, Shigeyuki Kuratsu, Nobuhito Araki, Yasuaki Aoki, and Hideki Yoshikawa

Abstract

Objective: The purpose of this study is to evaluate the efficacy of a four-drug regimen neoadjuvant chemotherapy for osteosarcoma with doxorubicin, cisplatin, methotrexate, and ifosfamide for patients ≤40 years of age with nonmetastatic osteosarcoma of the extremity.

Methods: From 1997 to 2012, 82 patients were evaluated. Treatment consisted of ten courses of chemotherapy and wide local excision. Preoperatively, patients received two courses of doxorubicin (90 mg/m^2)/cisplatin (120 mg/m^2) combination and high-dose ifosfamide (15 g/m^2). Postoperatively, patients received two courses of doxorubicin/cisplatin combination, high-dose ifosfamide, and high-dose methotrexate (12 g/m^2 on consecutive weeks).

Results: There were 2 patients with local recurrence, 17 patients with lung metastasis, and 1 patient with bone metastasis. At the last follow-up, 61 patients were continuously disease-free, 11 patients had no evidence of disease, 3 patients

S. Kakunaga (✉)
Osaka University Orthopaedic Oncology Group, Department of Orthopaedic Surgery, Osaka National Hospital, 2-1-14 Hoenzaka Chuo-ku, Osaka 540-0006, Japan
e-mail: kakunaga@onh.go.jp

T. Ueda
Department of Orthopaedic Surgery, Osaka National Hospital, Osaka, Japan

N. Naka • H. Yoshikawa
Department of Orthopaedic Surgery, Osaka University Graduate School of Medicine, Suita, Japan

S. Kuratsu
Department of Orthopaedic Surgery, Bellland General Hospital, Sakai, Japan

N. Araki
Musculoskeletal Oncology Service, Osaka Medical Center for Cancer and Cardiovascular Diseases, Osaka, Japan

Y. Aoki
Department of Orthopaedic Surgery, Himeji Red Cross Hospital, Himeji, Japan

T. Ueda, A. Kawai (eds.), *Osteosarcoma*, DOI 10.1007/978-4-431-55696-1_8

were alive with disease, 6 patients died of disease, and 1 patient died of treatment-related toxicity. The 5-year and 10-year event-free survival rates were 77 % and 73 %, respectively. The 5-year and 10-year overall survival rates were 95 % and 90 %, respectively.

Conclusion: A four-drug regimen neoadjuvant chemotherapy for osteosarcoma with doxorubicin, cisplatin, methotrexate, and ifosfamide was feasible. The survival rates were similar or better than previous studies. This study shows that this four-drug ten-course regimen can be an effective treatment for osteosarcoma.

Keywords

Osteosarcoma • Chemotherapy • High-dose ifosfamide • Histological response • Cumulative dose

8.1 Introduction

The prognosis for patients with osteosarcoma has greatly improved with the introduction of multidrug chemotherapy [1–3]. It is generally accepted that there are four active drugs against osteosarcoma: doxorubicin (DOX), cisplatin (CDDP), methotrexate (MTX), and ifosfamide (IFM) [4, 5]. However, there is a controversy as to which combination is the most effective. IFM has been used mainly in regimen for poor responders or relapse [6, 7]. Also, IFM has been used as a single agent or with a combination of other agents such as DOX, CDDP, or etoposide [8–11]. When used as a single agent, the dose of IFM varied from 10 to 15 g/m^2 [12–14].

At Osaka University Orthopaedic Oncology Group, neoadjuvant chemotherapy with high-dose MTX (HD-MTX) and DOX followed by adjuvant chemotherapy with the same drugs was first introduced in 1976 for the treatment of osteosarcoma (OOS-A regimen). In 1982, CDDP was added and DOX was administered intra-arterially (OOS-B regimen) to achieve a higher intratumor concentration. Standard-dose IFM (10 g/m^2) was added to the OOS-B regimen (OOS-C regimen) in 1989 [12]. From 1997, the OOS-D regimen consisting of DOX/CDDP, HD-MTX, and high-dose IFM (HD-IFM) (15 g/m^2) was introduced. The purpose of this study is to evaluate the efficacy of the OOS-D regimen neoadjuvant chemotherapy for patients $\leq$40 years of age with nonmetastatic osteosarcoma of the extremity.

8.2 Patients and Methods

Patients were enrolled in our group of five institutions (Osaka University Graduate School of Medicine and four affiliated cancer centers). Eligibility criteria were biopsy-proven diagnosis of primary conventional high-grade osteosarcoma of the extremity with no known metastasis at presentation; under 40 years of age; normal hepatic, renal, cardiac function; and no prior therapy. Primary tumor was evaluated

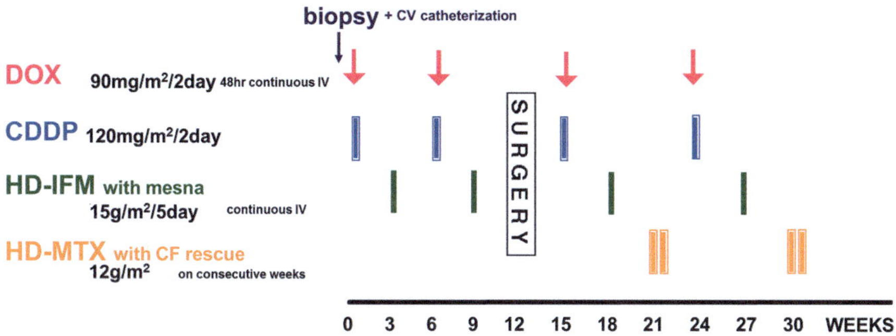

Fig 8.1 OOS-D regimen

by plain radiograms, magnetic resonance imaging (MRI) scans, and/or computed tomography (CT) scans. Screening for metastasis was evaluated by chest plain CT scan and bone scintigraphy.

OOS-D regimen: Chemotherapy consisted of DOX/CDDP (courses 1, 3, 5, 8), HD-IFM (courses 2, 4, 6, 9), and HD-MTX (courses 7, 10) according to the schedule and dose shown in Fig. 8.1. Each course was administered every 3 weeks. DOX was administered as a 48-h continuous infusion with a dose of 90 mg/m^2, and CDDP was administered intravenously for 4 h for 2 days at a daily dose of 60 mg/m^2. IFM was administered as a 5-day continuous intravenous infusion with a total dose of 15 g/m^2 with mesna uroprotection. MTX was administered as a 6-h infusion with citrovorum factor rescue every 6 h beginning 24 h after the start of MTX infusion. Sodium bicarbonate was administered for adequate alkalinization to keep urinary pH more than 7.0. One course of HD-MTX included two weekly administration of MTX. All the treatment was done as inpatient.

Complete blood count (CBC) and renal and hepatic functions were monitored before and after each chemotherapy administration. Granulocyte colony-stimulating factor was given to patients with grade 3 or 4 leukopenia. Chemotherapy was delayed or dose reduction (80 %) was allowed if granulocyte count was less than 1,000/mL, or platelet count was less than 100,000/mL, or there was renal or hepatic disorder. Normal renal function was required before each chemotherapy administration.

Surgical resection of tumor was scheduled after four courses of chemotherapy. All patients received limb salvage surgery. In principle, en bloc wide margin resection of the tumor was performed. Reconstruction was performed with either prosthetic replacement or intraoperative radiated autologous bone graft (IORBG) [15]. Postoperative chemotherapy was to start 3 weeks after surgery.

Toxicities were graded according to the Common Terminology Criteria for Adverse Events version 4.0. Histological response to chemotherapy was evaluated in resected tumor specimens. Good response was defined as total or more than 90 % necrosis of the tumor. Poor response was defined as lesser than 90 % necrosis of tumor [16].

8.2.1 Statistics

The event-free survival (EFS) was calculated from the date of start of chemotherapy until the date of first event including recurrence (local or distant) or chemotherapy-related death or the date of last follow-up examination. The overall survival (OS) was calculated from the date of start of chemotherapy until the date of death or the date of last follow-up examination. Survival curves were estimated using the Kaplan-Meier method and were compared by means of the log-rank test. Statistical analyses were performed using JMP ver. 10.0 software (SAS institute, North Carolina).

8.3 Results

From 1997 to 2012, out of 271 patients treated for osteosarcoma at our institute, 82 patients were eligible for this study. The patient characteristics are listed in Table 8.1. The median follow-up period for surviving patients was 113 months (range 29–193 months).

Table 8.1 Patient characteristics

	No.	%
Age (years)		
Median	16	
Mean	17.2	
Range	7–37	
Gender		
Male	54	66
Female	28	34
Surgical stage		
IIA	7	9
IIB	75	91
Site		
Femur	43	52
Tibia	22	27
Humerus	11	13
Fibula	6	7
Histological subtype		
Osteoblastic	51	62
Chondroblastic	9	11
Fibroblastic	6	7
Telangiectatic	5	6
Small round cell	1	1
Not specified	10	12

8.3.1 Chemotherapy Compliance and Toxicity

Of the 82 patients, 59 (72 %) completed all ten courses of chemotherapy. Of the courses uncompleted, HD-MTX was skipped the most at eight times. This was due to delayed excretion of MTX in the first week of HD-MTX, and the second week was skipped. HD-IFM was skipped four times due to severe prolonged hematological toxicity from the previous course. Other causes for discontinuation were renal disorder, wound infection, and patient's request.

One patient died as a result of chemotherapy-related toxicity. A 15-year-old boy died from acute heart failure 2 months after completion of therapy. There were no other patients who reported with cardiomyopathy. All patient experienced grade 4 hematologic toxicity.

8.3.2 Histological Response

During the preoperative chemotherapy, no clinical or radiological progression of disease was confirmed. Histological response to chemotherapy was good in 39 patients (56 %) and poor in 31 patients. The histological response of 12 patients could not be obtained because histological examination of the whole tumor was not available.

8.3.3 Patient Outcome

At the last follow-up, 61 (74 %) patients were continuously disease-free, 11 (13 %) patients were alive with no evidence of disease, 3 (4 %) patients were alive with disease, 6 (7 %) patients died of disease, and 1 (2 %) patient died of treatment-related toxicity. The 5-year and 10-year EFS rates were 77 % (95 % CI, 67–84 %) and 73 % (95 % CI, 62–82 %), respectively (Fig. 8.2). The 5-year and 10-year OS

Fig 8.2 Event-free survival of all patients

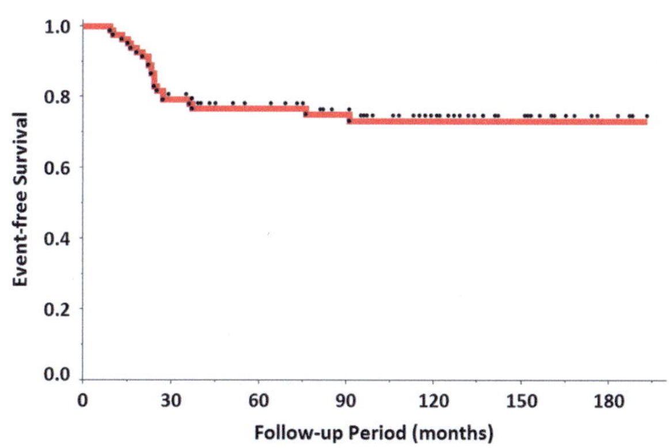

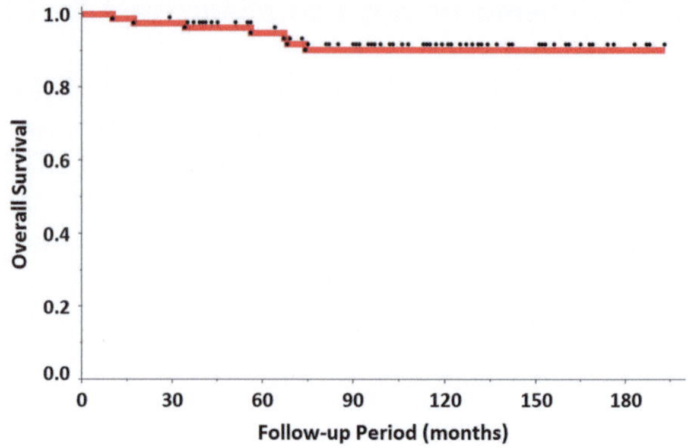

Fig 8.3 Overall survival of all patients

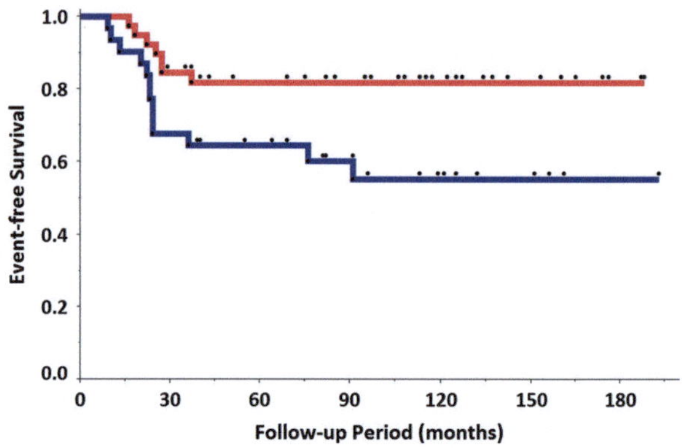

Fig 8.4 Event-free survival: good responder (*red*); poor responder (*blue*): $p = 0.025$

rates were 95 % (95 % CI, 87–97 %) and 90 % (95 % CI, 81–95 %), respectively (Fig. 8.3).

Two patients (2 %) had local recurrence 23 and 24 months after the start of treatment. Both patients had amputation of the affected limb. Seventeen patients (21 %) had lung metastasis and one patient (1 %) had bone metastasis. Median time to metastasis was 23.5 months (range 9–91 months). All patients underwent metastasectomy. The 3-year and 5-year post-relapse survival rates were 84 % and 67 %, respectively.

For good responders, the 5-year and 10-year EFS rates were both 82 % and were significantly better than poor responders at 65 % and 55 % ($p = 0.025$), respectively (Fig. 8.4). The 5-year and 10-year OS rates for good responders were 100 % and 94 % and were better than those for poor responders at 87 and 82 % though not statistically significant ($p = 0.11$) (Fig. 8.5).

Fig 8.5 Overall survival: good responder (*red*); poor responder (*blue*): $p = 0.11$

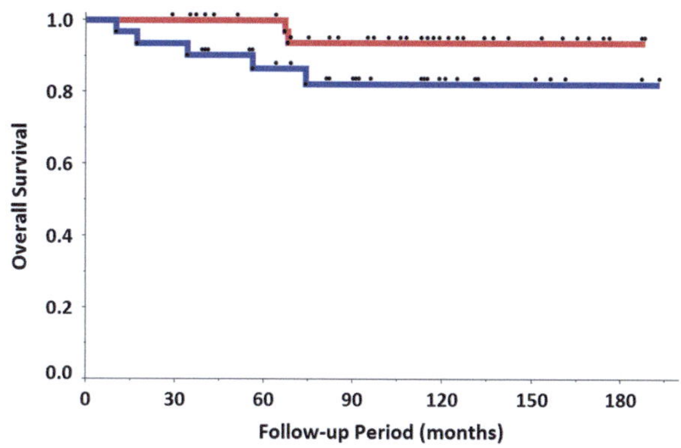

8.4 Discussion

The prognosis for patients with osteosarcoma has greatly improved with the introduction of multidrug chemotherapy. At our institution, since the introduction of chemotherapy, the 5-year OS has improved from 13 % to 49 % (OOS-A) to 72 % (OOS-B) to 78 % (OOS-C) [12]. The current OOS-D regimen has improved the 5-year OS to 95 % (Table 8.2). In planning for the OOS-D regimen, there were discussions on whether MTX should be included in preoperative chemotherapy. Previously at our institute, we had two cases of severe MTX excretion delay which led to the delay of chemotherapy and progression of disease. Because of this experience, we decided to omit HD-MTX from the preoperative regimen and include it only in the postoperative regimen. The histological response rate of this study was 56 % which was about equal to other studies even without MTX [14, 17].

IFM is widely used in the treatment of osteosarcoma. But IFM has been used mainly in patients for poor responders or relapse. Also, IFM has been used as a single agent or with a combination of other agents such as DOX, CDDP, or etoposide. When used as a single agent, the dose of IFM varied from 10 to 15 g/m^2. There are only a few studies with HD-IFM given first line in a preoperative phase [13, 14, 18]. Bacci et al. first reported in a pilot study that HD-IFM had a better EFS and OS than previous protocols, but in the ISG/SSG 1 study, Ferrari et al. reported that there was no benefit in oncological results [13, 14]. In this study, we report a 5-year EFS of 77 % and a 5-year OS of 95 %. There was a significant difference between the EFS rates for histological response. The oncological results were better than reports by other groups, even though the response rate was about the same with other reports (Table 8.3). Even the EFS and OS rates of poor responder were in the same range as other reports. This could be because of the contribution of HD-MTX and HD-IFM given postoperatively.

The addition of HD-IFM has been reported to have an increase in toxicity. The acute toxicity, mainly hematological and renal toxicity with Fanconi-like syndrome, has been reported [14]. In our study all patients experienced grade

Table 8.2 Overall survival of OOS regimens [12]

	5-year OS
No chemotherapy (~1976)	13 %
OOS-A (~1982)	49 %
OOS-B (~1989)	72 %
OOS-C (~1996)	78 %
OOS-D (1997~)	95 %

Table 8.3 Survival rates of regimen that include ifosfamide

Study group	Patients	Period	Regimen	5Y-EFS (%)	5Y-OS (%)
EOI [11]	43	1986–1990	DOX+CDDP+IFM 6 g/m^2	56	62
COG [17]	662	1993–1997	HD-MTX+DOX+CDDP (MAP)	64[a]	71[a]
			MAP+MTP-PE	63[a]	75[a]
			MAP+IFM 9 g/m^2	58[a]	70[a]
			MAP+IFM+MTP-PE	71[a]	81[a]
ISG/SSG 1 [14]	182	1997–2000	MAP+HD-IFM 15 g/m^2	64	77
OOS-D	82	1997–2012	MAP+HD-IFM 15 g/m^2	77	95

EOI European Osteosarcoma Intergroup, *COG* Children's Oncology Group, *ISG/SSG* Italian Sarcoma Group/Scandinavian Sarcoma Group
[a]6Y EFS/OS

4 hematologic toxicity, but we did not have any patient with severe renal toxicity. This could be because all the treatment was done inpatient, and there could be careful monitoring of hydration and urine output. Another toxicity associated with HD-IFM is infertility in males [19]. We have not analyzed the sperms of the patients, but two patients (both age 16 at diagnosis) have fathered children. The only fatal toxicity experienced was one patient with acute heart failure. Cumulative dose of DOX has been considered a risk for cardiomyopathy, but in this regimen, the total dose of DOX (360 mg/m^2) was considered low risk [20]. Another risk for severe toxicity is the cumulative dose of all the drugs. In this regimen, the cumulative dose of DOX was 360 mg/m^2, CDDP was 480 mg/m^2, MTX was 48 g/m^2, and IFM was 60 g/m^2. It compared to have a better balance of the four drugs than other regimens (Table 8.4).

In conclusion, the OOS-D regimen had an excellent outcome for patients with osteosarcoma of the extremities. This regimen consists of a well-balanced use of the four key drugs and was feasible and well tolerated. This study was not randomized and the sample size was not large. A larger study and longer follow-up will be important to assess benefits and long-term toxicity of this regimen.

Table 8.4 Cumulative dose

Study group	Subgroup	DOX (mg/m^2)	CDDP (mg/m^2)	MTX (g/m^2)	IFM (g/m^2)
EOI, 1999 [11]		450	300		18
COG, 2008 [16]	MAP	450	480	144	
	MAP+IFM	450	480	144	45
ISG/SSG 1, 2005 [14]	Good responder	330	480	48	60
	Poor responder	330	690	60	75
OOS-D		360	480	48	60

EOI European Osteosarcoma Intergroup, *COG* Children's Oncology Group, *ISG/SSG* Italian Sarcoma Group/Scandinavian Sarcoma Group

Acknowledgments We acknowledge all the members of the Osaka University Orthopaedic Oncology Group for their input in this study: Hideki Hamada, Atsumasa Uchida, Ikuo Kudawara, Akihiko Matsumine, Akira Myoui, Shigeki Mori, Hideto Obata, Susumu Joyama, Noriyuki Tamai, Tsukasa Sotobori, Tetsuho Fujimoto, Kenichiro Hamada, Kazuya Oshima, Satoshi Tanenaka, Hidetatsu Outani, and Yoshinori Imura.

References

1. Jaffe N, Frei III E, Traggis D, Bishop Y. Adjuvant methotrexate-citrovorum factor treatment of osteogenic sarcoma. N Engl J Med. 1974;291:994–7.
2. Rosen G, Marcove RC, Caparros B, Nirenberg A, Kosloff C, Huvos AG. Primary osteogenic sarcoma. The rationale for preoperative chemotherapy and delayed surgery. Cancer. 1979;43: 2163–77.
3. Link MP, Goorin AM, Miser AW, Green AA, Pratt CB, Belasco JB, et al. The effect of adjuvant chemotherapy on relapse-free survival in patients with osteosarcoma of the extremity. N Engl J Med. 1986;314:1600–6.
4. Meyers PA, Gorlick R, Heller G, Casper E, Lane J, Huvos AG, et al. Intensification of preoperative chemotherapy for osteogenic sarcoma: results of the Memorial Sloan-Kettering (T-12) protocol. J Clin Oncol. 1998;16:2452–8.
5. Pratt CB, Horowitz ME, Meyer WH, Etcubanas E, Thompson EI, Douglass EC, et al. Phase II trial of ifosfamide in children with malignant solid tumors. Cancer Treat Rep. 1987;71:131–5.
6. Marti C, Kroner T, Remagen W, Berchtold W, Cserhati M, Varini M. High-dose ifosfamide in advanced osteosarcoma. Cancer Treat Rep. 1985;69:115–7.
7. Patel SR, Vadhan-Raj S, Papadopolous N, Plager C, Burgess MA, Hays C, et al. High-dose ifosfamide in bone and soft tissue sarcomas: results of phase II and pilot studies dose response and schedule dependence. J Clin Oncol. 1997;15:2378–84.
8. Winkler K, Beron G, Delling G, Heise U, Kabisch H, Purfurst C, et al. Neoadjuvant chemotherapy of osteosarcoma: results of a randomized cooperative trail (COSS-82) with salvage chemotherapy based on histological tumor response. J Clin Oncol. 1988;6:329–37.
9. Winkler K, Bielack S, Delling G, Salzer-Kuntschik M, Kotz R, Greenshaw C, et al. Effect of intraarterial versus intravenous cisplatin in addition to systemic doxorubicin, high-dose methotrexate, and ifosfamide on histologic tumor response in osteosarcoma (study COSS-86). Cancer. 1990;66:1703–10.

10. Bacci G, Picci P, Avella M, Dallari D, Ferrari S, Prasad R, et al. The importance of dose-intensity in neoadjuvant chemotherapy of osteosarcoma: a retrospective analysis of high-dose methotrexate, cisplatinum and adriamycin used preoperatively. J Chemother. 1990;2:127–35.
11. Voute PA, Souhami RL, Nooji M, Somers R, Cortes-Funes H, van der Eijken JW, et al. A phase II study of cisplatin, ifosfamide and doxorubicin in operable primary, axial skeletal and metastatic osteosarcoma. Ann Oncol. 1999;10:1211–8.
12. Uchida A, Myoui A, Araki N, Yoshikawa H, Shinto Y, Ueda T. Neoadjuvant chemotherapy for pediatric osteosarcoma patients. Cancer. 1997;79:411–5.
13. Bacci G, Ferrari S, Longhi A, Picci P, Mercuri M, Alvegard TA, et al. High dose ifosfamide in combination with high dose methotrexate, adriamycin and cisplatin in the neoadjuvant treatment of extremity osteosarcoma: preliminary results of an Italian Sarcoma Group/Scandinavian Sarcoma Group pilot study. J Chemother. 2002;14:198–206.
14. Ferrari S, Smeland S, Mercuri M, Bertoni F, Longhi A, Ruggieri P, et al. Neoadjuvant chemotherapy with high-dose ifosfamide, high-dose methotrexate, cisplatin, and doxorubicin for patients with localized osteosarcoma of the extremity: a joint study by the Italian and Scandinavian Sarcoma Groups. J Clin Oncol. 2005;23:8845–52.
15. Araki N, Myoui A, Kuratsu S, Hashimoto N, Inoue T, Kudawara I, et al. Intraoperative extracorporeal autogeneous irradiated bone grafts in tumor surgery. Clin Orthop Relat Res. 1999;368:196–206.
16. Huvos AG, Rosen G, Marcove RC. Primary osteogenic sarcoma: pathologic aspects in 20 patients after treatment with chemotherapy en bloc resection, and prosthetic bone replacement. Arch Pathol Lab Med. 1977;101:14–8.
17. Meyers PA, Schwartz CL, Krailo MD, Healey JH, Bernstein ML, Betcher D, et al. Osteosarcoma: the addition of muramyl tripeptide to chemotherapy improves overall survival—a report from the Children's Oncology Group. J Clin Oncol. 2008;26:633–8.
18. Kudawara I, Aoki Y, Ueda T, Araki N, Naka N, Nakanishi H, et al. Neoadjuvant and adjuvant chemotherapy with high-dose ifosfamide, doxorubicin, cisplatin and high-dose methotrexate in non-metastatic osteosarcoma of the extremities: a phase II trial in Japan. J Chemother. 2013; 25:41–8.
19. Longhi A, Macchiagodena M, Vitali G, Bacci G. Fertility in male patients treated with neoadjuvant chemotherapy for osteosarcoma. J Pediatr Hematol Oncol. 2003;25:292–6.
20. Von Hoff DD, Layard MW, Basa P, Davis HL, Von Hoff AV, et al. Risk factors for doxorubicin-induced congestive heart failure. Ann Intern Med. 1979;91:710–7.

Part IV

Surgery

Endoprosthetic Reconstruction for Extremity Osteosarcoma

9

Akihiko Matsumine

Abstract
Recent progress in multidisciplinary therapies for osteosarcoma promises the ability to perform successful limb salvage surgery. Endoprosthetic reconstruction following resection of a bone tumor has a history of more than 70 years, and modern endoprosthesis provides intraoperative flexibility to fill the bony defect and structural stability to allow for immediate weight bearing. Although prosthetic reconstruction has become a standard surgical technique, there remain many unresolved problems.

Keywords
Osteosarcoma • Limb salvage surgery • Endoprosthesis • Reconstruction

9.1 Introduction

Osteosarcoma is an aggressive malignant neoplasm that exhibits osteoblastic differentiation and produces malignant osteoid [1]. It is most prevalent in children and young adults. Because of the advances in imaging, surgical techniques, and adjuvant chemotherapy protocols, osteosarcoma patients have had a considerable improvement in prognosis during the past 25 years [2–5]. Recent progress in these multidisciplinary therapies had made it possible to perform successful limb salvage surgery, which is considered to be the standard procedure for the majority of patients with osteosarcoma involving the extremities (Fig. 9.1) [2, 6–9].

In this chapter, I review the advantages of endoprosthetic reconstruction and the history of endoprosthesis in Europe, the USA, and Japan and point out issues and

A. Matsumine, M.D. (✉)
Department of Orthopaedic Surgery, Mie University School of Medicine, 2-174, Edobashi, Tsu-City, Mie 514-8507, Japan
e-mail: matsumin@clin.medic.mie-u.ac.jp

T. Ueda, A. Kawai (eds.), *Osteosarcoma*, DOI 10.1007/978-4-431-55696-1_9

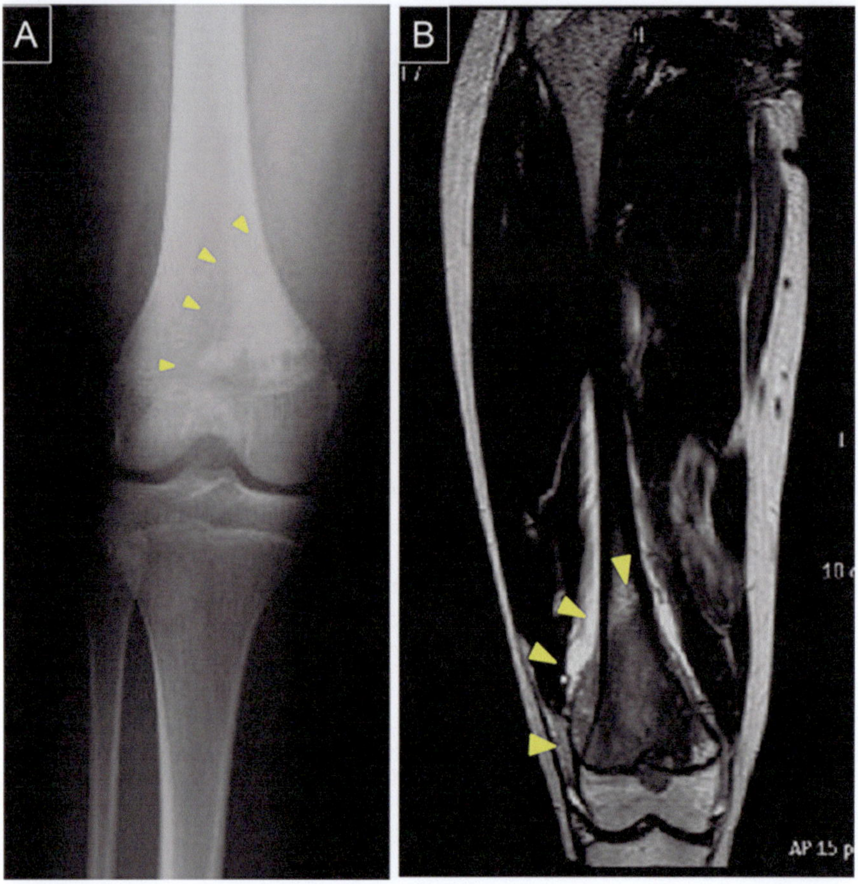

Fig. 9.1 Overview of the endoprosthetic reconstruction for extremity osteosarcoma. A radiography (**a**) and a MR image (**b**) indicated the osteosarcoma of the distal femur (*yellow triangle*). Osteosarcoma of the distal femur was resected with wide margin including surrounding muscles (**c**) and reconstructed using distal femoral endoprosthesis (**d**). Postoperative radiographic finding showed the good alignment of the reconstructed lower extremity without aseptic loosening (**e**)

perspectives associated with endoprosthetic reconstruction following the wide excision of osteosarcoma located in the extremities.

9.2 Advantages of Endoprosthetic Reconstruction

There are three types of reconstruction strategies used for the massive bone defect that is left following the resection of osteosarcoma. The first strategy is biological reconstruction, including allogeneic bone grafting, autologous recycled bone grafting, and vascularized bone grafting [10]. The second reconstructive strategy is prosthetic reconstruction, and the third is reconstruction using recycled bone/

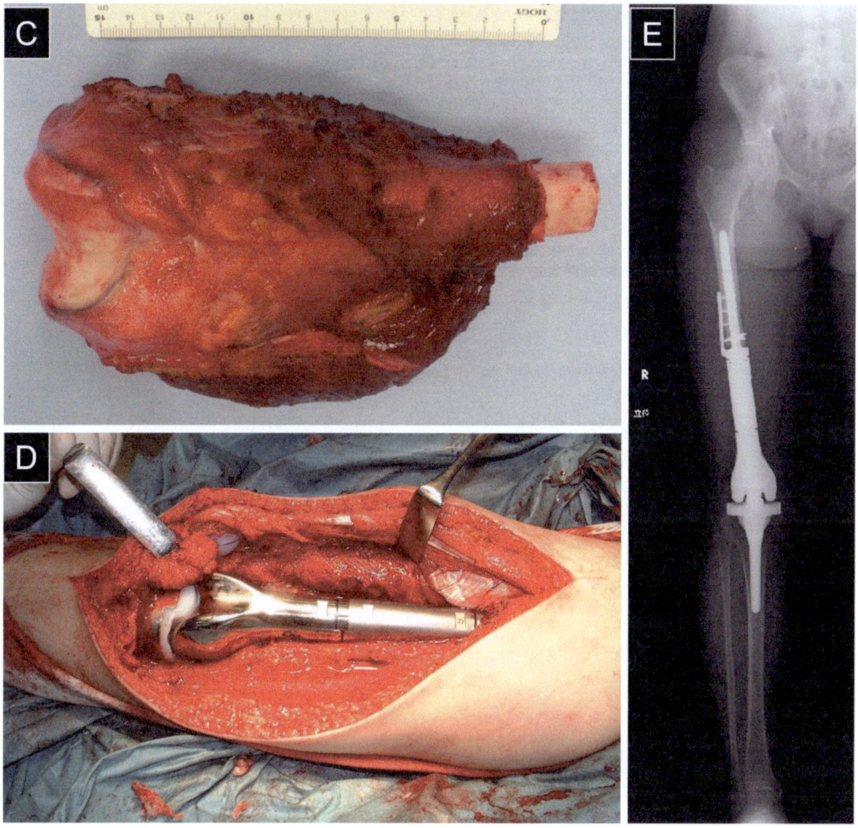

Fig. 9.1 (continued)

allograft-endoprosthesis composite [11]. Biological reconstruction has a major advantage with respect to durability, when the graft bone is implanted into the intercalary defect of the long bone after resection of a diaphyseal bone tumor [10]. However, because most osteosarcoma arises in the meta-diaphysis of the long bones, the surgical indications for biological reconstruction are limited to special cases of osteosarcoma patients [1]. Thus, prosthetic reconstruction has become the standard surgical technique in developed countries.

Various types of prostheses have been developed and applied for the reconstruction of a bone defect after tumor resection. The current models of prostheses include modular segments, a wrought stem, a kinetic rotating hinge around the knee, circumferential porous coating around the endoprosthesis at the bone–prosthesis junction, and loopholes for soft-tissue attachment [12]. The advantages of the current modular prostheses include durability, intraoperative flexibility to fill the bony defect, and structural stability to allow for immediate weight bearing [12–15] (Fig. 9.1).

9.3 History of Endoprostheses in Europe and the USA

In 1943, the first metallic endoprosthesis was implanted into the proximal femur after resection of a giant cell tumor of bone by Austin Moore and Harold Bohlman in the USA [16]. This first endoprosthesis was made of a cobalt–chromium (Co–Cr) alloy. The Stanmore endoprosthesis also has a long clinical history of development and was first implanted in 1949 [17, 18]. It was a custom-made endoprosthesis with cemented fixation. The GUEPAR endoprosthesis (Benoit-Gerrard Company, Caen, France) was a custom-made Co–Cr cemented tumor endoprosthesis with a single-axis hinged knee which was used in France beginning in 1972 [19].

During the subsequent decades, many exploratory treatments were performed using endoprostheses made from cobalt–chromium alloy [20–23] and other materials, including stainless steel [24], polythene [25], and acrylic [26, 27] for treating bone defects after tumor resection. Although orthopedic oncologists had been interested in these tumor prostheses, these prostheses were only considered for the treatment of patients who refused amputation, because of their low reliability [28].

It was not until the late 1970s that endoprosthetic implants began to emerge as a valuable treatment option in orthopedic oncology. The late 1970s was an epoch-making turning point in the treatment of osteosarcoma. First, because of the development of antineoplastic drugs, including high-dose methotrexate and adriamycin, orthopedic oncologists began to use chemotherapy for osteosarcoma [29]. Chemotherapy was initially performed as adjuvant therapy following the removal of the primary tumor in order to kill the microscopic residual disease. Currently, the standard chemotherapeutic treatment for osteosarcoma is a combination of neoadjuvant and adjuvant chemotherapy [29].

Second, new diagnostic imaging modalities had become available in the field of musculoskeletal tumors. Although plain radiography is an essential modality in the early diagnosis of bone tumors, it was not sufficient to visualize the intraosseous/soft-tissue extent of bone tumors. Owing to the developments and popularization of computed tomography (CT) [30] in the late 1970s and magnetic resonance imaging (MRI) in the mid-1980s [31], orthopedic tumor surgeons could correctly evaluate the bony and soft-tissue extension of tumors [13, 30, 31]. Progress in limb salvage surgery and endoprosthetic reconstruction of bone defect was based on the advances in imaging modalities and chemotherapy protocols.

Because the advances in imaging modalities and chemotherapy protocols enabled the safe tumor excision in the latter 1970s, limb-sparing surgery using endoprosthetic reconstruction was expected to become a realistic surgical procedure. To provide patient-specific endoprostheses that could be modified during surgery without the cost and delay of a custom endoprosthesis, modular systems were developed. Prior to the development of modular systems, physicians were unable to provide an optimal-fitting endoprosthesis during surgery. Modular systems allowed surgeons to use components with the best size and length for each patient (Fig. 9.2).

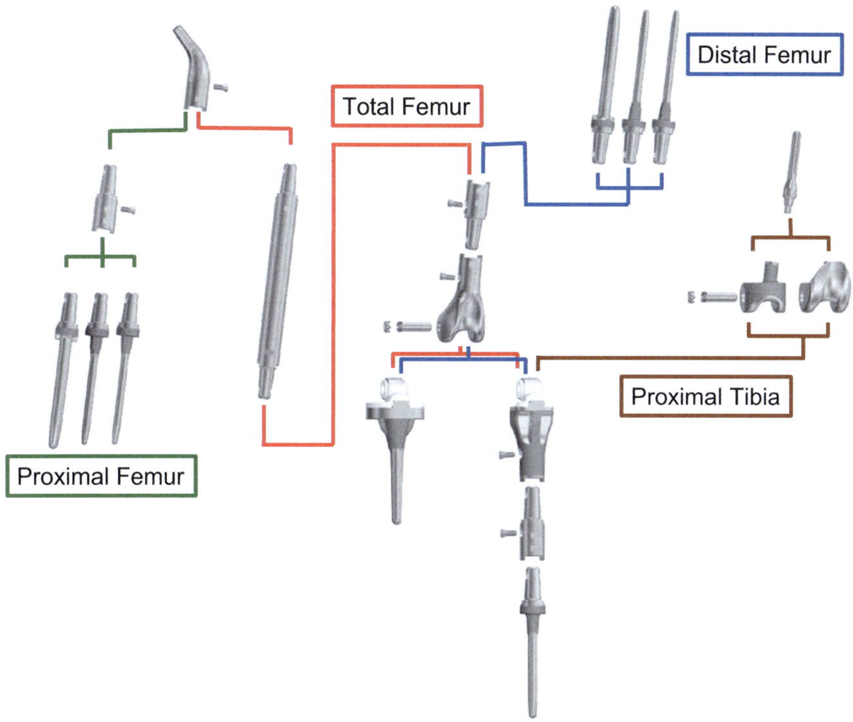

Fig. 9.2 Modular prosthesis for the reconstruction of the bone defect following the resection of extremity bone tumor. Owing to the development of modular prosthesis, physicians can provide an optimal-fitting prosthesis during surgery. The indicated system is the Kyocera Modular Limb Salvage system (KMLS system)

The first clinical application of a modular ceramic endoprosthesis was indicated for a humeral bone tumor by Salzer et al. [31]. The first modular knee prosthetic systems were developed by Kotz in 1982 and were published as the Kotz modular femur tibia reconstruction system (KMFTR) in 1986 [32]. Although the KMFTR showed good clinical outcomes, the KMFTR was developed into the Howmedica Modular Resection System (HMRS) in 1988. The HMRS had several new features, including a porous coating on the metal surface to promote extracortical bone bridging and one side plate on the femoral stem, and in 1996, a rotating hinge knee was added to the system [13]. Based on the clinical success of the rotating hinge mechanism, a new Global Modular Replacement System (GMRS), which is the next generation of both HMRS and MRS (modular replacement system), was developed in 2002. The GMRS has a unique cementless titanium stem made of titanium alloy with titanium plasma spray, and its proximal 3 cm is coated with hydroxyapatite.

Modular endoprosthetic systems thereby simplified reconstructive surgical procedures. Stanmore Implants produced the METS proximal femur replacement system and METS distal femoral replacement system (designed as a modular system) in 2001 and 2002, respectively. Since 1992, the MUTARS (Modular Universal Tumour and Revision System, Implantcast, Buxtehude, Germany) has been used for the treatment of major bone defects of the lower and upper extremities. The fixation is achieved with an intramedullary stem, which can be inserted either cementless or cemented. In the cementless version, the stem is inserted press-fit in order to achieve sufficient primary stability. The stem has a rough surface with a pore size of 100 μm to allow the bone to grow onto the surface. The stem has a hexagonal cross section and is made of titanium alloy (TiAl6V4) in the cementless version and of Co–Cr–Mo alloy in the cemented version [33].

9.4 History of Endoprosthesis in Japan

In Japan, the first prosthetic reconstruction was performed by Dr. Katayama at Jikei University School of Medicine in January 1962, for a chondrosarcoma patient using an acrylic hinge-type knee endoprosthesis, which was manufactured at Nemoto Shokai (Tokyo, Japan) [27, 34]. This custom-made endoprosthesis was made from stainless steel, with the surface covered with an acrylate resin, including the metallic hinge axis, in order to reduce the intermetallic friction (Fig. 9.3a). The judgment whether or not bone cement should be used for the stem fixation was left to the surgeon's discretion. These acrylic hinge-type knee prostheses were applied in 35 patients between 1961 and 1969 and, thereafter, were used for more than 600 patients until 1998 after modifying the implant design and the material from stainless steel to titanium alloy (Fig. 9.3b). Although there have been no systemic long-term follow-up studies of this endoprosthesis, Yamawaki et al. reported a patient who retained the endoprosthesis 40 years after the initial surgery [34].

In 1984, the KMFTR was approved by the Japanese Ministry of Health, Labour and Welfare and was widely used for the reconstruction of bone defects after resection of a bone tumor. However, the KMFTR was designed for Caucasian physical constitution and was sometimes too large in size [35–40] and too heavy in weight for Asia-Pacific patients. Therefore, Kyocera Corp. (Kyoto, Japan) made two types of prostheses. One type of Kyocera endoprosthesis is a full ceramic custom-made endoprosthesis, the C-TKP (Fig. 9.4a), and the other is a metallic endoprosthesis, the PHK series (Fig. 9.4b–d). The C-TKP was a unique endoprosthesis in that the extraosseous component was made of aluminum, and the stem component was made of sapphire. Although the C-TKP was used from 1988 to 1994, it showed a risk of stem breakage.

In 1987, the Japanese Musculoskeletal Oncology Group (JMOG) developed an initial prosthetic system with a unique loose hinge for distal femoral bone replacement, the KYOCERA Physio Hinge Total Knee System Type I (PHK I) (KYOCERA Corp. Kyoto, Japan) (Fig. 9.4b). However, several mechanical defects in the hinge joint of the PHK I led to the development of the PHK II (Fig. 9.4c) with a conventional hinge joint in May 1990. Although the PHK II had good clinical performance, new modular endoprosthesis with a rotating hinge joint, the PHK III, was introduced in April 1997 (Fig. 9.4d) [12]. The PHK III was designed for Asian

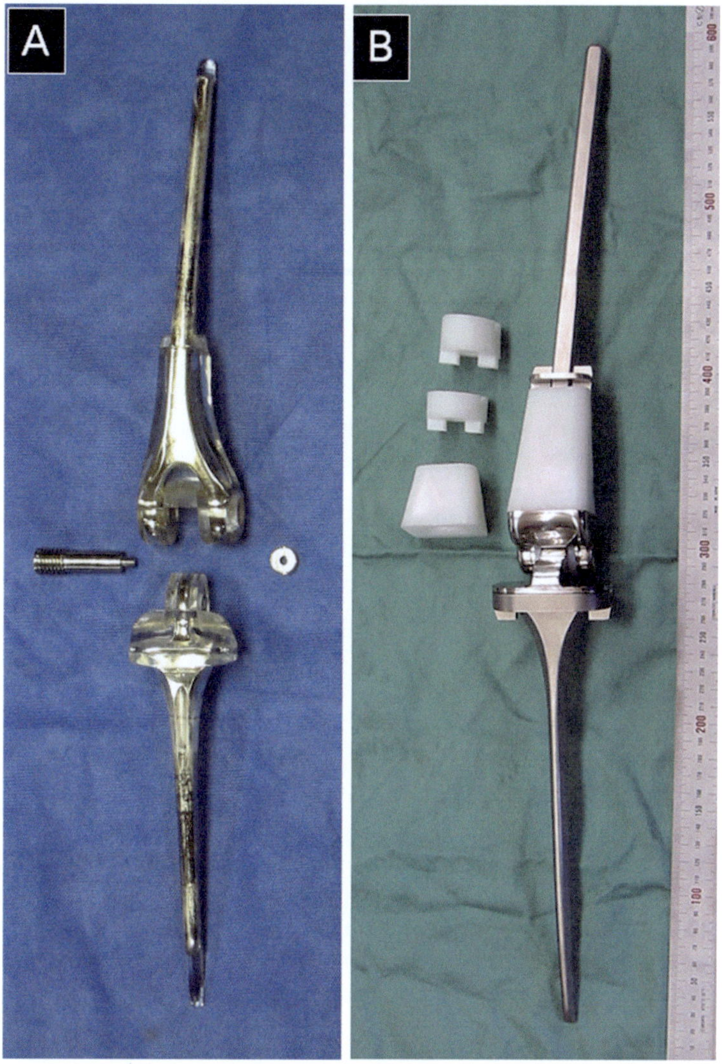

Fig. 9.3 The hinge-type knee prosthesis manufactured at Nemoto Shokai (Tokyo, Japan). The first endoprosthetic reconstruction in Japan was performed in January 1962 at Jikei University School of Medicine. The prosthesis was acrylic hinge-type knee prosthesis (**a**). These Jikei-type hinge knee prostheses were used until 1998 modifying the implant design and the material from stainless steel to titanium alloy (**b**)

patients, including Japanese, who have a smaller anatomical architecture of the knee joint. PHK III was expected to have various advantages in contrast to widely used endoprosthesis.

The PHK III has a unique semi-rotator hinge joint which allows maximal flexion of 142° and internal/external rotation of 5° [12]. The metallic parts of the PHK III

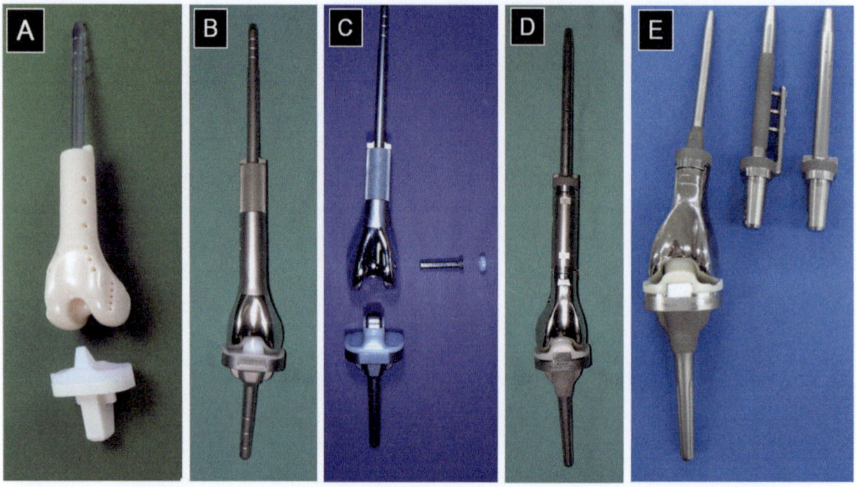

Fig. 9.4 Tumor endoprostheses manufactured by KYOCERA Medical Corporation. The first prosthesis was a full ceramic custom-made prosthesis, the C-TKP (**a**), which was used from 1988 to 1994. After the development of Physio Hinge Total Knee System Type I (PHK I) (**b**) and PHK II (**c**), PHK III (**d**) was introduced in 1997. In April 2002, the Kyocera Medical Limb Salvage system (KMLS system) was developed by a collaboration between the JMOG and KYOCERA Medical Corp. (**e**). The PHK III remains a distal femoral prosthesis with a cement fixation stem in the product line of the KMLS system

are made of lightweight and high-strength titanium alloy with good biocompatibility and bio-stability and allow scanning by magnetic resonance imaging (MRI). As a result, the PHK III is extremely lightweight. For example, when the PHK III was used for an 11 cm bony defect of the distal femur, the total weight was about 660 g, whereas reconstruction of a 12 cm bony defect using the HMRS reaches a weight of about 1200 g. The metallic surface of the hinge shaft and the rotator, which creates friction between high-density polyethylenes, was fabricated using surface-hardening treatment by azote-ionic inpouring to obtain greater durability of the hinge joint. The rotation sleeve, plate, and shaft sleeve were made of ultrahigh molecular weight polyethylene. A multi-institutional cooperative study by the JMOG showed that the 5-year overall prosthetic survival rates, prosthetic survival rate without aseptic loosening, and limb preservation rate were 85 %, 90 %, and 86 %, respectively. The mean functional score according to the classification system of the Musculoskeletal Tumor Society was 20.5 points (68 %) [12].

In April 2002, the Kyocera Modular Limb Salvage system (KMLS system) was developed by a collaboration between the JMOG and KYOCERA Medical Corp. (Figs. 9.4e and 9.5) [15]. The KMLS system is a modular endoprosthesis system which was developed for the reconstruction of a defect after resection of a tumor located at the proximal humerus, proximal femur, distal femur, proximal tibia, or distal humerus. The distal femoral endoprosthesis of the KMLS system has the same mechanical construction of the prosthetic component as the PHK III

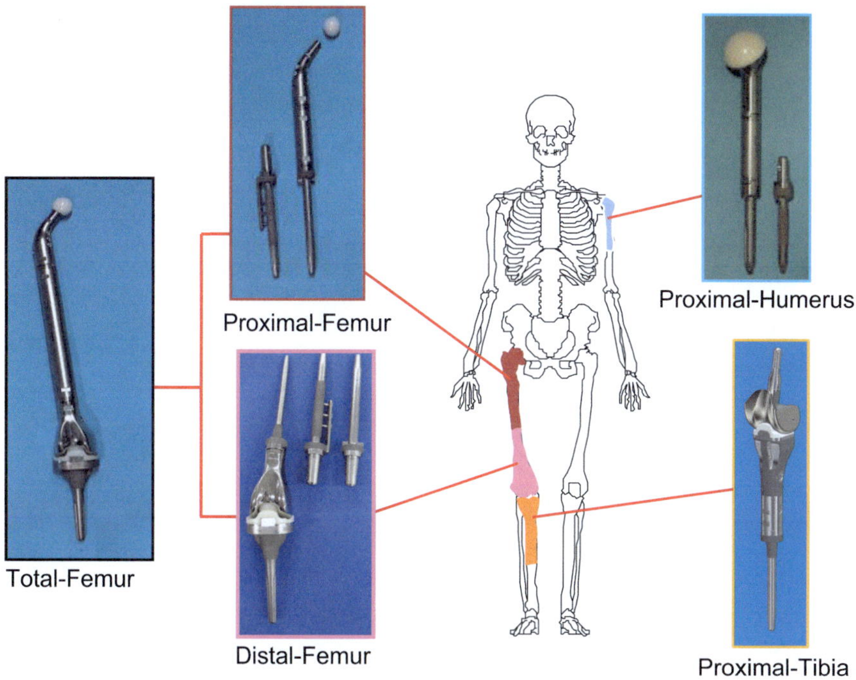

Fig. 9.5 The overview of the KMLS system. The KMLS system is a modular endoprosthesis system which was developed for the reconstruction of a defect after resection of a tumor located at the proximal humerus, proximal femur, distal femur, proximal tibia, or distal humerus

(Fig. 9.4d, e), but is characterized by the addition of a cementless stem component. The PHK III remains a distal femoral endoprosthesis with a cement fixation stem in the product line of the KMLS system. A multi-institutional cooperative study by the JMOG showed that the 5-year overall endoprosthetic survival rate was 80.0 %, and the 5-year limb salvage rate was 94.5 %. The mean function score according to the scoring system of the Musculoskeletal Tumour Society was 21.8 points (72.5 %) [15]. This modular system provided patient-specific endoprostheses that could be modified during surgery without the cost and delay of a custom endoprosthesis (Fig. 9.2).

Kobe Steel, Material Ltd. (Kobe, Japan) also developed a tumor endoprosthesis made from titanium alloy, mainly in collaboration with Kyoto University. The K-MAX Hip System H-1 (Fig. 9.6a) was applied for the reconstruction of a proximal femoral bone defect in 1990, and the K-MAX Knee System K-2 (Fig. 9.6b) was used for the reconstruction of a distal femoral bone defect in 1994. The K-MAX Hip System H-1 was the world's first tumor prostheses made of titanium alloy. Although these simple prostheses promised stable clinical outcomes, the medical material businesses of Kobe Steel, Ltd. Material and Kyocera Corporation was integrated, and the processing technologies of for ceramics and metals were inherited by KYOCERA Medical Corporation.

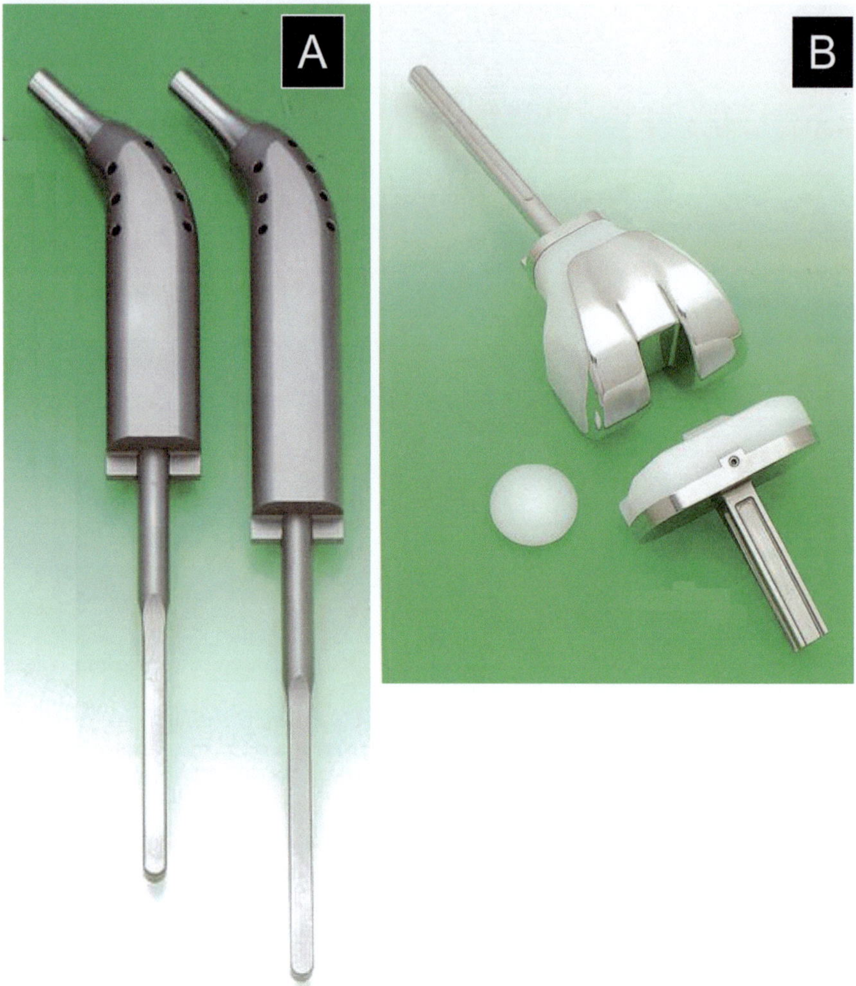

Fig. 9.6 The K-MAX Hip System H-1(**a**) and the K-MAX Knee System K-2 (**b**). Kobe Steel, Material Ltd. (Kobe, Japan), also developed tumor endoprostheses made from titanium alloy

9.5 Problems with the Modern Endoprostheses and Future Perspectives

Although endoprosthetic reconstruction of a massive bone defect following tumor resection has become a standard surgical technique, there remain many unresolved problems which may require revision surgery. The prosthetic 5- and 10-year survival rate for distal femoral prostheses in previous studies ranged from 57 %

to 93 % and 0 %–88 %, respectively. The 5-year limb preservation rates were 86–96 % [14, 17, 18, 41–49]. These results mean that about 10 % of patients required limb amputation due to an endoprosthesis-related complication. Thus, orthopedic tumor surgeons require endoprostheses with better durability.

Breakage of the components, including the stem components and hinge mechanism, sometimes lead to revision surgery (Fig. 9.7a). The thin stem is especially associated with a high risk of stem breakage. In the PHK III series, breakage of the femoral stem could be attributed to the fact that all four broken stems reported were small-sized stems with a 10 mm diameter [12]. Therefore, small stems less than 10 mm in diameter should be avoided. However, the patients with osteosarcoma are mainly children with a small physique. Moreover, the average size of Japanese knees was found to be 5–10 % smaller than that of Caucasians [50, 51]. Thus, further metallurgical improvement of the metal strength is warranted.

Infection is currently the most common serious complication of endoprostheses, because patients who undergo surgery for a neoplastic condition are often subjected to extensive soft-tissue dissection and long operations and are immunosuppressed [47, 52] (Fig. 9.7b). Several reports have indicated that the endoprosthesis-associated infection rates were 2–15 % [14, 17, 18, 44–49, 52–59]. Infections may result in the amputation of the patients' limbs. In addition, the cost of treating an infected endoprosthesis is considerable, and infections often recur.

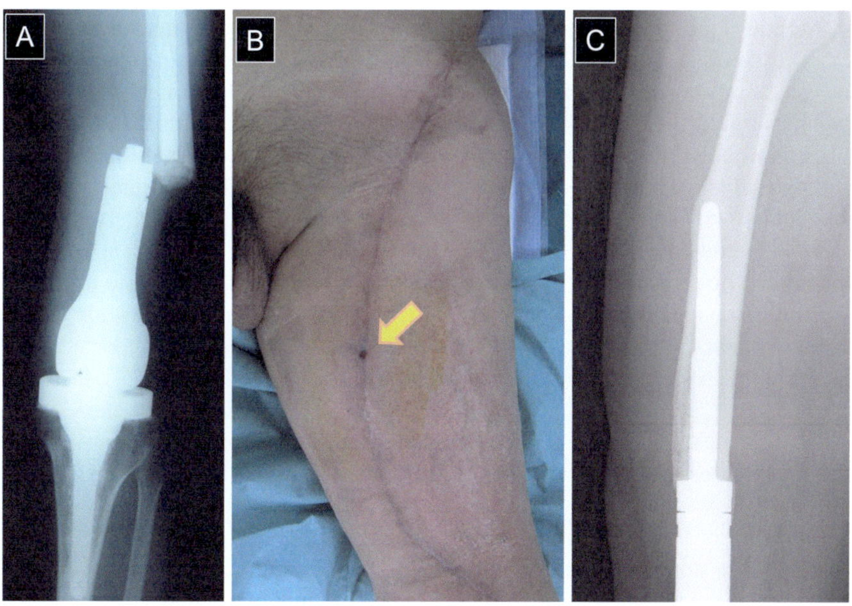

Fig. 9.7 Complication after endoprosthetic reconstruction. Breakage of component (**a**), infection (**b**), and stem loosening (**c**) are major complications after endoprosthetic reconstruction. An *arrow* in B shows the fistula

An analysis of clinical factors which caused endoprosthesis loss or amputation suggested that the soft-tissue condition significantly influenced the duration of the infection control period and likelihood of limb salvage [60]. The use of muscle rotation flaps or a vascularized musculocutaneous flap should be considered when only the rectus femoris muscle has been preserved [14].

Several promising technologies are aimed at decreasing the risk of infection following limb preservation. Recently, it was reported that the use of silver-coated prostheses reduced the infection rate [61]. In 2012, a European CE mark was awarded to the ionic silver-treated massive endoprosthesis tumor system ("METS") as a modular implant system from Stanmore Implants. Silver-coated prostheses are also produced by MUTARS (Implantcast Ltd, Buxtehude, Germany). Hardes et al. reported that the use of silver-coated megaprostheses resulted in a reduced infection rate by analyzing a total of 51 patients who were treated with a silver-coated proximal femur replacement or proximal tibia replacement [61]. Another option to prevent endoprosthetic infection is the use of iodine-coated prostheses. Shirai et al. performed a clinical trial of iodine-coated endoprostheses in 47 patients with malignant bone tumors or pyogenic arthritis [62]. The iodine-coated endoprostheses were used to prevent infection in 21 patients and to treat active infections in 26 patients. Infections were prevented in 20 out of 21 patients. In 26 treatment cases involving one- or two-stage revision surgery, the infection subsided without any additional surgery in all cases. An iodine-coated endoprosthesis may play an important role not only in prophylaxis for infections but also in the treatment of an infected endoprosthesis.

Aseptic loosening of the endoprosthesis is one of common reasons for endoprosthesis revision [12, 14, 15, 17, 54, 58, 63] (Fig. 9.7c). Most endoprostheses have a stem component with a round cross section and circumferential porous coating around the endoprosthesis at the bone–prosthesis junction. To promote the initial bone formation at the bone–prosthesis junction, several technical improvements have been introduced in the tumor prosthesis. Since 1991, a cementless version of the Stanmore endoprosthesis has been available with a hydroxyapatite-coated titanium stem. Additionally, parts of the implant body are HA-coated to enhance the extracortical bone bridging [33]. Some types of cementless endoprostheses, including the KMFTR/HMRS and KMLS, had a side plate to obtain the initial stem stability [13, 15, 32, 57]. However, it appeared that these side plates caused the stress shielding of the cortical bone at the end of the residual bone and led to stem loosening [13, 15, 32, 57]. Therefore, the GMRS, which is the next generation of both HMRS and MRS, has a proximally arranged fin at the cementless press-fit stem to obtain rotational stability. The stems are made of titanium alloy with titanium plasma spray, and the proximal 3 cm of the endoprosthesis is coated with hydroxyapatite. Although the shape of the cross section of the stem component is important to prevent intramedullary stem loosening, most of the prostheses had a stem component with a round cross section. The cementless stem of the MUTARS has a hexagonal cross section and is inserted press-fit in order to achieve sufficient primary stability [33].

The rotating hinge mechanism was associated with better function and was expected to achieve lower rates of loosening in the previous reports [14, 59, 64–66]. In a follow-up study, Kawai et al. [14] compared a fixed hinge knee endoprosthesis, the HSS (Hospital for Special Surgery: Biomet, Warsaw, IN), with a rotating hinge knee, the FINN endoprosthesis (Biomet). The HSS showed aseptic loosening in 31.4 % of cases compared to 6.5 % in the FINN group. The 5-year survivorship was 64 % for the HSS endoprosthesis and 82 % for the FINN endoprosthesis. Thus, a rotating hinge mechanism can reduce the mechanical stress, thus reducing the intramedullary stress.

Most limb salvage procedures performed today are reconstructed using modular tumor endoprostheses with long cemented stems and uncemented stems. Compressive osseointegration fixation (Compress: Biomet) is a new technology for the fixation of tumor endoprostheses [67]. The principal potential advantages of this technique include preservation of the bone stock, prevention of stress shielding, and a short working length of bone necessary for fixation of the implant. Using compressive osseointegration technology, a compressive force is continuously loaded across the bone–implant interface and the bone at the bone–implant interface hypertrophies with time. Although there have been no long-term follow-up studies of this technology yet, Monument et al. indicated that the overall survival rate was 67 % and the endoprosthesis-related implant survival was 89 % after a minimum of 5 years of clinical follow-up. To more accurately assess this fixation strategy, longer clinical follow-up studies are needed.

In conclusion, because of the advances in imaging, surgical techniques, and adjuvant chemotherapy protocols, osteosarcoma patients have had a considerable improvement in prognosis during the past 25 years [2–5]. Recent progress made in these multidisciplinary therapies has made it possible to perform successful limb salvage surgery, and this is now considered to be the standard procedure for the majority of the patients with osteosarcoma involving the extremities. Endoprosthetic reconstruction promises intraoperative flexibility to fill the bony defect and immediate structural stability to allow for weight bearing. Although prosthetic reconstruction has become a standard surgical technique, there remain a lot of unresolved problems which may lead to the need for revision surgery. Thus, orthopedic tumor surgeons are urgently seeking endoprostheses with better durability.

References

1. Fletcher CDM, DM, Bridge JA, Hogendoorn P, Mertens F. WHO classification of tumours of soft tissue and bone. 4th ed. Lyon: International Agency for Research on Cancer; 2013.
2. Veth R, van Hoesel R, Pruszczynski M, Hoogenhout J, Schreuder B, Wobbes T. Limb salvage in musculoskeletal oncology. Lancet Oncol. 2003;4(6):343–50.
3. Ferrari S, Palmerini E. Adjuvant and neoadjuvant combination chemotherapy for osteogenic sarcoma. Curr Opin Oncol. 2007;19(4):341–6.
4. Whelan J, Seddon B, Perisoglou M. Management of osteosarcoma. Curr Treat Options Oncol. 2006;7(6):444–55.

5. Onikul E, Fletcher BD, Parham DM, Chen G. Accuracy of MR imaging for estimating intraosseous extent of osteosarcoma. Am J Roentgenol. 1996;167(5):1211–5.
6. Kneisl JS, Finn HA, Simon MA. Mobile knee reconstructions after resection of malignant tumors of the distal femur. Orthop Clin North Am. 1991;22(1):105–19.
7. Skaliczki G, Antal I, Kiss J, Szalay K, Skaliczki J, Szendri M. Functional outcome and life quality after endoprosthetic reconstruction following malignant tumours around the knee. Int Orthop. 2005;29(3):174–8. Epub 2005 Apr 14.
8. Marulanda GA, Henderson ER, Johnson DA, Letson GD, Cheong D. Orthopedic surgery options for the treatment of primary osteosarcoma. Cancer Control. 2008;15(1):13–20.
9. Swallow CJ, Catton CN. Local management of adult soft tissue sarcomas. Semin Oncol. 2007;34(3):256–69.
10. Kunz P, Bernd L. Methods of biological reconstruction for bone sarcoma: indications and limits. Recent Results Cancer Res. 2009;179:113–40.
11. Benedetti MG, Bonatti E, Malfitano C, Donati D. Comparison of allograft-prosthetic composite reconstruction and modular prosthetic replacement in proximal femur bone tumors: functional assessment by gait analysis in 20 patients. Acta Orthop. 2013;84(2):218–23.
12. Matsumine A, Ueda T, Sugita T, Yazawa Y, Isu K, Kawai A, Japanese Musculoskeletal Oncology Group, et al. Clinical outcomes of the KYOCERA physio hinge total knee system type III after the resection of a bone and soft tissue tumor of the distal part of the femur. J Surg Oncol. 2011;103(3):257–63.
13. Kotz RI. Progress in musculoskeletal oncology from 1922–2012. Int Orthop. 2014;38 (5):1113–22.
14. Kawai A, Lin PP, Boland PJ, et al. Relationship between magnitude of resection, complication, and prosthetic survival after prosthetic knee reconstructions for distal femoral tumors. J Surg Oncol. 1999;70(2):109–15.
15. Nakamura T, Matsumine A, Uchida A, Kawai A, Nishida Y, Kunisada T, et al. Clinical outcomes of Kyocera modular limb salvage system after resection of bone sarcoma of the distal part of the femur: the Japanese Musculoskeletal Oncology Group study. Int Orthop. 2014;38(4):825–30.
16. Moore AT, Bohlman HR. Metal hip joint: a case report. J Bone Joint Surg Am. 1943;25 (3):688–92.
17. Unwin PS, Cannon SR, Grimer RJ, Kemp HB, Sneath RS, Walker PS. Aseptic loosening in cemented custom-made prosthetic replacements for bone tumours of the lower limb. J Bone Joint Surg Br. 1996;78(1):5–13.
18. Unwin PS, Cobb JP, Walker PS. Distal femoral arthroplasty using custom-made prostheses. The first 218 cases. J Arthroplasty. 1993;8(3):259–68.
19. Mascard E, Anract P, Touchene A, Pouillart P, Tomeno B, Mascard E, et al. Complications from the hinged GUEPAR prosthesis after resection of knee tumor. 102 cases. Rev Chir Orthop Reparatrice Appar Mot. 1998;84:628–37.
20. Brav EA, Mc FJ, Miller JA. The replacement of shaft defects of long bones by metallic prostheses. Am J Surg. 1958;95(5):752–60.
21. Loomis LK. Internal prosthesis for upper portion of femur; a case report. J Bone Joint Surg Am. 1950;32(A:4):944–6.
22. Venable CS. An elbow and an elbow prosthesis; case of complete loss of the lower third of the humerus. Am J Surg. 1952;83(3):271–5.
23. Moore AT. The self-locking metal hip prosthesis. J Bone Joint Surg Am. 1957;39-A (4):811–27.
24. Horwitz T. Use of a shaft prosthesis in the treatment of surgically resistant nonunion of the humerus. Bull Hosp Joint Dis. 1955;16(1):37–44.
25. Seddon HJ, Scales JT. A polythene substitute for the upper two-thirds of the shaft of the femur. Lancet. 1949;2(6583):795.
26. Macausland WR. Replacement of the lower end of the humerus with a prosthesis; a report of four cases. West J Surg Obstet Gynecol. 1954;62(11):557–66.

27. Katayama R, Maezawa T. Total replacement of the knee joint by prosthesis: the first report. J Jpn Orthop Assoc. 1968;42:187–92.
28. Hwang JS, Mehta AD, Yoon RS, Beebe KS. From amputation to limb salvage reconstruction: evolution and role of the endoprosthesis in musculoskeletal oncology. J Orthop Traumatol. 2014;15(2):81–6.
29. Rosen G, Murphy ML, Huvos AG, Gutierrez M, Marcove RC. Chemotherapy, en bloc resection, and prosthetic bone replacement in the treatment of osteogenic sarcoma. Cancer. 1976;37(1):1–11.
30. Destouet JM, Gilula LA, Murphy WA. Computed tomography of long-bone osteosarcoma. Radiology. 1979;131(2):439–45.
31. Zimmer WD, Berquist TH, McLeod RA, Sim FH, Pritchard DJ, Shives TC, Wold LE, May GR. Magnetic resonance imaging of osteosarcomas. Comparison with computed tomography. Clin Orthop Relat Res. 1986;208:289–99.
32. Kotz R, Ritschl P, Trachtenbrodt J. A modular femur-tibia reconstruction-system. Orthopedics. 1986;9:1639–52.
33. Heisel C, Kinkel S, Bernd L, Ewerbeck V. Megaprostheses for the treatment of malignant bone tumours of the lower limbs. Int Orthop. 2006;30(6):452–7.
34. Yamawaki K, Aoki H, Shimizu K, Mori T, Kidokoro K. Revision of acrylic hinge-type knee prosthesis after a follow-up of almost 40 years. J Orthop Sci. 2006;11(1):97–102.
35. Siu D, Rudan J, Wevers HW, Griffiths P. Femoral articular shape and geometry. A three-dimensional computerized analysis of the knee. J Arthroplasty. 1996;11(2):166–73.
36. Hitt K, Shurman 2nd JR, Greene K, McCarthy J, Moskal J, Hoeman T, et al. Anthropometric measurements of the human knee: correlation to the sizing of current knee arthroplasty systems. J Bone Joint Surg Am. 2003;85-A Suppl 4:115–22.
37. Wang SW, Feng CH, Lu HS. A study of Chinese knee joint geometry for prosthesis design. Chin Med J (Engl). 1992;105(3):227–33.
38. Uehara K, Kadoya Y, Kobayashi A, Ohashi H, Yamano Y. Anthropometry of the proximal tibia to design a total knee prosthesis for the Japanese population. J Arthroplasty. 2002;17 (8):1028–32.
39. Bhudhikanok GS, Wang MC, Eckert K, Matkin C, Marcus R, Bachrach LK. Differences in bone mineral in young Asian and Caucasian Americans may reflect differences in bone size. J Bone Miner Res. 1996;11(10):1545–56.
40. Low FH, Khoo LP, Chua CK, Lo NN. Kinematic analysis of total knee prosthesis designed for Asian population. Crit Rev Biomed Eng. 2000;28(1–2):33–40.
41. Torbert JT, Fox EJ, Hosalkar HS, Ogilvie CM, Lackman RD. Endoprosthetic reconstructions: results of long-term followup of 139 patients. Clin Orthop Relat Res. 2005;438:51–9.
42. Kawai A, Healey JH, Boland PJ, Athanasian EA, Jeon DG. A rotating-hinge knee replacement for malignant tumors of the femur and tibia. J Arthroplasty. 1999;14(2):187–96.
43. Mittermayer F, Krepler P, Dominkus M, Schwameis E, Sluga M, Heinzl H, et al. Long-term followup of uncemented tumor endoprostheses for the lower extremity. Clin Orthop Relat Res. 2001;388:167–77.
44. Roberts P, Chan D, Grimer RJ, Sneath RS, Scales JT. Prosthetic replacement of the distal femur for primary bone tumours. J Bone Joint Surg Br. 1991;73(5):762–9.
45. Muschler GF, Ihara K, Lane JM, Healey JH, Levine MJ, Otis JC, et al. A custom distal femoral prosthesis for reconstruction of large defects following wide excision for sarcoma: results and prognostic factors. Orthopedics. 1995;18(6):527–38.
46. Ham SJ, Schraffordt Koops H, Veth RP, van Horn JR, Molenaar WM, Hoekstra HJ. Limb salvage surgery for primary bone sarcoma of the lower extremities: long-term consequences of endoprosthetic reconstructions. Ann Surg Oncol. 1998;5(5):423–36.
47. Griffin AM, Parsons JA, Davis AM, Bell RS, Wunder JS. Uncemented tumor endoprostheses at the knee: root causes of failure. Clin Orthop Relat Res. 2005;438:71–9.

48. Biau D, Faure F, Katsahian S, Jeanrot C, Tomeno B, Anract P. Survival of total knee replacement with a megaprosthesis after bone tumor resection. J Bone Joint Surg Am. 2006;88(6):1285–93.
49. Sharma S, Turcotte RE, Isler MH, Wong C. Cemented rotating hinge endoprosthesis for limb salvage of distal femur tumors. Clin Orthop Relat Res. 2006;450:28–32.
50. Mensch JS, Amstutz HC. Knee morphology as a guide to knee replacement. Clin Orthop Relat Res. 1975;112:231–41.
51. Miyake T. Studies on the sizes and shapes of Japanese knee and their applications to the design of knee prosthesis. J Jpn Orthop Assoc. 1978;52:865–79.
52. Jeys LM, Grimer RJ, Carter SR, Tillman RM. Periprosthetic infection in patients treated for an orthopaedic oncological condition. J Bone Joint Surg Am. 2005;87(4):842–9.
53. Jeys LM, Grimer RJ, Carter SR, Tillman RM. Risk of amputation following limb salvage surgery with endoprosthetic replacement, in a consecutive series of 1261 patients. Int Orthop. 2003;27(3):160–3. Epub 2003 Feb 8.
54. Heisel C, Breusch SJ, Schmid G, Bernd L. Lower limb salvage surgery with MUTARS endoprostheses: 2 to 7 year results. Acta Orthop Belg. 2004;70(2):142–7.
55. Hardes J, Gebert C, Schwappach A, et al. Characteristics and outcome of infections associated with tumor endoprostheses. Arch Orthop Trauma Surg. 2006;26:289–96.
56. Shin DS, Weber KL, Chao EY, et al. Reoperation for failed prosthetic replacement used for limb salvage. Clin Orthop Relat Res. 1999;358:53–63.
57. Capanna R, Morris HG, Campanacci D, Del Ben M, Campanacci M. Modular uncemented prosthetic reconstruction after resection of tumours of the distal femur. J Bone Joint Surg Br. 1994;76(2):178–86.
58. Kawai A, Muschler GF, Lane JM, Otis JC, Healey JH. Prosthetic knee replacement after resection of a malignant tumor of the distal part of the femur. Medium to long-term results. J Bone Joint Surg Am. 1998;80(5):636–47.
59. Bickels J, Wittig JC, Kollender Y, Henshaw RM, Kellar-Graney KL, Meller I, et al. Distal femur resection with endoprosthetic reconstruction: a long-term followup study. Clin Orthop Relat Res. 2002;400:225–35.
60. Morii T, Morioka H, Ueda T, Araki N, Hashimoto N, Kawai A, et al. Deep infection in tumor endoprosthesis around the knee: a multi-institutional study by the Japanese musculoskeletal oncology group. BMC Musculoskelet Disord. 2013;14:51.
61. Hardes J, von Eiff C, Streitbuerger A, Balke M, Budny T, Henrichs MP, et al. Reduction of periprosthetic infection with silver-coated megaprostheses in patients with bone sarcoma. J Surg Oncol. 2010;101(5):389–95.
62. Shirai T, Tsuchiya H, Nishida H, Yamamoto N, Watanabe K, Nakase J, et al. Antimicrobial megaprostheses supported with iodine. J Biomater Appl. 2014;29(4):617–23.
63. Zeegen EN, Aponte-Tinao LA, Hornicek FJ, Gebhardt MC, Mankin HJ. Survivorship analysis of 141 modular metallic endoprostheses at early followup. Clin Orthop Relat Res. 2004;420:239–50.
64. Choong PF, Sim FH, Pritchard DJ, Rock MG, Chao EY. Megaprostheses after resection of distal femoral tumors. A rotating hinge design in 30 patients followed for 2–7 years. Acta Orthop Scand. 1996;67(4):345–51.
65. Myers GJ, Abudu AT, Carter SR, Tillman RM, Grimer RJ. Endoprosthetic replacement of the distal femur for bone tumours: long-term results. J Bone Joint Surg Br. 2007;89(4):521–6.
66. Myers GJ, Abudu AT, Carter SR, Tillman RM, Grimer RJ. Erratum. J Bone Joint Surg Br. 2007;89(5):706.
67. Monument MJ, Bernthal NM, Bowles AJ, Jones KB, Randall RL. What are the 5-year survivorship outcomes of compressive endoprosthetic osseointegration fixation of the femur? Clin Orthop Relat Res. 19 June 2014 [Epub ahead of print].

Limb-Salvage Surgery and Reconstruction for Skeletally Immature Childhood Osteosarcoma: Extendible Endoprosthesis

10

Hiroyuki Futani and Shinichi Yoshiya

Abstract

The purpose of this article is to report on the development, indication, and clinical outcome of extendible endoprostheses for the management of osteosarcomas in the skeletally immature patients after resection of major growth plates in conjunction with limb-salvage surgery. The first generation of extendible endoprostheses appeared in the late 1970s. They were invasive, and open lengthening procedures were required. Several subsequent modifications have yielded the endoprostheses capable of lengthening through less invasive methods to minimize the risk of complications. An extendible endoprosthesis should be applied for the skeletally immature patients when the estimated leg length discrepancy at skeletal maturity is expected to be more than 3 cm or when the arm length discrepancy will be more than 5 cm. Prosthetic reconstruction is well received emotionally and cosmetically. Furthermore, even if additional revision surgeries are required, extendible endoprostheses provide good functional outcome in skeletally immature children with osteosarcomas. However, the patients and their families must be carefully selected with an emphasis on motivation and acceptance, since rather frequent and substantial treatment during follow-up is inevitably required. In the future, improvements in the surgical techniques and endoprosthetic designs are needed to diminish the number of complications.

Keywords

Limb salvage • Children • Skeletally immature • Extendible prosthesis • Malignant bone tumors

H. Futani (✉) • S. Yoshiya
Departments of Orthopedic Surgery, Hyogo College of Medicine, 1-1 Mukogawa, Nishinomiya, Hyogo 663-8501, Japan
e-mail: h-futani@hyo-med.ac.jp

T. Ueda, A. Kawai (eds.), *Osteosarcoma*, DOI 10.1007/978-4-431-55696-1_10

10.1 Introduction

Limb-salvage surgery has been a widely accepted alternative to amputation in patients with osteosarcomas since limb-salvage provides better function and quality of life without a reduction in survival [1, 2]. This is the result of the advances in the understanding of the biology and staging of tumors, the improvement in reconstructive techniques, and the development of effective chemotherapy. Particularly, chemotherapy has dramatically changed the cure rate of osteosarcomas [3, 4]. Since the introduction of effective neoadjuvant chemotherapy in the 1980s, more than 80 % of patients with osteosarcoma of the extremity have been considered treatable with limb-salvage surgery [5].

Osteosarcomas commonly involve the most rapidly growing parts of the skeleton, such as the metaphysis of the distal femur and proximal tibia. In the skeletally immature patients, the eventual functional impairment due to subsequent growth inhibition and limb length discrepancy must be considered after resection of major growth plates in conjunction with limb-salvage surgery.

This author reported that the functional assessment was significantly better in those patients who underwent lengthening procedures compared to those who did not (Fig. 10.1). This finding indicated that lengthening procedures are required to obtain better function for the skeletally immature patients [6]. A limb length discrepancy of 2 cm or more has been considered significant enough to require corrective surgery or accommodated through shoe modification [7]. Several techniques have been applied to address limb length discrepancy, such as extendible endoprostheses, distraction osteogenesis [8–10], allograft [11, 12], and the use of a shoe lift [13].

The purpose of this article is to report on the development, indication, and clinical outcome of extendible endoprostheses for the management of osteosarcoma in the skeletally immature patients.

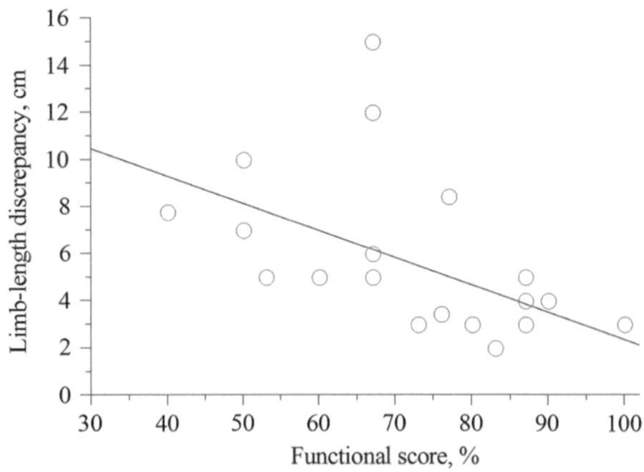

Fig. 10.1 Regression plot between limb length discrepancy and functional score. There was a significant negative correlation between these parameters with an r-value of 0.53 and $p = 0.0091$ (Quotation from Futani et al. [6])

10.2 Evolution of Extendible Endoprostheses

The first generation of extendible endoprostheses appeared in the late 1970s. They were invasive, and open lengthening procedures were required. Several subsequent modifications have yielded the endoprostheses capable of lengthening through less invasive methods [14]. The initial part of the first generation was lengthened by means of a ball-bearing mechanism. It was replaced by a system which required insertion of a "C" collar in 1988 [15]. The Lewis Expandable Adjustable Prosthesis (Dow Corning Wright Corporation, Arlington, Tennessee) was also introduced in 1983. It used a fixed stem with a screw extension mechanism that expanded the endoprosthesis [16]. These endoprostheses had a high failure rate over the time required for multiple lengthening procedures [6].

The second generation of extendible endoprostheses was minimally invasive. Lengthening was achieved with an elongating screw mechanism that was rotated via a small incision. The need for soft tissue dissection was dramatically reduced, and joint motion was better, even though they also required an open procedure [15]. In 1987, the minimally invasive Growing Kotz prosthesis was introduced [4] (Fig. 10.2).

Third-generation extendible endoprostheses were noninvasive; lengthening was achieved without open surgery, and the risk of complications due to repeated surgeries was minimized [4, 17, 18]. The noninvasive extendible endoprosthesis (Wright Medical Technology, Inc, Arlington, Tennessee), originally known as the Repiphysis or Phenix prosthesis (Phenix Medical, Paris, France) [17, 19], and the Stanmore noninvasive extendible prosthesis (Stanmore, Middlesex, UK) were also introduced by the use of an external electromagnetic or rotating magnetic field for lengthening. Once implanted, these noninvasive extendible endoprostheses require no further surgical procedure during lengthening, thus allowing maximum extension without additional surgery.

10.3 Indications for Extendible Endoprostheses

Osteosarcomas predominantly occur in the metaphyseal region close to the growth plate. The distal end of the femur is the most common site for an osteosarcoma in children [20, 21]. When major growth plates are completely removed during limb-salvage surgery, the growth of the affected limb is seized before skeletal maturity.

Skeletal maturity is expected by the age of 16 years in boys and 14 years in girls [22, 23]. The amount of bone growth that can be expected from each growth plate has been described [24]. Up to 67 % of the lower limb growth occurs around the knee (distal femur and proximal tibia) [25]. The distal femoral physis presumably contributes to approximately 10 mm of growth per year until skeletal maturity [22, 23]. Significant leg length discrepancy results in gait abnormalities, leg pain, and back pain [26]. Kenan et al. reported that leg lengthening was necessary in patients younger than 13 years of age at the time of limb-salvage surgery [27].

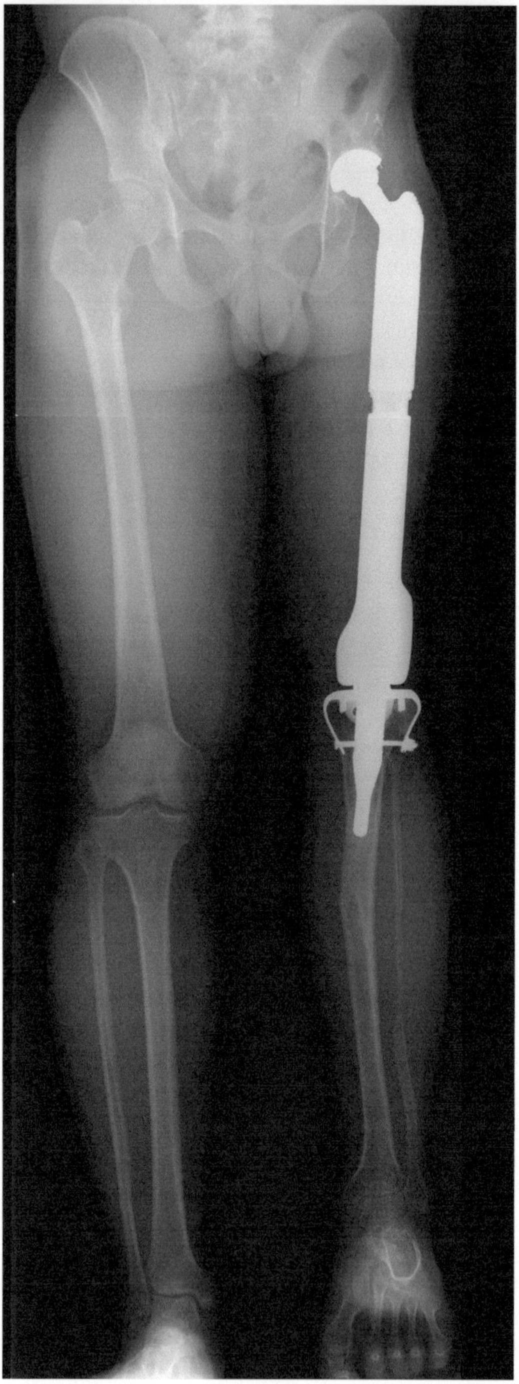

Fig. 10.2 Limb length discrepancy in a patient after total femoral replacement. This patient had an osteosarcoma located in the distal femur that also extended into the proximal part of femur. Consequently, a total femur replacement was required. At first, this patient had a custom-made endoprosthesis followed by distraction osteogenesis of the tibia. Then the endoprosthesis was exchanged for an extendible one, and finally he needed limb lengthening through endoprosthetic expansion (Quotation from Futani et al. [6])

As for the humerus, 80 % of total growth occurs in the proximal growth plate [25]. Ayoub et al. [28] mentioned that the main problem of arm length discrepancy is cosmetic. Functionally, lengthening of the humerus gains less functional advantage in comparison to the femur or tibia.

The necessity for an extendible endoprosthesis is based on the estimated growth remaining in the resected growth plate, calculated using the growth charts [22] after an estimation of bone age based on interpretation of a radiograph of the hand [29]. However, accurate prediction of future growth often becomes problematic. Dominkus et al. reported that the patients in their series required a mean expansion that was 24.3 % larger than the expansion anticipated after careful preoperative assessment of growth potential [30]. Implementation of a permanent solution at the time of the initial surgery may therefore lead to a discrepancy of unforeseen proportions. For this reason, an extendible endoprosthesis should be applied for the pediatric patient when the estimated leg length discrepancy at skeletal maturity is expected to be more than 3 cm or when the arm length discrepancy will be more than 5 cm [14, 28].

10.4 Function

Several investigators have reported on patient functional scores after extendible endoprostheses. It has been widely accepted that extendible endoprostheses result in superior satisfaction and functional scores compared with those of amputation. Prosthetic reconstruction is well received emotionally and cosmetically by patients and their parents. Furthermore, the clinical and functional outcome correlates to that reported for adult patients [27, 31–33].

This author reported that the final functional score for endoprosthetic reconstruction was 74 %, in spite of the frequent necessity for additional operations, such as limb-lengthening procedures and revisions [6]. Function in the endoprosthetic group was comparable to the study of Schindler, in which the Musculoskeletal Tumor Society (MSTS) functional score was 77 % in 12 children with Stanmore custom-made extendible distal femoral endoprostheses [34]. Ruggieri et al. [35] reported that the mean MSTS score was 79 % (range, 30–100 %) by the use of the second and third generation of extendible endoprostheses; the mean MSTS score was 81 % (range, 63–93 %) for the Kotz Growing prostheses, 78 % (range, 33–100 %) for the Repiphysis, and 79 % (range, 30–100 %) for the Stanmore prostheses, without a significant difference between the type of endoprostheses.

Emotional satisfaction is an important factor for improved quality of life for young patients with extendible endoprostheses [36]. The Pediatric Outcomes Data Collection Instrument (PODCI) was developed to measure body image, social acceptance, as well as physical function and satisfaction after treatment for musculoskeletal disorders specifically in the pediatric population [36]. Henderson et al. [37] showed high emotional satisfaction for pediatric patients with extendible endoprostheses according to PODCI. Overall, patients reported excellent perceptions of body image and physical attractiveness. In addition, frequent social interactions and no difficulty in making new friends were also found.

10.5 Complications

Complications related to surgery, such as infection, aseptic loosening, implant breakage, dislocation, and skin necrosis, are frequent.

This author reported that 45 % of the skeletally immature patients with endoprosthetic reconstruction had experienced complications at 5 years, and the complication rate increased to 69 % at 10 years [6].

Deep infection was the most common complication. In the previous literature, the rate of deep infection in the femur varies from 4 % (1 of 24 patients) in the series by Cool [24] to 40 % (2 of 5 patients) in Schiller's series [4]. Comparable results have been reported by others [34, 38–40].

Aseptic loosening has been reported as a major problem [4, 6, 35, 41], accounting for 10 % (4 of 39 patients) of complications in the series by Ruggieri P [36] up to 50 % (6 of 12 patients) reported by Schindler [34]. Picardo et al. [40] reported only 1 of 44 patients (2 %) with aseptic loosening by the use of the Stanmore noninvasive extendible endoprosthesis. Cannon et al. [42] reported that in distal femoral and proximal tibial resections, the rate of failure was higher when >60 % of bone was removed.

10.6 Survival of Prostheses

Previous studies have reported revision rates from a minimum of 20 % (5 of 24 patients) in the series by Cool [24] up to 100 % (12 of 12 patients) by Schindler [34]. Comparable results have been reported by others [4, 15, 24, 35, 39]. Unwin reported that 105 patients with distal femoral extendible endoprostheses had a probability of survival of 80 % at 4 years 29. This author reported on the long-term results of endoprosthetic survival: 77 % at 5 years and 51 % at 10 years, respectively [6]. Recently, Ruggieri et al. showed comparable results of 32 primary endoprostheses: 78 % survival at 5 years and 66 % at 10 years, respectively [35].

10.7 Future Direction

Novel surgical techniques and endoprosthetic designs will provide the longevity of the devices and fewer complications. New endoprosthetic designs of coating with silver [43] and other antimicrobial substance such as iodine [44] will decrease the rate of periprosthetic infections.

Composite reconstruction with allograft or recycled bone will provide better soft tissue attachments with anatomical site, which will enhance the articulation and stability of limb and endoprosthesis. The new invention of bone ingrowth stems will increase longevity and decrease need for bone cement. The computer-assisted techniques might contribute to less invasive surgery.

References

1. Simon MA, Aschliman MA, Thomas N, Mankin HJ. Limb-salvage treatment versus amputation for osteosarcoma of the distal end of the femur. J Bone Joint Surg Am. 1986;68:1331–7.
2. Rougraff BT, Simon MA, Kneisl JS, Greenberg DB, Mankin HJ. Limb salvage compared with amputation for osteosarcoma of the distal end of the femur. A long-term oncological, functional, and quality-of-life study. J Bone Joint Surg Am. 1994;76:649–56.
3. Link MP, Goorin AM, Horowitz M, Meyer WH, Belasco J, Baker A, Ayala A, Shuster J. Adjuvant chemotherapy of high-grade osteosarcoma of the extremity. Updated results of the Multi-Institutional Osteosarcoma Study. Clin Orthop. 1991;270:8–14.
4. Schiller C, Windhager R, Fellinger EJ, Salzer-Kuntschik M, Kaider A, Kotz R. Extendable tumour endoprostheses for the leg in children. J Bone Joint Surg (Br). 1995;77:608–14.
5. Bacci G, Picci P, Ferrari S, Ruggieri P, Casadei R, Tienghi A, Brach el Prever A, Gherlinzoni F, Mercuri M, Monti C. Primary chemotherapy and delayed surgery for nonmetastatic osteosarcoma of the extremities. Results in 164 patients preoperatively treated with high doses of methotrexate followed by cisplatin and doxorubicin. Cancer. 1993;72:3227–38.
6. Futani H, Minamizaki T, Nishimoto Y, Abe S, Yabe H, Ueda T. Long-term follow-up after limb salvage in skeletally immature children with a primary malignant tumor of the distal end of the femur. J Bone Joint Surg Am. 2006;88:595–603.
7. Gross RH. Leg length discrepancy: how much is too much? Orthopedics. 1978;1:307–10.
8. Gonzalez-Herranz P, Burgos-Flores J, Ocete-Guzman JG, Lopez-Mondejar JA, Amaya S. The management of limb-length discrepancies in children after treatment of osteosarcoma and Ewing's sarcoma. J Pediatr Orthop. 1995;15:561–5.
9. Tsuchiya H, Abdel-Wanis ME, Sakurakichi K, Yamashiro T, Tomita K. Osteosarcoma around the knee. Intraepiphyseal excision and biological reconstruction with distraction osteogenesis. J Bone Joint Surg (Br). 2002;84:1162–6.
10. Erler K, Yildiz C, Baykal B, Atesalp AS, Ozdemir MT, Basbozkurt M. Reconstruction of defects following bone tumor resections by distraction osteogenesis. Arch Orthop Trauma Surg. 2005;125:177–83.
11. Brigman BE, Hornicek FJ, Gebhardt MC, Mankin HJ. Allografts about the knee in young patients with high-grade sarcoma. Clin Orthop Relat Res. 2004;421:232–9.
12. Campanacci L, Manfrini M, Colangeli M, Alí N, Mercuri M. Long-term results in children with massive bone osteoarticular allografts of the knee for high-grade osteosarcoma. J Pediatr Orthop. 2010;30:919–27.
13. Stanitski DF. Limb-length inequality: assessment and treatment options. J Am Acad Orthop Surg. 1999;7:143–53.
14. Marulanda GA, Henderson ER, Palumbo BT, Alexander GE, Cheong D, Letson GD. Use of extendable prostheses: a limb-salvaging alternative for patients with malignant bone tumors. Expert Rev Med Devices. 2008;5:467–74.
15. Unwin PS, Walker PS. Extendible endoprostheses for the skeletally immature. Clin Orthop. 1996;322:179–93.
16. Lewis MM, Bloom N, Esquieres EM, Kenan S, Ryniker DM. The expandable prosthesis. An alternative to amputation for children with malignant bone tumors. AORN J. 1987;46:457–70.
17. Neel MD, Wilkins RM, Rao BN, Kelly CM. Early multicenter experience with a noninvasive expandable prosthesis. Clin Orthop Relat Res. 2003;415:72–81.
18. Wilkins RM, Miller CM. Reoperation after limb preservation surgery for sarcomas of the knee in children. Clin Orthop. 2003;412:153–61.

19. Wilkins RM, Soubeiran A. The Phenix expandable prosthesis: early American experience. Clin Orthop Relat Res. 2001;382:51–8.
20. O'Flanagan SJ, Stack JP, McGee HM, Dervan P, Hurson B. Imaging of intramedullary tumour spread in osteosarcoma. A comparison of techniques. J Bone Joint Surg (Br). 1991;73:998–1001.
21. Finn HA, Simon MA. Limb-salvage surgery in the treatment of osteosarcoma in skeletally immature individuals. Clin Orthop. 1991;262:108–18.
22. Anderson M, Green WT, Messner MB. Growth and predictions of growth in the lower extremities. J Bone Joint Surg Am. 1963;45:1–14.
23. Westh RN, Menelaus MB. A simple calculation for the timing of epiphysial arrest. A further report. J Bone Joint Surg (Br). 1981;63:117–9.
24. Cool WP, Carter SR, Grimer RJ, Tillman RM, Walker PS. Growth after extendible endoprosthetic replacement of the distal femur. J Bone Joint Surg (Br). 1997;79:938–42.
25. Pritchett JW. Longitudinal growth and growth-plate activity in the lower extremity. Clin Orthop Relat Res. 1992;275:274–9.
26. Song KM, Halliday SE, Little DG. The effect of limb length on gait. J Bone Joint Surg Am. 1997;79:1690–8.
27. Kenan S, Lewis MM. Limb salvage in pediatric surgery. The use of the expandable prosthesis. Orthop Clin North Am. 1991;22:121–31.
28. Ayoub KS, Fiorenza F, Grimer RJ, Tillman RM, Carter SR. Extensible endoprostheses of the humerus after resection of bone tumours. J Bone Joint Surg (Br). 1999;81:495–500.
29. Greulich WW, Pyle SI. Radiographic atlas of skeletal development of the hand and wrist. 2nd ed. Stanford: Stanford University Press; 1966.
30. Dominkus M, Krepler P, Schwameis E, Windhager R, Kotz R. Growth prediction in extendable tumor prostheses in children. Clin Orthop Relat Res. 2001;390:212–20.
31. Delepine G, Delepine N, Desbois JC, Goutallier D. Expanding prostheses in conservative surgery for lower limb sarcoma. Int Orthop. 1998;22:27–31.
32. Eckardt JJ, Kabo JM, Kelley CM, Ward Sr WG, Asavamongkolkul A, Wirganowicz PZ, Yang RS, Eilber FR. Expandable endoprosthesis reconstruction in skeletally immature patients with tumors. Clin Orthop. 2000;373:51–61.
33. Grimer RJ, Belthur M, Carter SR, Tillman RM, Cool P. Extendible replacements of the proximal tibia for bone tumours. J Bone Joint Surg (Br). 2000;82:255–60.
34. Schindler OS, Cannon SR, Briggs TW, Blunn GW. Stanmore custom-made extendible distal femoral replacements. J Bone Joint Surg (Br). 1997;79:927–37.
35. Ruggieri P, Mavrogenis AF, Pala E, Romantini M, Manfrini M, Mercuri M. Outcome of expandable prostheses in children. J Pediatr Orthop. 2013;33:244–53.
36. Daltroy LH, Liang MH, Fossel AH, Goldberg MJ. The POSNA pediatric musculoskeletal functional health questionnaire: report on reliability, validity, and sensitivity to change. Pediatric Outcomes Instrument Development Group. Pediatric Orthopaedic Society of North America. J Pediatr Orthop. 1998;18:561–71.
37. Henderson ER, Pepper AM, Marulanda GA, Millard JD, Letson GD. What is the emotional acceptance after limb salvage with an expandable prosthesis? Clin Orthop Relat Res. 2010;468:2933–8.
38. Cara JA, Canadell J. Limb salvage for malignant bone tumors in young children. J Pediatr Orthop. 1994;14:112–8.
39. Alman BA, De Bari A, Krajbich JI. Massive allografts in the treatment of osteosarcoma and Ewing sarcoma in children and adolescents. J Bone Joint Surg Am. 1995;77:54–64.
40. Picardo NE, Blunn GW, Shekkeris AS, Meswania J, Aston WJ, Pollock RC, Skinner JA, Cannon SR, Briggs TW. The medium-term results of the Stanmore non-invasive extendible endoprosthesis in the treatment of paediatric bone tumours. J Bone Joint Surg (Br). 2012;94:425–30.
41. Neel MD, Letson GD. Modular endoprostheses for children with malignant bone tumors. Cancer Control. 2001;8:344–8.

42. Cannon SR. Massive prostheses for malignant bone tumours of the limbs. J Bone Joint Surg (Br). 1997;79:497–506.
43. Gosheger G, Hardes J, Ahrens H, Streitburger A, Buerger H, Erren M, Gunsel A, Kemper FH, Winkelmann W, Von Eiff C. Silver-coated megaendoprostheses in a rabbit model – an analysis of the infection rate and toxicological side effects. Biomaterials. 2004;25:5547–56.
44. Shirai T, Tsuchiya H, Nishida H, Yamamoto N, Watanabe K, Nakase J, Terauchi R, Arai Y, Fujiwara H, Kubo T. Antimicrobial megaprostheses supported with iodine. J Biomater Appl. 2014;29:617–23.

Limb Salvage Surgery for Pelvic Osteosarcoma

11

Toshiyuki Kunisada, Ken Takeda, Tomohiro Fujiwara, Shinsuke Sugihara, and Toshifumi Ozaki

Abstract

Patients with pelvic osteosarcoma have a poor outcome; treatment is one of the most challenging problems for the orthopedic oncologist. The reconstructive approach varies according to anatomic location, extent of resection, the patient's functional demands, and individual surgeon preference. The choice of optimal technique for reconstruction after acetabular tumor resection depends on numerous parameters and includes iliofemoral arthrodesis or pseudoarthrodesis, combined use of hip arthroplasty with massive allograft or recycled autograft, and pelvic and saddle prosthesis. The type of reconstruction modality can influence the rate of infection. Hip transposition resulted in the least incidence of complications after resection of the acetabulum, compared to the use of prosthesis or prosthesis and allograft. The absence of large implants and allografts helps reduce surgical time, facilitates closure, and may decrease the incidence of infection and late revision due to implant failure. These can lead to early postoperative systemic treatment and functional recovery and are critical for patients with a high incidence of local recurrence and distant metastases.

T. Kunisada, M.D., Ph.D. (✉)
Department of Medical Materials for Musculoskeletal Reconstruction, Okayama University Graduate School of Medicine, Dentistry and Pharmaceutical Sciences, 2-5-1 Shikata-cho, Kita-ku, Okayama 700-8558, Japan

Department of Orthopaedic Surgery, Okayama University Graduate School of Medicine, Dentistry, and Pharmaceutical Sciences, 2-5-1 Shikata-cho, Kita-ku, Okayama 700-8558, Japan
e-mail: toshi-kunisada@umin.ac.jp

K. Takeda • T. Fujiwara • T. Ozaki
Department of Orthopaedic Surgery, Okayama University Graduate School of Medicine, Dentistry, and Pharmaceutical Sciences, 2-5-1 Shikata-cho, Kita-ku, Okayama 700-8558, Japan

S. Sugihara
Department of Orthopaedic Surgery, Shikoku Cancer Center, 160 Ko, Minamiumemoto-cho, Matsuyama 791-0280, Japan

T. Ueda, A. Kawai (eds.), *Osteosarcoma*, DOI 10.1007/978-4-431-55696-1_11

We believe that resection arthroplasty should be indicated for the patient with acetabular osteosarcoma.

Keywords
Osteosarcoma • Pelvis • Acetabular resection • Reconstruction • Resection arthroplasty

11.1 Osteosarcoma of the Pelvis

Pelvic osteosarcoma is rare and reportedly accounts for less than 10 % of all osteosarcoma [1–3]. The Japan bone tumor registry showed that the incidence of pelvic osteosarcoma was 9.8 % of all osteosarcoma registered between 2006 and 2011. In contrast to extremity osteosarcoma, pelvic osteosarcoma tends to occur in older individuals, arising secondary to other conditions such as radiation and Paget's disease [4, 5]. The tumors are often large and present late and may already have metastasized before the diagnosis is established. The 5-year overall survival rates of pelvic osteosarcoma range from 18 to 38 % [3–8], markedly poor compared with extremity osteosarcoma. The management of pelvic osteosarcoma is still one of the most challenging problems in orthopedic oncology. The keys to treatment success depend on an effective response to chemotherapy, accurate assessment of the true extent of the tumor, and the ability to achieve a complete surgical resection with adequate margins.

Pelvic osteosarcoma is often associated with a poor response to chemotherapy compared with extremity osteosarcoma. Ozaki et al. reported that 71 % of patients who underwent surgery after preoperative chemotherapy had a poor response [6]. Kawai et al. demonstrated that the histologic effect in resected specimens was poor in 76 % of patients who underwent preoperative chemotherapy [4]. First, the median age of patients with pelvic osteosarcoma is higher, so that chemotherapy dose intensity may be lower [6]. Second, pelvic osteosarcomas are often chondroblastic, a histologic subtype that responds poorly to chemotherapy [4, 5, 8]. Furthermore, the biologic character of pelvic osteosarcoma may differ from that of extremity osteosarcoma.

Many authors identified complete resection with an adequate surgical margin as a good prognostic factor for pelvic osteosarcoma [4–6, 8]. External hemipelvectomy has been the accepted surgical treatment for primary malignant pelvic tumors. This has cosmetic and functional disadvantages; the loss of the limb is associated with a high morbidity rate. In the last two decades, internal hemipelvectomy with tumor removal and sparing of the lower extremity has frequently been performed. The reconstructive procedure to restore the limb function is also challenging, with a reported high incidence of mechanical, infectious, and neurovascular complications after internal hemipelvectomy. We review the options for limb sparing reconstruction following resection of pelvic osteosarcoma.

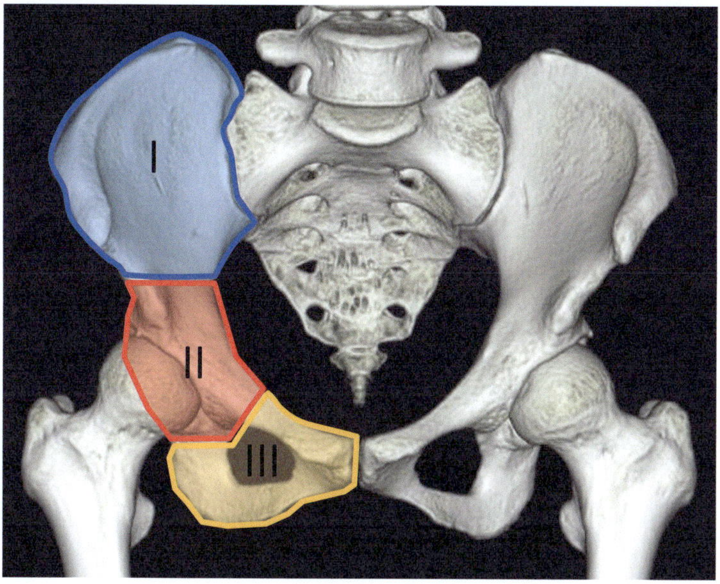

Fig. 11.1 Type of pelvic resection according to Enneking and Dunham. Type I involves the ilium, type II involves the periacetabulum, and type III involves the pubic rami

11.2 Classification of Pelvic Resection

The classification of pelvic resection type was proposed by Enneking and Dunham, describing the various subtypes based on the portion of bone removed [9]. Type I involves the ilium, type II involves the periacetabulum, and type III involves the pubic rami (Fig. 11.1). Resection may also include combinations of types. This classification scheme is still relevant today and is frequently referred to in the literature. Partial type I resections (when the pelvic ring remains in continuity) and type III resections typically do not require reconstruction. Type II or I+II periacetabular resections require restoration of hip joint function as well as extended bone and soft tissue defects, representing one of the most difficult situations in pelvic resection. For reconstruction after type II resection, either biologic methods or endoprosthetic options are established. We describe the reconstructive procedures for type II resection in the following text.

11.3 Prosthetic Reconstruction Methods

11.3.1 Constrained Total Hip Arthroplasty (C-THA)

Tumors extending into the pelvic cavity or buttock require the removal of the muscles that maintain hip joint stability, resulting in severe instability for hip prosthetic reconstruction. Constrained total hip prosthesis was developed in Japan

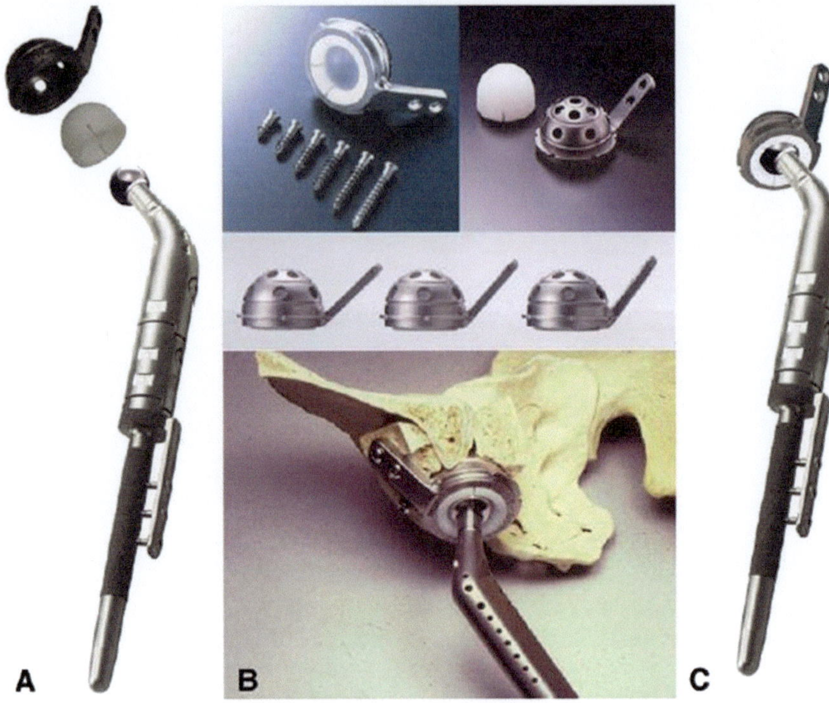

Fig. 11.2 Modular reconstruction system with a constrained total hip mechanism consists of three components (**a**). The original acetabular reconstruction cup system with a blade plate (**b**) and combined with these components (**c**)

for reconstruction after pelvic tumor resection and was easily fixed to the residual bone without restoration of pelvic continuity [10]. C-THA is composed of three parts (Fig. 11.2). The metallic outer head is fixed firmly with screws, bone cement, and bone grafting to the remaining ilium and sacrum. The inner head with a long neck and stem is cemented into the femoral shaft. These two components are connected by a high-density polyethylene-bearing insert, and the constrained total hip replacement is accomplished.

Reconstruction with the present C-THA model can lead to early rehabilitation due to immediate iliofemoral stabilization with a reduced risk of hip dislocation (Fig. 11.3). It is not necessary to reconstruct the pelvic ring disruption, resulting in a shorter operative time and fewer complications. Ueda et al. reviewed 25 patients treated with C-THA, demonstrating a mean MSTS (Musculoskeletal Tumor Society) functional score of 55 % and a 10-year implant survival rate of 67 % [11]. Major postoperative complications were seen in 32 %. They concluded that C-THA could provide pain-free hip reconstruction with immediate iliofemoral stability, suggesting this to be a useful reconstructive option for periacetabular tumors, despite serious postoperative complications.

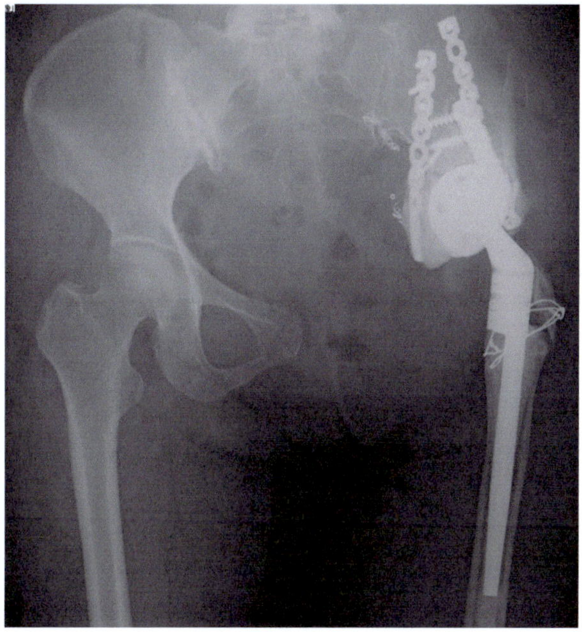

Fig. 11.3 Seven-year postoperative follow-up of constrained total hip arthroplasty after type II+III resection

11.3.2 Saddle Prosthesis

The saddle prosthesis initially was designed by Nieder et al. in 1979 for large acetabular defects in revision hip arthroplasty [12]. Since the end of the 1980s, it has been used primarily for hip reconstruction after periacetabular tumor resection (Fig. 11.4) [13]. The largest series is from Aljassir et al. (27 cases), and the average MSTS score in their 17 living patients is 51 %, similar to functional results in other series [14].

The benefit of a saddle prosthesis includes stable limb reconstruction for early weight bearing, equal leg length, acceptable function, and relative ease of prosthesis placement compared to arthrodesis or allograft-prosthetic composites [15]. However, many design-related complications such as loosening, loss of motion, dislocation, and fractures have been addressed. In Japan, we have much less experience with saddle prosthesis, and there are only a few case reports available, which are published only in Japanese. Recent papers with a long-term follow-up period demonstrated that saddle prosthesis showed poor clinical and functional results, although it was a simple method of pelvic reconstruction that reduced surgical time [16, 17].

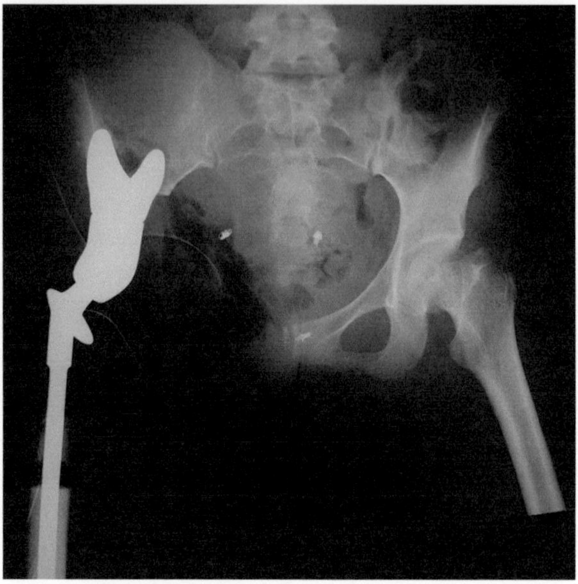

Fig. 11.4 Postoperative X-ray of saddle prosthesis after type II+III resection

11.3.3 Other Types of Pelvic Prosthesis

Various kinds of pelvic prostheses including custom-made or modular prosthesis have been reported in many countries [18–21], although reconstruction with pelvic megaprostheses was less popular for periacetabular tumors in Japan. Most papers regarding reconstruction with megaprostheses demonstrated that after good functional results in the beginning, the use of these mega-implants had a high complication rate: deep infection, dislocation, prosthesis loosening, broken screws, and prosthesis migration [2, 18, 19]. Due to its high complication rate, technical challenge, and implant expense, the concept of pelvic reconstruction has been changed. New types of pelvic replacement, such as "ice-cream cone" reconstruction or pedestal cup, were developed with promising early results [22, 23].

11.4 Biologic Reconstruction Methods

11.4.1 Recycled Autograft and Allograft Reconstruction

Reimplantation of recycled autograft has been a popular procedure for reconstruction following resection of bone and soft tissue sarcoma in Japan. Autografts have some advantages over allograft. Autografts do not contain foreign infectious or immunogenic agents. The fit at the host-graft junction and at the hip joint can always be perfect, and there is no need to maintain an extensive allograft bone bank. Since massive allografts such as pelvic bone are hardly available, surgical

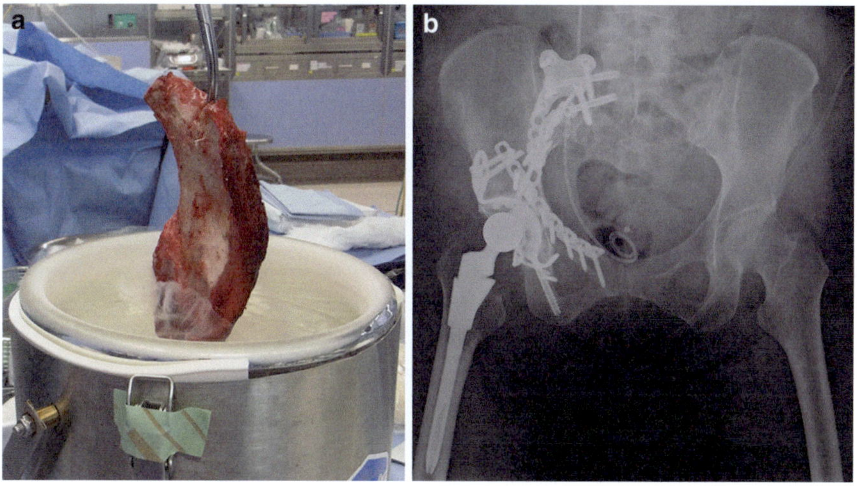

Fig. 11.5 Reconstruction using frozen autograft treated with liquid nitrogen (Figures courtesy of Dr. H. Tsuchiya and Dr. N. Yamamoto of Kanazawa University). (**a**) Resected bone (type I+II) containing tumor was treated with liquid nitrogen. (**b**) Postoperative X-ray of frozen autograft and prosthesis composite

reimplantation of irradiated [24, 25], thermally heated [26, 27], and liquid-nitrogen-treated bones [28] has been widely accepted in Japan.

Reconstruction with pelvic recycled autobone and prosthesis could result in improved function (Fig. 11.5). However, this procedure has been associated with nonunion, bone absorption, and deep infection. The series of 15 patients with pelvic reconstruction using irradiated autobone demonstrated complications in 13 patients (87 %), including three deep infections [29]. Koyanagi et al. reported the long-term results of pasteurized autograft, demonstrating that three of four pelvic reconstructions resulted in deep infection; two of them were finally removed [30]. Jeon et al. reported 5- and 10-year survival rates of pasteurized bone to be 64 % and 32 %, respectively, in 14 patients with periacetabular tumor [31]. Yamamoto et al. reported a 33 % infection rate following pelvic reconstruction using frozen autograft [32]. Allograft and prosthesis composites have been popular procedures for periacetabular tumors in Western countries; [33–36] we believe that there is a little difference between long-term outcomes of recycled autobone and allograft.

Reimplantation of recycled autobone will inevitably only be indicated for a small proportion of patients with pelvic tumors. Jeon et al. suggested that first, ilioischial and iliopectineal lines should be intact radiologically, and second, the tumor should be small in volume [31]. According to Wafa et al. [37], the key indication is for the patient with a type I+II tumor which can safely be resected with clear margins and in whom the bone is of sufficient quality and solid enough to reimplant. Furthermore, since it would take up to a year to complete bone healing

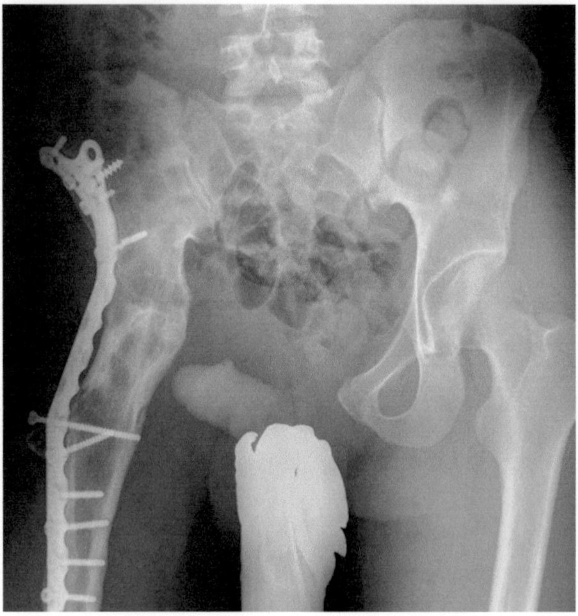

Fig. 11.6 Arthrodesis of the femoral head to the remaining ilium was made using plate and screws

and regain function, this procedure should ideally be used in patients with a reasonable prognosis.

11.4.2 Arthrodesis

Iliofemoral and ischiofemoral arthrodeses have been employed successfully for many years in limb salvage for malignant pelvic tumors. The basic principle of arthrodesis is to obtain continuity of the hip with the residual pelvis, improving pelvic stability and weight-bearing potential. Fixation of the proximal femur or femoral head to the remaining ilium is performed using plates (Fig. 11.6). Patients with a solid fusion clearly showed a 71 % MSTS score [38]. The iliofemoral arthrodesis is the reconstructive option of choice for young and active patients with more activity requirements, because it is stable and durable.

Furthermore, iliofemoral or sacrofemoral arthrodesis using microsurgical fibula grafting has been reported [39, 40]. This technique restored continuity of the pelvic ring with minimal limb length shortening (Fig. 11.7), despite being a technical demanding procedure with a relatively long operative time.

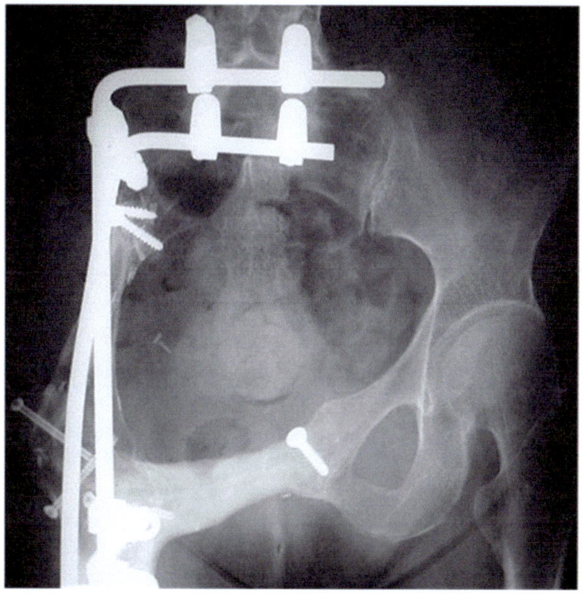

Fig. 11.7 X-ray 14 years after surgery of iliofemoral and ischiofemoral arthrodesis with vascularized-free fibula grafts (Figure courtesy of Dr. S. Nagoya of Sapporo Medical University)

11.4.3 Resection Arthroplasty (Flail Hip, Pseudoarthrosis, Hip Transposition)

An alternative to hindquarter amputation was reserving the leg after internal hemipelvectomy without reconstruction and leaving the remaining femur in place [41, 42]. Flail hip is at the opposite end of the spectrum of pelvic stability. Takami et al. demonstrated that the functional results of flail hip correlated with the amount of remaining ilium [43]. Schwartz et al. reported excellent results of flail hip with an average MSTS sore of 73 %, emphasizing the role of prolonged rehabilitation in its success [44]. Pseudoarthrosis may result as a failure after attempted fusion or an option of planned pseudoarthrosis, to preserve partial motion of the hip joint. Although the construct is less stable and the functional score is poorer than arthrodesis [38], pseudoarthrosis can maintain hip flexion, which is ideal for patients who sit more [22]. Surgical technique of hip transposition was described by Gebert et al. [45], where the femoral head is adjusted and fixed to the proximal osteotomy region with soft tissue or textile implants (Fig. 11.8). Hip transposition provided satisfactory quality of life and functional results, compared with other types of reconstruction [46].

Resection arthroplasty is usually shorter, technically less demanding, and possibly associated with a lower complication rate, compared with complex reconstructive procedures that carry high rates of postoperative complications (Table 11.1). The primary disadvantage of resection arthroplasty is the resulting shortening of the leg, which is not definitively associated with a poor functional outcome [46]. We currently do not usually conduct reconstruction with pelvic prostheses or autograft/allografts

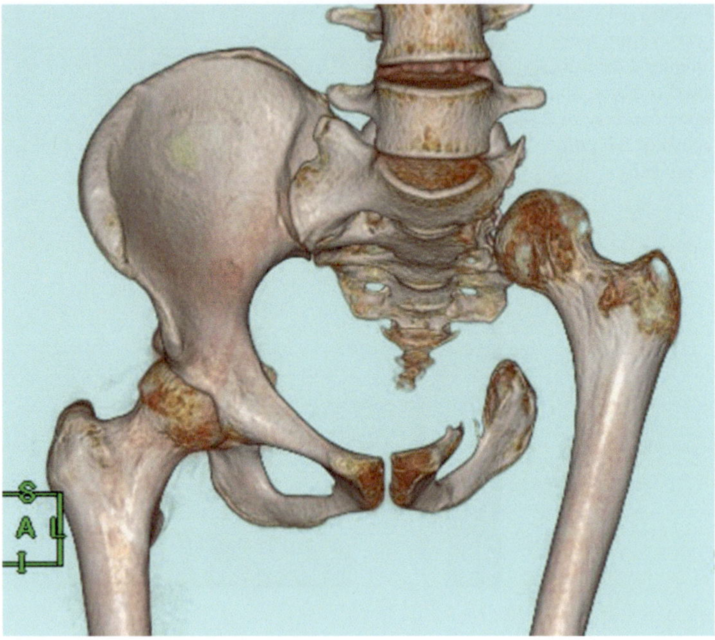

Fig. 11.8 3D-CT of hip transposition shows the femoral head attached to the osteotomy region of the sacrum

Table 11.1 Functional results and postoperative complications according to reconstructive approach

			Complication	
Type of reconstruction	*n*	MSTS score (%)	Infection	Additional surgery (total)
Hip transposition	20	61	0	0
Pelvic prosthesis	10	40	4	8
Allograft/autograft	4	63	2	2
No reconstruction	3	33	0	0
External hemipelvectomy	8	26	1	2

Reported by Hoffmann et al. [46]
MSTS (Musculoskeletal Tumor Society) score was evaluated according to Enneking et al. [50]

for type II resection and largely prefer resection arthroplasty such as pseudoarthrosis or hip transposition. We also believe that a temporal external fixation method is better than long-time bed rest, casting, or the use of a brace to maintain rigid fixation between the femoral head and the remaining pelvis [47, 48].

11.5 Summary

Patients with pelvic osteosarcoma have a poor outcome; treatment is one of the most challenging problems for the orthopedic oncologist. The reconstructive approach varies according to anatomic location, extent of resection, the patient's functional demands, and individual surgeon preference. The choice of optimal technique for reconstruction after acetabular tumor resection depends on numerous parameters and includes iliofemoral arthrodesis or pseudoarthrodesis, combined use of hip arthroplasty with massive allograft or recycled autograft, and pelvic and saddle prosthesis. The type of reconstruction modality can influence the rate of infection. Hillman et al. reported that hip transposition had the least incidence of complications after resection of the acetabulum, compared to the use of prosthesis or prosthesis and allograft [49]. The absence of large implants and allografts helps reduce surgical time, facilitates closure, and may decrease the incidence of infection and late revision due to implant failure. These can lead to early postoperative systemic treatment and functional recovery and are critical for patients with a high incidence of local recurrence and distant metastases. We believe that resection arthroplasty should be indicated for the patient with acetabular osteosarcoma.

References

1. Unni KK. Dahlin's bone tumors: general aspects and data on 11,087 cases. Philadelphia: Lippincott-Raven; 1996.
2. Ozaki T, Hoffmann C, Hillmann A, Gosheger G, Lindner N, Winkelmann W. Implantation of hemipelvic prosthesis after resection of sarcoma. Clin Orthop Relat Res. 2002;396:197–205.
3. Isakoff MS, Barkauskas DA, Ebb D, Morris C, Letson GD. Poor survival for osteosarcoma of the pelvis: a report from the Children's Oncology Group. Clin Orthop Relat Res. 2012;470:2007–13.
4. Kawai A, Huvos AG, Meyers PA, Healey JH. Osteosarcoma of the pelvis. Oncologic results of 40 patients. Clin Orthop Relat Res. 1998;348:196–207.
5. Grimer RJ, Carter SR, Tillman RM, Spooner D, Mangham DC, Kabukcuoglu Y. Osteosarcoma of the pelvis. J Bone Joint Surg (Br). 1999;81:796–802.
6. Ozaki T, Flege S, Kevric M, et al. Osteosarcoma of the pelvis: experience of the Cooperative Osteosarcoma Study Group. J Clin Oncol Off J Am Soc Clin Oncol. 2003;21:334–41.
7. Saab R, Rao BN, Rodriguez-Galindo C, Billups CA, Fortenberry TN, Daw NC. Osteosarcoma of the pelvis in children and young adults: the St. Jude Children's Research Hospital experience. Cancer. 2005;103:1468–74.
8. Fuchs B, Hoekzema N, Larson DR, Inwards CY, Sim FH. Osteosarcoma of the pelvis: outcome analysis of surgical treatment. Clin Orthop Relat Res. 2009;467:510–18.
9. Enneking WF, Dunham WK. Resection and reconstruction for primary neoplasms involving the innominate bone. J Bone Joint Surg Am. 1978;60:731–46.
10. Uchida A, Myoui A, Araki N, Yoshikawa H, Ueda T, Aoki Y. Prosthetic reconstruction for periacetabular malignant tumors. Clin Orthop Relat Res. 1996;326:238–45.
11. Ueda T, Kakunaga S, Takenaka S, Araki N, Yoshikawa H. Constrained total hip megaprosthesis for primary periacetabular tumors. Clin Orthop Relat Res. 2013;471:741–9.
12. Nieder E, Elson RA, Engelbrecht E, Kasselt MR, Keller A, Steinbrink K. The saddle prosthesis for salvage of the destroyed acetabulum. J Bone Joint Surg (Br). 1990;72:1014–22.

13. Aboulafia AJ, Buch R, Mathews J, Li W, Malawer MM. Reconstruction using the saddle prosthesis following excision of primary and metastatic periacetabular tumors. Clin Orthop Relat Res. 1995;314:203–13.
14. Aljassir F, Beadel GP, Turcotte RE, et al. Outcome after pelvic sarcoma resection reconstructed with saddle prosthesis. Clin Orthop Relat Res. 2005;438:36–41.
15. Kitagawa Y, Ek ET, Choong PF. Pelvic reconstruction using saddle prosthesis following limb salvage operation for periacetabular tumour. J Orthop Surg (Hong Kong). 2006;14:155–62.
16. Donati D, D'Apote G, Boschi M, Cevolani L, Benedetti MG. Clinical and functional outcomes of the saddle prosthesis. J Orthop Traumatol Off J Ital Soc Orthop Traumatol. 2012;13:79–88.
17. Jansen JA, van de Sande MA, Dijkstra PD. Poor long-term clinical results of saddle prosthesis after resection of periacetabular tumors. Clin Orthop Relat Res. 2013;471:324–31.
18. Bruns J, Luessenhop SL, Dahmen Sr G. Internal hemipelvectomy and endoprosthetic pelvic replacement: long-term follow-up results. Arch Orthop Trauma Surg. 1997;116:27–31.
19. Wirbel RJ, Schulte M, Maier B, Mutschler WE. Megaprosthetic replacement of the pelvis: function in 17 cases. Acta Orthop Scand. 1999;70:348–52.
20. Muller PE, Durr HR, Wegener B, Pellengahr C, Refior HJ, Jansson V. Internal hemipelvectomy and reconstruction with a megaprosthesis. Int Orthop. 2002;26:76–9.
21. Jaiswal PK, Aston WJ, Grimer RJ, et al. Peri-acetabular resection and endoprosthetic reconstruction for tumours of the acetabulum. J Bone Joint Surg (Br). 2008;90:1222–7.
22. Dominkus M, Darwish E, Funovics P. Reconstruction of the pelvis after resection of malignant bone tumours in children and adolescents. Recent Results Cancer Res Fortschr Krebsforschung Prog Rech Cancer. 2009;179:85–111.
23. Fisher NE, Patton JT, Grimer RJ, et al. Ice-cream cone reconstruction of the pelvis: a new type of pelvic replacement: early results. J Bone Joint Surg (Br). 2011;93:684–8.
24. Araki N, Myoui A, Kuratsu S, et al. Intraoperative extracorporeal autogenous irradiated bone grafts in tumor surgery. Clin Orthop Relat Res. 1999;368:196–206.
25. Hatano H, Ogose A, Hotta T, Endo N, Umezu H, Morita T. Extracorporeal irradiated autogenous osteochondral graft: a histological study. J Bone Joint Surg (Br). 2005;87:1006–11.
26. Manabe J, Ahmed AR, Kawaguchi N, Matsumoto S, Kuroda H. Pasteurized autologous bone graft in surgery for bone and soft tissue sarcoma. Clin Orthop Relat Res. 2004;419:258–66.
27. Sugiura H, Nishida Y, Nakashima H, Yamada Y, Tsukushi S, Yamada K. Evaluation of long-term outcomes of pasteurized autografts in limb salvage surgeries for bone and soft tissue sarcomas. Arch Orthop Trauma Surg. 2012;132:1685–95.
28. Tsuchiya H, Wan SL, Sakayama K, Yamamoto N, Nishida H, Tomita K. Reconstruction using an autograft containing tumour treated by liquid nitrogen. J Bone Joint Surg (Br). 2005;87:218–25.
29. Sys G, Uyttendaele D, Poffyn B, Verdonk R, Verstraete L. Extracorporeally irradiated autografts in pelvic reconstruction after malignant tumour resection. Int Orthop. 2002;26:174–8.
30. Koyanagi H, Matsumoto S, Shimoji T, et al. Long-term results from use of pasteurized bone. J Orthop Sci Off J Jpn Orthop Assoc. 2012;17:605–13.
31. Jeon DG, Kim MS, Cho WH, Song WS, Lee SY. Reconstruction with pasteurized autograft-total hip prosthesis composite for periacetabular tumors. J Surg Oncol. 2007;96:493–502.
32. Yamamoto N, Hayashi K, Tanzawa Y, Kimura H, Takeuchi A, Tsuchiya H. Clinical results of infection after reconstruction surgery using re-cycled autograft for malignant bone tumor (in Japanese). Cent Jpn J Orthop Trauma. 2012;55:1157–8.
33. Ozaki T, Hillmann A, Bettin D, Wuisman P, Winkelmann W. High complication rates with pelvic allografts. Experience of 22 sarcoma resections. Acta Orthop Scand. 1996;67:333–8.
34. Bell RS, Davis AM, Wunder JS, Buconjic T, McGoveran B, Gross AE. Allograft reconstruction of the acetabulum after resection of stage-IIB sarcoma. Intermediate-term results. J Bone Joint Surg Am. 1997;79:1663–74.
35. Langlais F, Lambotte JC, Thomazeau H. Long-term results of hemipelvis reconstruction with allografts. Clin Orthop Relat Res. 2001;388:178–86.

36. Delloye C, Banse X, Brichard B, Docquier PL, Cornu O. Pelvic reconstruction with a structural pelvic allograft after resection of a malignant bone tumor. J Bone Joint Surg Am. 2007;89:579–87.
37. Wafa H, Grimer RJ, Jeys L, Abudu AT, Carter SR, Tillman RM. The use of extracorporeally irradiated autografts in pelvic reconstruction following tumour resection. Bone Joint J. 2014;96-b:1404–10.
38. Fuchs B, O'Connor MI, Kaufman KR, Padgett DJ, Sim FH. Iliofemoral arthrodesis and pseudarthrosis: a long-term functional outcome evaluation. Clin Orthop Relat Res. 2002;397:29–35.
39. Nagoya S, Usui M, Wada T, Yamashita T, Ishii S. Reconstruction and limb salvage using a free vascularised fibular graft for periacetabular malignant bone tumours. J Bone Joint Surg (Br). 2000;82:1121–4.
40. Yu G, Zhang F, Zhou J, et al. Microsurgical fibular flap for pelvic ring reconstruction after periacetabular tumor resection. J Reconstr Microsurg. 2007;23:137–42.
41. Steel HH. Partial or complete resection of the hemipelvis. An alternative to hindquarter amputation for periacetabular chondrosarcoma of the pelvis. J Bone Joint Surg Am. 1978;60:719–30.
42. Eilber FR, Grant TT, Sakai D, Morton DL. Internal hemipelvectomy – excision of the hemipelvis with limb preservation. An alternative to hemipelvectomy. Cancer. 1979;43:806–9.
43. Takami M, Ieguchi M, Takamatsu K, et al. Functional evaluation of flail hip joint after periacetabular resection of the pelvis. Osaka City Med J. 1997;43:173–83.
44. Schwartz AJ, Kiatisevi P, Eilber FC, Eilber FR, Eckardt JJ. The Friedman-Eilber resection arthroplasty of the pelvis. Clin Orthop Relat Res. 2009;467:2825–30.
45. Gebert C, Gosheger G, Winkelmann W. Hip transposition as a universal surgical procedure for periacetabular tumors of the pelvis. J Surg Oncol. 2009;99:169–72.
46. Hoffmann C, Gosheger G, Gebert C, Jurgens H, Winkelmann W. Functional results and quality of life after treatment of pelvic sarcomas involving the acetabulum. J Bone Joint Surg Am. 2006;88:575–82.
47. Kusuzaki K, Shinjo H, Kim W, Nakamura S, Murata H, Hirasawa Y. Resection hip arthroplasty for malignant pelvic tumor. Outcome in 5 patients followed more than 2 years. Acta Orthop Scand. 1998;69:617–21.
48. Kunisada T, Katayama Y, Takeda K, Hasei J, Senda M, Ozaki T. Early rehabilitation using temporal external fixation following resection of pelvic sarcoma. 17th general meeting of International Society of Limb Salvage. Bologna; 2013.
49. Hillmann A, Hoffmann C, Gosheger G, Rodl R, Winkelmann W, Ozaki T. Tumors of the pelvis: complications after reconstruction. Arch Orthop Trauma Surg. 2003;123:340–4.
50. Enneking WF, Dunham W, Gebhardt MC, Malawar M, Pritchard DJ. A system for the functional evaluation of reconstructive procedures after surgical treatment of tumors of the musculoskeletal system. Clin Orthop Relat Res. 1993;286:241–6.

Management of Postoperative Infection After Limb Salvage Surgery in Osteosarcoma Patients

12

Takeshi Morii

Abstract

Postoperative infection is one of the most severe complications associated with limb salvage surgery in osteosarcoma patients. The incidence of infection is approximately ten times higher than that of conventional orthopedic surgery, and the impact of infection on limb survival and functional loss is significant. Due to the paucity of the surrounding soft tissue, the local conditions of limb salvage surgery for osteosarcoma patients and the pathophysiological mechanisms of infection are specific. Accordingly, preventative strategies should be based both on general guidelines on surgical site infection and on the specific properties of infection associated with orthopedic oncological surgery. Various treatment modalities and their success rates have been reported, and it has been found that the selection of management strategy should be based on both soft tissue conditions and infection conditions, with particular focus on the intensity, establishment period, and extension area of an infection.

Keywords

Limb salvage • Surgical site infection • Osteosarcoma

12.1 Introduction

Osteosarcoma patients are subject to a number of risk factors for postoperative infection, such as a lack of soft tissue, an immunocompromised host condition, and the use of endoprosthetics in reconstruction. Postoperative infection can result in

T. Morii (✉)
Department of Orthopaedic Surgery, Faculty of Medicine, Kyorin University, 6-20-2, Shinkawa, Mitaka, Tokyo 181-8611, Japan
e-mail: t-morii@gb3.so-net.ne.jp

T. Ueda, A. Kawai (eds.), *Osteosarcoma*, DOI 10.1007/978-4-431-55696-1_12

long-term hospitalization, a requirement for multistep operations for recovery, a reduced quality of life, and in some cases failure of limb salvage [1].

In this chapter the etiology, management practices for prevention and treatment, and perspectives on postoperative infection are reviewed. The evidence presented here comes from studies of osteosarcoma patients and from studies of cohorts with other malignant bone tumors due to the rarity of studies focusing only on osteosarcoma. However, it should be recognized that the fundamental properties of osteosarcoma patients differ from those with other primary or metastatic malignant bone tumors in terms of age, tumor site, reconstruction modalities, and chemotherapy regimens.

12.2 Defining Surgical Site Infection

The importance of defining surgical site infection (SSI) in surveying, interpreting, forming consensus on, or comparing infection characteristics is emphasized in the Guideline for Prevention of Surgical Site Infection from the US Centers for Disease Control and Prevention (CDC), and failure to use objective criteria has been shown to substantially affect reported SSI rates [2]. In this guideline, SSI is classified into three types: superficial incisional, deep incisional, and organ/space. Deep incisional infection involves deep soft tissues (e.g., facial tissue and muscle layers), whereas organ/space infection occurs in a part of the anatomy other than the incision site or any area that was manipulated during surgery. For all categories, SSI is defined as an infection that occurs within 30 days of surgery without implants or within 1 year with implants (these are now processing of revision at 2013 June [3]). However, these definitions cannot be clearly applied to the field of orthopedic oncology, where infections are often reported over a year post-surgery [1, 4]. As infections associated with limb salvage operations for osteosarcoma have different properties to ordinary SSIs, including those with prosthesis placement for joint reconstruction in degenerative diseases, infection after a prolonged period post-surgery could be accepted as a treatment-related infection if the specific case of osteosarcoma was clearly defined in the reports.

Clinical curing of infections is also difficult to define as recurrence is sometimes seen. Hardes et al. defined a clinical cure of infection as "no clinical signs of inflammation and negative C-reactive protein assessed by the treating clinician at the date of the last available follow-up" [5]. In previous reports, we have applied the same definition [1, 6].

12.3 Etiology

12.3.1 Incidence

The infection rate associated with surgery for malignant bone tumor resection is approximately ten times higher than that for conventional orthopedic surgery, including osteosynthesis, spine surgery, and arthroplasty [1, 7, 8].

For endoprosthesis placement, a recent systematic review of 48 studies, including a total of 4838 patients, concluded that the overall pooled weighted infection rate for lower-extremity limb salvage surgery with endoprosthetic reconstruction was approximately 10 % (95 % CI, 8–11 %) [9]. In addition, several recent studies on reconstruction following resection of a malignant bone tumor, using both biological materials and prostheses, have shown similar values for the incidence of infection at approximately 10 % (Fig. 12.1) [1, 4, 5, 10–33].

12.3.2 Time to Infection Presentation

Hardes et al. have reported that time to infection after insertion of a prosthesis can range from 1 to 70 months (mean, 16 months) [5]. I, along with my colleagues, have previously reported on 57 cases of infection following tumor-related endoprosthetic placement surgery, where time to infection from initial surgery ranged from 1 to

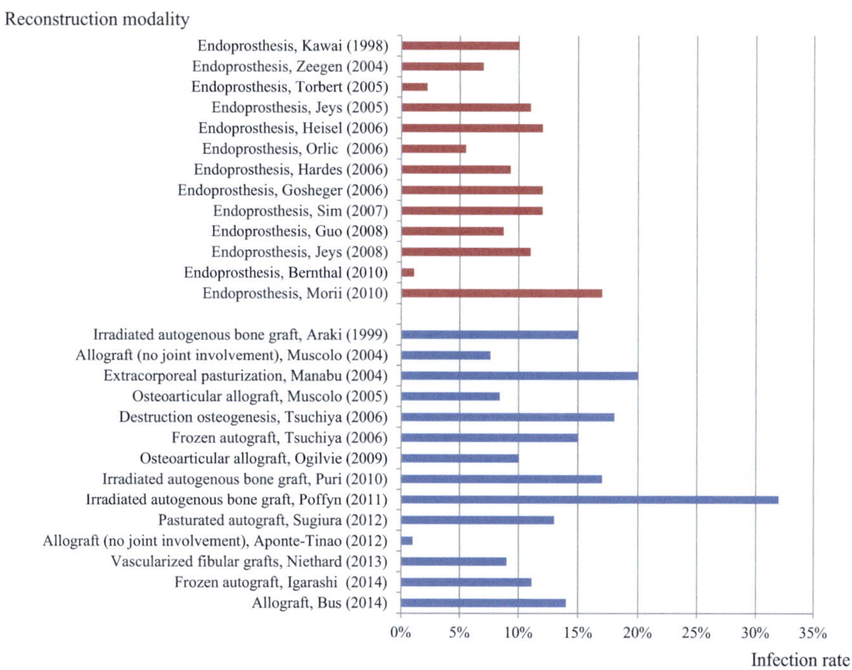

Fig. 12.1 Incidence of surgical site infection by reconstruction modality [1, 4, 5, 10–33]

85 months. In this study, the mean period and median period to infection were 12.8 and 4 months, respectively, and of the total infections 26.3 % occurred more than 12 months after initial surgery [6].

In a study of 76 patients with allografts, six contracted infection. Of these infections, four developed during the early postoperative period, while the other two developed later and were considered to be chemotherapy-related [19]. Meanwhile, in another study of 108 patients undergoing biological reconstruction using irradiated autogenous bone grafts, there were 17 cases of early and 18 cases of late infection [15], suggesting a considerably higher rate of late infection compared with prosthetic reconstruction.

12.3.3 Risk Factors

The incidence of infection seems to be regulated by factors such as tumor site and adjuvant therapy, including neoadjuvant chemotherapy and perioperative radiotherapy. Theoretically, immunological changes due to malignancy or chemotherapy, lack of soft tissue as a result of wide resection, prolonged surgery duration, a large volume of blood loss, a large amount of avascular material in reconstruction, and radiotherapy are all risks for infection in patients with osteosarcoma. Many studies have suggested that tumor site is an obvious risk factor for infection. Figure 12.2

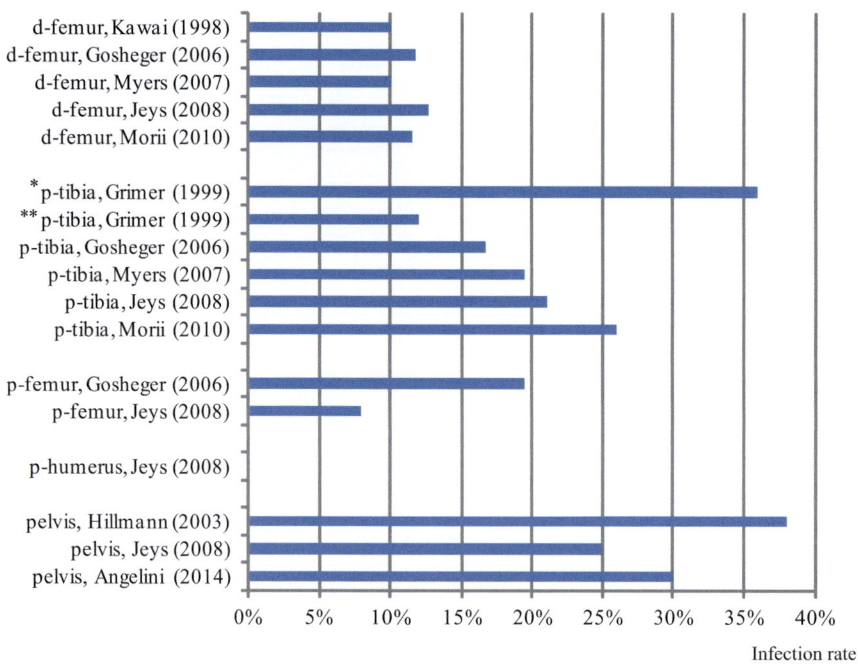

Fig. 12.2 Association between infection rate and the site of endoprosthetic reconstruction. The infection rate with tumor-associated endoprosthetic placement in the proximal tibia is higher in cases without a flap of the medial gastrocnemius* than with** [1, 24, 27, 32–37]

Table 12.1 Risk factors for infection in orthopedic oncological surgery

Significant risks	References
Proximal tibia tumor	[4, 27]
Pelvic tumor	[4, 34]
Proximal femur tumor	[27]
Chemotherapy	[37]
Radiotherapy	[4, 38]
Subsequent patellar resurfacing	[4]
Use of extendable prosthesis	[4]
Subsequent surgery to replace bushing	[4]
Extra-articular resection	[27]
Composite allograft reconstruction (vs. allograft without prosthesis)	[10]
Not using a gastrocnemius flap (for proximal tibia tumors)	[32]
Skin necrosis	[1]
Prior skin infection	[1, 39]
Antibiotic administration <24 h (vs. >24 h)	[9]
Pseudarthrosis in irradiated autograft	[5]
Nonsignificant factors	
Age	[1, 4, 32]
Sex	[1, 4]
Tumor type	[1, 4, 32]
Chemotherapy	[1, 4, 15, 32, 38]
Bone resection length	[1, 32]
Local recurrence	[4]

shows the infection rate with endoprosthesis placement in relation to tumor site [1, 24, 27, 32–37]. Here there is an obviously higher incidence of infection for the pelvis and proximal tibia. In previous reports of infection with malignant bone tumor resection, several significant risk factors for infection have been identified, although some remain controversial (Table 12.1) [1, 4, 9, 10, 15, 27, 32, 34, 37–39]. Some of these factors, such as extra-articular resection and not using a gastrocnemius flap, suggest a close relationship between SSI and a lack of soft tissue, while other factors such as skin necrosis and radiotherapy suggest that the condition of soft tissue is significant in SSI establishment.

12.3.4 Clinical Characteristics

12.3.4.1 Symptoms

Common clinical symptoms of deep infection include pain, local heat, discharge/pus, local redness, and an elevation of body temperature [2]. In my previously described study, discharge/pus around the prosthesis and loosening of the endoprosthesis were detected in 56.1 % and 8.7 % of cases, respectively, and

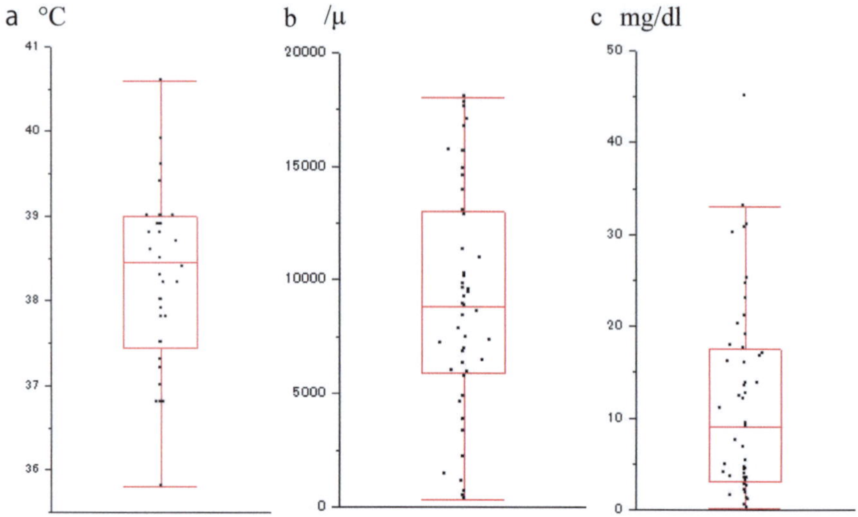

Fig. 12.3 Clinical parameters at the establishment of infection in tumor-associated endoprosthetic placement ([6] and unpublished data from T. Morii), showing (**a**) body temperature, (**b**) white blood cell count, and (**c**) C-reactive protein

body temperature at the time of presentation ranged from 35.8 to 40.6 °C (mean, 38.3 °C; median, 38.5 °C, Fig. 12.3a) [6].

With tumor-related endoprosthetic placement, clinical symptoms are sometimes representative of patient condition. For example, infection has been shown to occur significantly earlier in those with discharge/pus as opposed to those without and significantly later in cases with loosening of the endoprosthesis than in those without. Additionally, discharge/pus was significantly more likely among cases with extra-articular resection [6].

12.3.4.2 Laboratory Data

As for other infections, blood tests including erythrocyte sedimentation rate, C-reactive protein level, and white blood cell counts are used in the diagnosis of SSIs [40]. Grimer et al. reported an elevated erythrocyte sedimentation rate ranging from 31 to 140 mm/h (normal rate <15 mm/h) for patients with endoprosthesis-associated infections [40]. In my previous study, white blood cell counts (per mm^3) ranged from 300 to 18,000 (mean, 9,023; median, 8,800) (Fig. 12.3b) [6]. However, for some immunocompromised patients undergoing systemic chemotherapy, the white blood cell number was below the normal range. In their study, Grimer et al. suggested that white blood cell count was not actually helpful, as it was above 11,000 (per mm^3) for only 12 of the 34 patients [40]. C-reactive protein levels in our study ranged from 0.2 to 45.1 mg/dL (mean, 11.4 mg/dL; median, 9.0 mg/dL, Fig. 12.3c) [6]. In endoprosthesis-associated infection, analysis of synovial fluid, such as synovial fluid white blood cell counts and the calculation of neutrophil percentage, could be useful for diagnosis [41]. However, technetium bone scans, gallium scans, or white blood cell scans were reported not to be useful [40].

12.3.4.3 Pathogens

In endoprosthesis-associated infection, the infecting organism is isolated in approximately 75.4–93 % of cases [4–6], with coagulase-negative staphylococcus, *Staphylococcus aureus*, and *Staphylococcus epidermidis* infections being common [5, 6, 32, 38, 40]. *Enterococci*, *Pseudomonas aeruginosa*, *Acinetobacter baumannii*, *Proteus mirabilis*, and *Streptococcus pyogenes* are found to a lesser extent [5]. In my study, 37 % of *S. aureus* cases were methicillin resistant, and we noted that methicillin-resistant *S. aureus* infection is significantly associated with extra-articular resection and prolonged surgery [6].

In allograft studies, *S. epidermidis*, *S. aureus*, alpha-hemolytic streptococcus, *Pseudomonas* species, *Enterococci*, and *Enterobacter* species have been reported as of the most common postoperative pathogens [19].

12.3.5 Impact of Infection on Patient Outcomes

12.3.5.1 Oncological Outcomes

In general, once infection occurs during the treatment of osteosarcoma, adjuvant chemotherapy is interrupted because of its immunosuppressive effects. Thus, postoperative infection might worsen oncological outcome, especially overall survival. However, others and I have seen no association between infection and oncological outcome [1]. Interestingly, a paper by Jeys et al. reported increased survival after deep postoperative infection in osteosarcoma patients [38]. They speculated that the underlying mechanisms might include stimulation of tumor necrosis factor alpha (TNFα), tumor suppression through cell-mediated cytotoxicity, and prevention of tumor neovascularization due to infection conditions.

12.3.5.2 Limb Survival

Infections associated with endoprosthesis placement following limb salvage surgery for malignant bone tumors have been reported as a risk factor for amputation. Grimer et al. reported a risk of amputation due to infection following tumor-associated endoprosthesis placement in the proximal tibia [32]. Likewise, I have found that in addition to extracapsular resection, infection leads to an increased risk of amputation with prosthetics around the knee, although this was not found to be an independent risk factor in multivariate analysis [42].

12.3.5.3 Prosthesis Survival

Infection following endoprosthesis placement has been reported to impact prosthesis survival. Zeegen et al. reported that, along with prosthesis location, infection was an independent risk factor for prosthesis loss [31]. In my research, I have also found infection to be a significant risk for prosthesis loss [1]. In this series, resection of extended part of the quadriceps muscle, i.e., loss of soft tissue, was reported to be a risk for deep infection of the proximal femur tumor endoprosthesis. Interestingly, Hardes et al. have emphasized the importance of soft tissue condition in salvaging an infected limb along with prosthesis reconstruction, suggesting a protective role of soft tissue around the prosthesis against infection [5].

12.3.5.4 Limb Function

Zeegen et al. [31] reported that prosthesis infection was an independent risk for functional loss. I have found that functional score can be significantly different between the infected limb and the limb without infection. However, there is no clinical difference in the average scores, at 19.3 and 21.6, respectively, for patients with and without infection [42] using the Musculoskeletal Tumor Society scoring system. These findings suggest that once amputation is avoided through effective treatment of infection, there is no clinical difference in functionality.

12.4 Management

12.4.1 Prevention

12.4.1.1 General Approaches to the Prevention of Surgical Site Infection

Recently there have been many studies on the prevention of SSIs. These include studies on the administration of preoperative antimicrobial agents timed such that serum and tissue concentrations are established at the start of surgery, the implementation of glycemic control in diabetic patients to ensure perioperative blood glucose levels are <200 mg/dL [2], the maintenance of perioperative normothermia [43], and the administration of a higher fraction of inspired oxygen (FiO2) both intraoperatively and in the immediate postoperative period [44]. The findings of these studies have been incorporated into guidelines on the prevention of SSIs by the CDC and others. In general, I believe that most of these findings are relevant to infections in osteosarcoma patients. However, in some aspects, there must be differences in the pathophysiological conditions of SSI establishment between conventional orthopedic surgery and surgery for orthopedic malignancy. This is discussed in the next section.

12.4.1.2 Properties of Infections in Orthopedic Oncology

The most obvious risk for infection in osteosarcoma patients is the lack of soft tissue resulting from the wide margin used in tumor resection, and there is a large amount of evidence directly or indirectly suggesting the significance of soft tissue preservation in the management of infection. A study by Grimer et al. in 1999 on the management of proximal tibia osteosarcoma showed an infection rate of 12 % and 36 %, respectively, in cases with and without a gastrocnemius flap [32]. In a study of SSI following proximal tibia reconstruction with prosthesis due to malignancy, patients with gastrocnemius muscle flap coverage at initial surgery needed

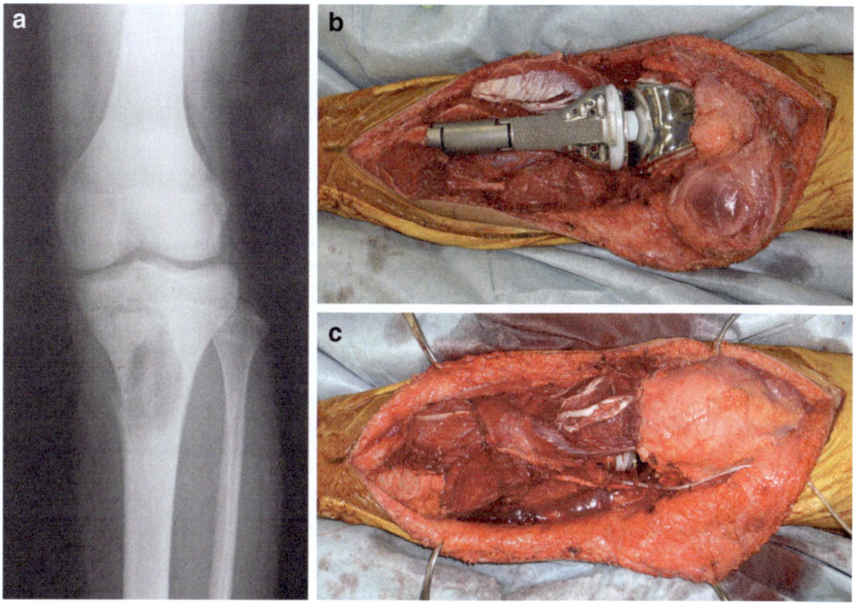

Fig. 12.4 Application of a gastrocnemius flap in the reconstruction of the proximal tibia in osteosarcoma. (**a**) Radiographs at presentation, (**b**) a wide resection of the proximal tibia followed by endoprosthetic reconstruction in a 16-year-old boy with osteosarcoma, and **c** gastrocnemius flap application with blood flow from the posterior tibia vessels

significantly fewer surgical procedures to control subsequent infection than those without a flap [6]. Thus, the routine application of a muscle flap, both with prosthetic and biological reconstruction, is currently recommended for infection control (Fig. 12.4) [10]. Likewise, in a previous study, I have shown that extended resection of the quadriceps in distal femur cases increased the risk for deep infection following prosthetic reconstruction [1]. Patients with extracompartmental resection tend to lose more soft tissue, as a larger margin is resected with the tumor. In infected patients, the final infection control rate is better for intracompartmental rather than extracompartmental resection [6]. Moreover, the risk of amputation is elevated with extracompartmental resection [6]. Although the preservation of soft tissue is practically dependent on the tumor extension, I would refer to the routine use of gastrocnemius muscle flap coverage in proximal tibia cases. In addition, if extended resection of soft tissue is required and a severe lack of soft tissue is expected due to surgery at another site, plastic surgery should be considered at the initial surgery for soft tissue coverage.

These findings highlight the differences in surgical conditions between oncological resection for osteosarcoma and conventional orthopedic surgery. A recent study on SSI in orthopedic surgery recommends a shorter period of single antimicrobial prophylaxis to prevent the emergence of antibiotic-resistant bacterial infection [45]. So far, there have been few studies of antimicrobial prophylaxis modality in orthopedic oncology. In 2013, Racano et al. conducted a systematic review of articles published in English between 1980 and July 2011 on clinical studies of infection rates in adults with primary bony malignancies of the lower extremities that were treated with surgery and endoprosthetic reconstruction. The pooled weighted infection rate was 13 % after short-term (<24 h) postoperative antibiotic administration and 8 % after long-term (>24 h) postoperative antibiotic administration [9], suggesting that long-term antibiotic prophylaxis reduces the risk of deep infection. Likewise, a considerably lower rate of postoperative infection with long-term antibiotic administration has been recently reported [46]. In addition, others and I have found that the use of one instead of two antibiotics during orthopedic oncological resection and endoprosthetic reconstruction surgery conferred a significant risk of amputation [6]. This shows that the prevention of SSI during conventional procedures is not always applicable to SSI in osteosarcoma surgery. Although the low case number and heterogeneity in terms of tumor location, surgery duration, tumor size, and reconstruction modality, in addition to immunological suppression in patients would make it difficult, concrete guidelines on the prevention of SSI in orthopedic oncology should be established.

12.4.2 Treatment Strategy

Surgical modalities in the control of SSIs involve the preservation of reconstruction materials, or either temporary or permanent removal of reconstruction material. As shown in Fig. 12.5, there is a large variation in the invasiveness of each modality. In general, a higher level of infection control is achieved with more invasive procedures; however, these require more time, surgical procedures, and cost and sometimes incur more functional loss than less invasive procedures. Currently,

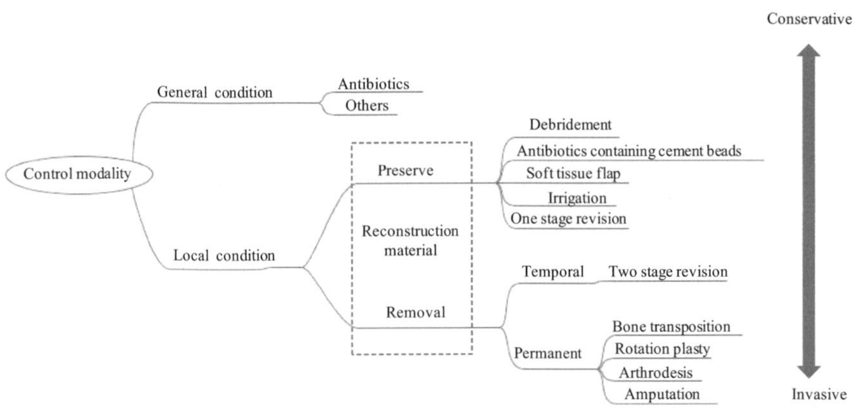

Fig. 12.5 Management modalities for surgical site infection. Surgical modalities involve either the preservation or removal of reconstruction materials. As indicated in the figure, surgery with material removal is more invasive

there are few principles on which to base selection of an appropriate modality. Both patients and surgeons tend to select those in which reconstruction materials such as endoprosthetics are preserved. Recent evidence shows that infection control is more effective with surgical procedures than conservative therapy, and that surgical procedures in which reconstruction material is removed are more effective than those in which it is preserved. For example, in the management of postoperative infection following limb salvage surgery with prosthetic reconstruction, prosthesis removal resulted in better infection control than conservative or prosthesis preserving therapy [4–6].

12.4.2.1 Conservative Therapy

Antibiotic administration is easy to perform and less invasive and is used in the management of most SSIs in the early stages of disease. As mentioned above, infection control with antibiotics alone occurs for $<10\ \%$ cases with both endoprosthetic [4] and biological reconstruction (Table 12.2) [10, 12–14, 19, 47–49]; however, for both patients and surgeons, this is the best option. Thus, I analyzed the properties of cases from a previous study with tumor-associated endoprosthetic reconstruction around the knee, in which conservative therapy was effective in SSI control, and found that conservative therapy was significantly more successful in cases with prostheses in the tibia than the femur and more successful in cases without discharge/pus at infection presentation [6]. In addition, Hardes et al. reviewed 30 such patients and found that only one patient with a late, low-grade infection could be treated successfully with intravenous antibiotics [5]. In biological reconstruction, surface infection is more successfully controlled by conservative therapy [14, 47].

Table 12.2 Successful modalities for the control of surgical site infection following biological reconstruction

Lead author	Reconstruction modality	Infection control/case number	References
Bus	Allograft	Antibiotics 3	[10]
Aponte-Tinao	Allograft	Two-stage (allograft) 2	[13]
Muscolo	Allograft	Arthrodesis 4	[19]
		Two-stage (composite) 1	
		Two-stage (endoprosthesis) 1	
Niethard	Vascularized fibular grafts	Two-stage (autograft) 2	[12]
Puri	Irradiated autograft	Cement spacer 2	[49]
		Rotationplasty 1	
		Amputation 1	
Sugiura	Pasteurized autograft	Debridement 2	[14]
		Graft removal 2	
Tsuchiya	Distraction osteogenesis	Antibiotics 1	[47]
		Two-stage (bone transport) 1	

12.4.2.2 Surgery Without Reconstruction Material Removal

Infection control modalities that do not involve the removal of reconstruction material include debridement, the use of antibiotic containing cement beads, soft tissue flap, and wound irrigation, either alone or in combination. The principle of these is to alter conditions so that they are less favorable for bacterial growth and more favorable for local immunity, without removing reconstruction materials. It has been shown that soft tissue is critical in the prevention of infection following malignant bone tumor resection [1, 32]; this would suggest that soft tissue reconstruction, such as flap application, should be used as part of the treatment regimen for infection following limb salvage surgery. Obviously, a large amount of good quality soft tissue with a blood supply would improve defenses against bacterial growth. However, in many cases this modality is not sufficient to control infection if conditions around the reconstruction materials are bad, such as an infected bone graft or biofilm formation on an endoprosthesis. Theoretically, once an infection has extended into the medullary area of the bone, these modalities would not be effective in its control because of the weakness of bone against infection. Thus, they should only be used in the early stages of infection. Indeed, the infection control rates associated with these modalities are unacceptable. In my previous study on endoprosthetic infection, infection control rates with soft tissue flap application, irrigation, debridement, and antibiotic containing beads were 43 %, 29 %, 21 %, and 20 %, respectively [6].

Compared with two-stage revision, one-stage revision has advantages such as the avoidance of temporary gross instability, less suffering for the patient, a shorter period of hospitalization, and lower costs [50]. In fact, this type of procedure is successful under limited conditions [4, 5, 50, 51], and, in general, can be used for short-term infections or patients with extreme comorbidities. Hardes et al. reported that debridement with prosthesis retention and one-stage reimplantation without changing stems can be successful in early infections (one superinfected seroma patient); however, they did not recommend one-stage revision in the case of late, high-grade infection [5]. Holzer et al. analyzed their one-stage revision cases and concluded that the procedure should be conducted when infection is localized within the scar tube and does not invade the medullary canal [50]. If anchorage components are well fixed to the bone and the infection does not involve the medullary bone, one-stage revision seems to be more successful. On the other hand, the procedure is not recommended if there is a lack of sufficient soft tissue or in patients with antibiotic-resistant infections. Likewise, for infection control with biological reconstruction, a limited number of cases with one-stage revision have been reported to date (Table 12.2).

12.4.2.3 Two-Stage Revision

The concept of two-stage revision is based on the hypothesis that once an infection becomes chronic and the medullary bone is involved, the removal of bacterial growth cannot be achieved without total resection of the infected material. Taking into consideration the pathophysiological mechanisms of chronic osteomyelitis, this hypothesis seems to be reasonable. Once these conditions are established, improving the surrounding conditions alone would not sufficiently control infection.

Two-stage revision has been reported to successfully control SSIs around tumor-associated endoprosthetic implants [40]. The process, as described by Grimer et al. [40], includes complete removal of the prosthesis, debridement, and insertion of a sufficiently sized spacer made of cement with gentamicin or vancomycin; this is followed by waiting period (minimum 6 weeks, usually ranging from 10 to 34 weeks) before insertion of the new endoprosthesis. In 24 out of 34 patients, infections were completely controlled using this method [40]. In contrast, Hardes et al. [5] reported that one-stage revision was successful in only one out of three cases, and only in acute, early infections, and they emphasized the importance of the removal of the old stems. In their study, 24 patients underwent two-stage revision and 15 of these underwent reimplantation 3 weeks to 10 months after the initial removal procedure [5]. They emphasized the importance of soft tissue conditions in limb salvage with this process. Likewise for biological reconstruction materials, total removal of infected bone seems to be required. Thus, based on the literature, this modality is frequently successful in infection control, especially for deep and chronic infections (Table 12.2) [12, 13, 19, 47], although the reconstruction modality used for revision surgery shows wide variation including allografts, composites of grafts and prosthetics, endoprosthetics, or bone transposition. Thus, for infection control following limb salvage procedures, two-stage revision is the most reliable method, despite the prolonged treatment period and high costs.

12.4.2.4 Amputation and Other Modalities with Permanent Removal of Reconstruction Materials

Amputation is the final solution in the process of SSI control. Although the functional loss and psychological impact is significant, infection is totally eradicated [6]. For other modalities involving the permanent removal of reconstruction materials, success rates are quite high as the most profound source of infection for late-occurring infections is completely removed. Both for tumor-associated endoprosthesis placement and biological reconstruction, rotationplasty and arthrodesis are limb salvage options in infection control [5, 19, 49].

The decision to amputate is difficult for both patients and surgeons. Thus, amputation at an early stage of the infection control process is unlikely unless there is a specific condition, such as a limited prognosis, in which early hospital discharge is desired. I, together with my colleagues, analyzed the risk factors for amputation in controlling infections following tumor-associated endoprosthesis placement and found that, in the case of metastatic bone tumors, extra-articular resection at initial surgery, the use of a single antibiotic post-surgery, and the presence of discharge/pus at the diagnosis of infection were significant risks [6, 42].

12.5 Perspectives

SSI is a universal complication in surgery. In this chapter, I have emphasized the significance of soft tissue conditions in the establishment of SSIs following orthopedic osteosarcoma resection based on the previous findings. Thus, the most important factors in SSI control seem to be the reconstruction materials used and the soft tissue surrounding them. Here I discuss perspectives in SSI control focusing on these two factors.

12.5.1 Reconstruction Modality

The surface of reconstruction materials is a critical factor in infection as they lack blood supply. The eradication of biofilm-producing bacteria from prosthetic surfaces is difficult, and in these cases, the removal of the medical device seems to be the only way to resolve infection [52, 53]. Thus, the pretreatment of prosthesis surface with antibacterial materials such as silver or iodine has been conducted. Currently, endoprosthetics coated with antibacterial materials are being used in practice [52, 54, 55].

Hardes et al. compared silver-coated endoprosthetics to conventional titanium prosthetics and found a reduction in infection rate from 17.6 % to 5.9 % for the titanium and silver groups, respectively. Moreover, 38.5 % of patients in the titanium group ultimately had to undergo amputation following the development of periprosthetic infection. However, these mutilating surgical procedures were not necessary in the silver group [55].

Tsuchiya and his group at Kanazawa University (Kanazawa, Japan) developed an antimicrobial coating system using titanium implants coated with iodine (Fig. 12.6) and used them in clinical practice [54]. Among the high-risk 158 cases, such as those with cancer, with diabetes mellitus, or undergoing steroid treatment or chemotherapy, postoperative infection occurred in only 3 cases, most of which were cured conservatively. This implies that one of the main factors in preventing SSI in oncological reconstruction is the surface of the prosthesis.

12.5.2 Oncological Management: Preservation of Soft Tissue by Narrowing the Surgical Margin

There is a lot of evidence to show that preservation of soft tissue is critical in the prevention and management of postoperative infection for osteosarcoma [1, 5, 53]. Obviously, a decrease in the wide resection margins is challenging due to the fear of recurrence. Thus, enhancing the effects of adjuvant therapy might decrease the frequency of infection in these patients. Since 1987, Tsuchiya et al. have published reports on the possibility of marginal excision for osteosarcoma in conjunction with caffeine-assisted chemotherapy [56]. Caffeine can enhance the cytocidal effects of anticancer drugs safely through its inhibitory effects on DNA

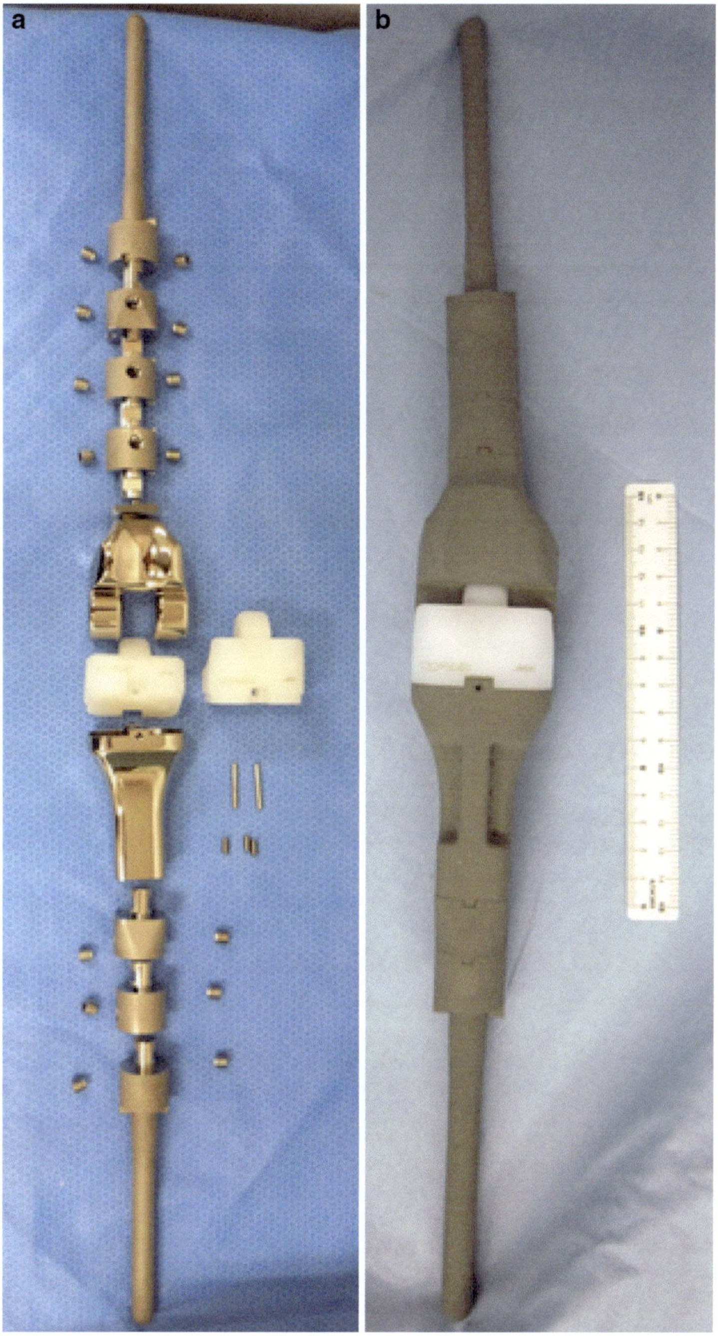

Fig. 12.6 Surface anodization of titanium implants. Povidone-iodine was used as an electrolyte to form an adhesive, porous anodic oxide with the antiseptic properties of iodine. (**a**) Before and (**b**) after modification (Figure kindly provided by Prof. Hiroyuki Tsuchiya, Department of Orthopaedic Surgery, Graduate School of Medical Science, Kanazawa University, Kanazawa Japan)

repair and as a result, the wide resection margins for osteosarcoma can be decreased practically and safely. They reported an infection rate in the treatment of osteosarcoma of 9.5 %. Another candidate for decreasing margins is photodynamic therapy using acridine orange with/without low-dose radiation as proposed by Kusuzaki et al. [57, 58]. Acridine orange has a strong cytocidal effect after it is illuminated with blue light or treated with low-dose X-ray radiation and with local administration has been reported to be equal to conventional wide resection in controlling high-grade sarcoma [59]. In terms of infection control, limited data has been reported on these modalities; however, at least theoretically, their widespread use could reduce infection rates following osteosarcoma surgery.

12.6 Summary

Considering its high incidence compared to conventional orthopedic surgery, the risk of SSI in limb salvage surgery for osteosarcoma should be recognized throughout the treatment period. Although general guidelines on SSI should be understood and reviewed by surgeons, the specific properties of infection in orthopedic oncological patients should be recognized, as the pathophysiological mechanisms of infection are different. Both the reconstruction material used and the surrounding soft tissue are significant in the establishment of infection, in addition to the general condition of patients, and should be well considered in the prevention, treatment, and development of management strategies for postoperative infection after limb salvage surgery in osteosarcoma patients.

This study was supported in part by the Health and Labour Sciences Research Expenses for Commission, Applied Research for Innovative Treatment of Cancer from the Ministry of Health, Labour and Welfare (H26-084).

References

1. Morii T, Yabe H, Morioka H, Beppu Y, Chuman H, Kawai A, et al. Postoperative deep infection in tumor endoprosthesis reconstruction around the knee. J Orthop Sci. 2010;15:331–9.
2. Mangram AJ, Horan TC, Pearson ML, Silver LC, Jarvis WR. Guideline for prevention of surgical site infection, 1999. Centers for Disease Control and Prevention (CDC) Hospital Infection Control Practices Advisory Committee. Am J Infect Control. 1999;27:97–132.
3. Centers for Disease Control and Prevention. National Healthcare Safety Network. Surgical Site Infection (SSI) Event. 2013. http://www.cdc.gov/nhsn/pdfs/pscmanual/9pscssicurrent.pdf. Accessed 17 June 2013.
4. Jeys LM, Grimer RJ, Carter SR, Tillman RM. Periprosthetic infection in patients treated for an orthopaedic oncological condition. J Bone Joint Surg Am. 2005;87:842–9.
5. Hardes J, Gebert C, Schwappach A, Ahrens H, Streitburger A, Winkelmann W, et al. Characteristics and outcome of infections associated with tumor endoprostheses. Arch Orthop Trauma Surg. 2006;126:289–96.

6. Morii T, Morioka H, Ueda T, Araki N, Hashimoto N, Kawai A, et al. Deep infection in tumor endoprosthesis around the knee: a multi-institutional study by the Japanese musculoskeletal oncology group. BMC Musculoskelet Disord. 2013;14:51.
7. Minnema B, Vearncombe M, Augustin A, Gollish J, Simor AE. Risk factors for surgical-site infection following primary total knee arthroplasty. Infect Control Hosp Epidemiol. 2004;25:477–80.
8. Berbari EF, Hanssen AD, Duffy MC, Steckelberg JM, Ilstrup DM, Harmsen WS, et al. Risk factors for prosthetic joint infection: case-control study. Clin Infect Dis. 1998;27:1247–54.
9. Racano A, Pazionis T, Farrokhyar F, Deheshi B, Ghert M. High infection rate outcomes in long-bone tumor surgery with endoprosthetic reconstruction in adults: a systematic review. Clin Orthop Relat Res. 2013;471:2017–27.
10. Bus MP, Dijkstra PD, van de Sande MA, Taminiau AH, Schreuder HW, Jutte PC, et al. Intercalary allograft reconstructions following resection of primary bone tumors: a nationwide multicenter study. J Bone Joint Surg Am. 2014;96:e26.
11. Igarashi K, Yamamoto N, Shirai T, Hayashi K, Nishida H, Kimura H, et al. The long-term outcome following the use of frozen autograft treated with liquid nitrogen in the management of bone and soft-tissue sarcomas. Bone Joint J. 2014;96-B:555–61.
12. Niethard M, Tiedke C, Andreou D, Traub F, Kuhnert M, Werner M, et al. Bilateral fibular graft: biological reconstruction after resection of primary malignant bone tumors of the lower limb. Sarcoma. 2013;2013:205832.
13. Aponte Tinao L, Farfalli GL, Ritacco LE, Ayerza MA, Muscolo DL. Intercalary femur allografts are an acceptable alternative after tumor resection. Clin Orthop Relat Res. 2012;470:728–34.
14. Sugiura H, Nishida Y, Nakashima H, Yamada Y, Tsukushi S, Yamada K. Evaluation of long-term outcomes of pasteurized autografts in limb salvage surgeries for bone and soft tissue sarcomas. Arch Orthop Trauma Surg. 2012;132:1685–95.
15. Poffyn B, Sys G, Mulliez A, Van Maele G, Van Hoorebeke L, Forsyth R, et al. Extracorporeally irradiated autografts for the treatment of bone tumours: tips and tricks. Int Orthop. 2011;35:889–95.
16. Puri A, Gulia A, Agarwal M, Jambhekar N, Laskar S. Extracorporeal irradiated tumor bone: a reconstruction option in diaphyseal Ewing's sarcomas. Indian J Orthop. 2010;44:390–6.
17. Ogilvie CM, Crawford EA, Hosalkar HS, King JJ, Lackman RD. Long-term results for limb salvage with osteoarticular allograft reconstruction. Clin Orthop Relat Res. 2009;467:2685–90.
18. Tsuchiya H, Abdel Wanis ME, Tomita K. Biological reconstruction after excision of juxta-articular osteosarcoma around the knee: a new classification system. Anticancer Res. 2006;26:447–53.
19. Muscolo DL, Ayerza MA, Aponte Tinao LA, Ranalletta M. Use of distal femoral osteoarticular allografts in limb salvage surgery. J Bone Joint Surg Am. 2005;87:2449–55.
20. Manabe J, Ahmed AR, Kawaguchi N, Matsumoto S, Kuroda H. Pasteurized autologous bone graft in surgery for bone and soft tissue sarcoma. Clin Orthop Relat Res. 2004;419:258–66.
21. Muscolo DL, Ayerza MA, Aponte Tinao LA, Ranalletta M. Partial epiphyseal preservation and intercalary allograft reconstruction in high-grade metaphyseal osteosarcoma of the knee. J Bone Joint Surg Am. 2004;86-A:2686–93.
22. Araki N, Myoui A, Kuratsu S, Hashimoto N, Inoue T, Kudawara I et al. Intraoperative extracorporeal autogenous irradiated bone grafts in tumor surgery. Clin Orthop Relat Res. 1999;368:196–206.
23. Bernthal NM, Schwartz AJ, Oakes DA, Kabo JM, Eckardt JJ. How long do endoprosthetic reconstructions for proximal femoral tumors last? Clin Orthop Relat Res. 2010;468:2867–74.
24. Jeys LM, Kulkarni A, Grimer RJ, Carter SR, Tillman RM, Abudu A. Endoprosthetic reconstruction for the treatment of musculoskeletal tumors of the appendicular skeleton and pelvis. J Bone Joint Surg Am. 2008;90:1265–71.

25. Guo W, Ji T, Yang R, Tang X, Yang Y. Endoprosthetic replacement for primary tumours around the knee: experience from Peking University. J Bone Joint Surg Br. 2008;90:1084–9.
26. Sim IW, Tse LF, Ek ET, Powell GJ, Choong PF. Salvaging the limb salvage: management of complications following endoprosthetic reconstruction for tumours around the knee. Eur J Surg Oncol. 2007;33:796–802.
27. Gosheger G, Gebert C, Ahrens H, Streitbuerger A, Winkelmann W, Hardes J. Endoprosthetic reconstruction in 250 patients with sarcoma. Clin Orthop Relat Res. 2006;450:164–71.
28. Orlic D, Smerdelj M, Kolundzic R, Bergovec M. Lower limb salvage surgery: modular endoprosthesis in bone tumour treatment. Int Orthop. 2006;30:458–64.
29. Heisel C, Kinkel S, Bernd L, Ewerbeck V. Megaprostheses for the treatment of malignant bone tumours of the lower limbs. Int Orthop. 2006;30:452–7.
30. Torbert JT, Fox EJ, Hosalkar HS, Ogilvie CM, Lackman RD. Endoprosthetic reconstructions: results of long-term followup of 139 patients. Clin Orthop Relat Res. 2005;438:51–9.
31. Zeegen EN, Aponte-Tinao LA, Hornicek FJ, Gebhardt MC, Mankin HJ. Survivorship analysis of 141 modular metallic endoprostheses at early followup. Clin Orthop Relat Res. 2004;420:239–50.
32. Grimer RJ, Carter SR, Tillman RM, Sneath RS, Walker PS, Unwin PS, et al. Endoprosthetic replacement of the proximal tibia. J Bone Joint Surg Br. 1999;81:488–94.
33. Kawai A, Muschler GF, Lane JM, Otis JC, Healey JH. Prosthetic knee replacement after resection of a malignant tumor of the distal part of the femur. Medium to long-term results. J Bone Joint Surg Am. 1998;80:636–47.
34. Angelini A, Drago G, Trovarelli G, Calabro T, Ruggieri P. Infection after surgical resection for pelvic bone tumors: an analysis of 270 patients from one institution. Clin Orthop Relat Res. 2014;472:349–59.
35. Hillmann A, Hoffmann C, Gosheger G, Rodl R, Winkelmann W, Ozaki T. Tumors of the pelvis: complications after reconstruction. Arch Orthop Trauma Surg. 2003;123:340–4.
36. Myers GJ, Abudu AT, Carter SR, Tillman RM, Grimer RJ. The long-term results of endoprosthetic replacement of the proximal tibia for bone tumours. J Bone Joint Surg Br. 2007;89:1632–7.
37. Myers GJ, Abudu AT, Carter SR, Tillman RM, Grimer RJ. Endoprosthetic replacement of the distal femur for bone tumours: long-term results. J Bone Joint Surg Br. 2007;89:521–6.
38. Jeys LM, Grimer RJ, Carter SR, Tillman RM, Abudu A. Post operative infection and increased survival in osteosarcoma patients: are they associated? Ann Surg Oncol. 2007;14:2887–95.
39. Shehadeh A, Noveau J, Malawer M, Henshaw R. Late complications and survival of endoprosthetic reconstruction after resection of bone tumors. Clin Orthop Relat Res. 2010;468:2885–95.
40. Grimer RJ, Belthur M, Chandrasekar C, Carter SR, Tillman RM. Two-stage revision for infected endoprostheses used in tumor surgery. Clin Orthop Relat Res. 2002;395:193–203.
41. Trampuz A, Hanssen AD, Osmon DR, Mandrekar J, Steckelberg JM, Patel R. Synovial fluid leukocyte count and differential for the diagnosis of prosthetic knee infection. Am J Med. 2004;117:556–62.
42. Morii T, Morioka H, Ueda T, Araki N, Hashimoto N, Kawai A, et al. Functional analysis of cases of tumor endoprostheses with deep infection around the knee: a multi institutional study by the Japanese Musculoskeletal Oncology Group (JMOG). J Orthop Sci. 2013;18:605–12.
43. Melling AC, Ali B, Scott EM, Leaper DJ. Effects of preoperative warming on the incidence of wound infection after clean surgery: a randomised controlled trial. Lancet. 2001;358:876–80.
44. Belda FJ, Aguilera L, Garcia de la Asuncion J, Alberti J, Vicente R, Ferrandiz L, et al. Supplemental perioperative oxygen and the risk of surgical wound infection: a randomized controlled trial. JAMA. 2005;294:2035–42.
45. Kanayama M, Hashimoto T, Shigenobu K, Oha F, Togawa D. Effective prevention of surgical site infection using a Centers for Disease Control and Prevention guideline-based antimicrobial prophylaxis in lumbar spine surgery. J Neurosurg Spine. 2007;6:327–9.

46. Li X, Moretti VM, Ashana AO, Lackman RD. Perioperative infection rate in patients with osteosarcomas treated with resection and prosthetic reconstruction. Clin Orthop Relat Res. 2011;469:2889–94.
47. Tsuchiya H, Abdel Wanis ME, Sakurakichi K, Yamashiro T, Tomita K. Osteosarcoma around the knee. Intraepiphyseal excision and biological reconstruction with distraction osteogenesis. J Bone Joint Surg Br. 2002;84:1162–6.
48. Sugiura H, Yamamura S, Sato K, Katagiri H, Nishida Y, Nakashima H, et al. Remodelling and healing process of moderately heat-treated bone grafts after wide resection of bone and soft-tissue tumors. Arch Orthop Trauma Surg. 2003;123:514–20.
49. Puri A, Gulia A, Jambhekar N, Laskar S. The outcome of the treatment of diaphyseal primary bone sarcoma by resection, irradiation and re-implantation of the host bone: extracorporeal irradiation as an option for reconstruction in diaphyseal bone sarcomas. J Bone Joint Surg Br. 2012;94:982–8.
50. Holzer G, Windhager R, Kotz R. One-stage revision surgery for infected megaprostheses. J Bone Joint Surg Br. 1997;79:31–5.
51. Funovics PT, Hipfl C, Hofstaetter JG, Puchner S, Kotz RI, Dominkus M. Management of septic complications following modular endoprosthetic reconstruction of the proximal femur. Int Orthop. 2011;35:1437–44.
52. Gosheger G, Hardes J, Ahrens H, Streitburger A, Buerger H, Erren M, et al. Silver-coated megaendoprostheses in a rabbit model – an analysis of the infection rate and toxicological side effects. Biomaterials. 2004;25:5547–56.
53. Capanna R, Morris HG, Campanacci D, Del Ben M, Campanacci M. Modular uncemented prosthetic reconstruction after resection of tumours of the distal femur. J Bone Joint Surg Br. 1994;76:178–86.
54. Tsuchiya H, Shirai T, Nishida H, Murakami H, Kabata T, Yamamoto N, et al. Innovative antimicrobial coating of titanium implants with iodine. J Orthop Sci. 2012;17:595–604.
55. Hardes J, von Eiff C, Streitbuerger A, Balke M, Budny T, Henrichs MP, et al. Reduction of periprosthetic infection with silver-coated megaprostheses in patients with bone sarcoma. J Surg Oncol. 2010;101:389–95.
56. Hayashi K, Tsuchiya H, Yamamoto N, Takeuchi A, Tomita K. Functional outcome in patients with osteosarcoma around the knee joint treated by minimised surgery. Int Orthop. 2008;32:63–8.
57. Kusuzaki K, Murata H, Matsubara T, Miyazaki S, Okamura A, Seto M, et al. Clinical trial of photodynamic therapy using acridine orange with/without low dose radiation as new limb salvage modality in musculoskeletal sarcomas. Anticancer Res. 2005;25:1225–35.
58. Satonaka H, Kusuzaki K, Matsubara T, Shintani K, Nakamura T, Matsumine A, et al. In vivo anti-tumor activity of photodynamic therapy with intravenous administration of acridine orange, followed by illumination with high-power flash wave light in a mouse osteosarcoma model. Oncol Lett. 2010;1:69–72.
59. Nakamura T, Kusuzaki K, Matsubara T, Matsumine A, Murata H, Uchida A. A new limb salvage surgery in cases of high-grade soft tissue sarcoma using photodynamic surgery, followed by photo- and radio dynamic therapy with acridine orange. J Surg Oncol. 2008;97:523–8.

Part V

Surgery: Biological Reconstruction

13 Biological Reconstruction for Extremity Osteosarcoma: Long-Term Results and Current Concept of Intraoperative Extracorporeal Irradiated Bone Graft (IORBG)

Nobuhito Araki and Osaka Orthopaedic Oncology Group

Abstract

Background: The improvement of survival in osteosarcoma has made a demand to get the long-term durability in the reconstruction method after wide resection.

Purpose: The long-term results of intraoperative extracorporeal irradiated bone graft (IORBG) for malignant bone tumors are analyzed to know the long-term durability of this method.

Method: Seventy-two bone tumor patients treated with IORBG for the last 25 years were reviewed. The oncological results, complication, reoperation-free survival, and graft survival were analyzed.

Results: Oncological 5-year and 10 year survival rates were 90 % and 81 %. Local recurrence was detected in one case outside the implanted bone. Major complications, namely, infection, collapse, fracture, and nonunion, were seen within a short term after initial operation. The reoperation rate was as high as 43 %. The graft survival rate was 81 % at 10 years.

Discussion: Although the reoperation rate was high, complications occurred rather in a shorter term compared with that of tumor knee prosthesis (TKR). This IORBG method is less troublesome than the prosthetic replacement which needs maintenance surgery particularly after long-term follow-up. However, as osteosarcoma occurs mostly in the second decade of life, we should continue to seek a better reconstruction method.

The Osaka Orthopaedic Oncology Group comprises doctors in Department of Orthopaedic Surgery of Osaka University, Osaka National Hospital, JRC Himeji Hospital, Bell Land General Hospital, Kawachi General Hospital and Nozaki Tokushukai Hospital.

N. Araki (✉)
Department of Orthopaedic Surgery, Osaka Medical Center for Cancer and Cardiovascular Disease, Nakamichi 1-Chome, Higashinari-ku, Osaka 537-8511, Japan
e-mail: nobaraki@nifty.com

T. Ueda, A. Kawai (eds.), *Osteosarcoma*, DOI 10.1007/978-4-431-55696-1_13

Keywords
Intraoperative extracorporeal irradiation • Autogenous bone graft • Treated recycled bone • Reconstruction method • Malignant bone tumor

13.1 Introduction

The prognosis of osteosarcoma has been improved to about 70–90 % [1, 2]. The reconstruction method of the affected limb after wide resection should be more stable and tolerable for a long term in concordance with prolonged survival. On one hand, the prosthetic reconstruction needs maintenance surgery for the wear of joint parts, loosening of the stem, and breakage after long-term usage. These maintenance surgeries have a risk of infection because of massive prosthesis and bad skin condition [3]. Moreover, in some prostheses, maintenance parts are already not available because of the economic conditions. On the other hand, in order to avoid the need for maintenance surgery, we started to reuse extracorporeally irradiated affected bones. In this paper, we report the long-term results and the current concept of IORBG method in malignant bone tumor patients.

13.2 Patients and Methods

13.2.1 Patients

From 1988 to 2013, 97 patients were treated by IORBG in our three institutions [4–6]. There were 57 males and 40 females. Bone tumor consisted of 72 cases, and soft tissue tumor comprised 25 cases. The mean age of bone tumor patients was younger at 25 years (median 19 years) compared with that of soft tissue tumor patients at 50 years (median 54 years). In this study, the 72 bone tumors were analyzed. The histological diagnoses of the 72 cases are osteosarcoma (48 cases), chondrosarcoma (6 cases), Ewing sarcoma (5 cases), malignant fibrous histiocytoma (MFH) of the bone (3 cases), metastatic carcinoma (3 cases), and others (7 cases). The distribution of the anatomical sites for the application of IORBG in bone tumor is shown in Table 13.1. The tibia was the most frequent site followed by the femur, humerus, etc. This distribution of IORBG is different from

Table 13.1 Anatomical sites of the 72 bone tumors

Tumor site	No. of cases
Tibia	30
Femur	18
Humerus	14
Pelvis	6
Scapula	2
Radius	1
Ulna	1

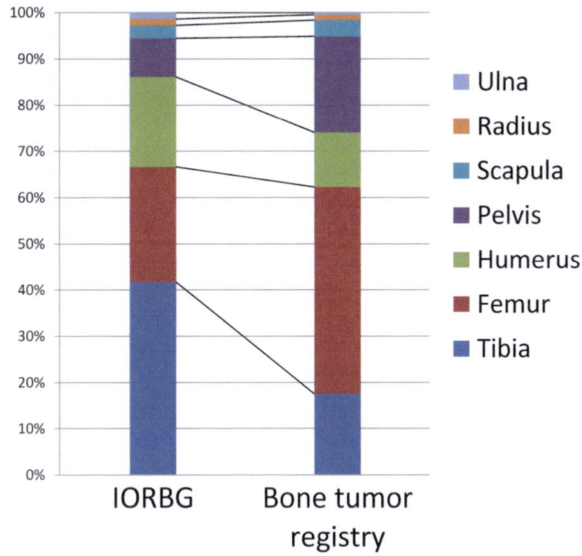

Fig. 13.1 Comparison of tumor site distribution of IORBG to that in the bone tumor registry. The humerus and tibia are preferred sites for the application of this method in order to reconstruct the rotator cuff and patellar tendon

those of the bone tumor registry in Japan [7] (Fig. 13.1). The cases on the tibia and humerus were preferred for this method in order to reconstruct the patellar ligaments and the rotator cuff in comparison to the other sites. Median follow-up interval after definitive surgery was 102 months (range 12–299 months).

13.2.2 Methods

The procedure of IORBG is shown in Fig. 13.2. Widely resected tumor material (Fig. 13.2a, b) was trimmed up to the bone and ligaments for reconstruction (Fig. 13.2c) and packed into a sterile plastic container filled with saline (Fig. 13.2d). Then, the bone was irradiated using Liniac with 6 or 10-MV photons (Fig. 13.2e). The irradiation dose was 50–80 Gy in one fraction to the whole wrapped container for about 40 min. After irradiation, the autogenous bone graft was reimplanted to the remaining bone (Fig. 13.2f) with intramedullary rods, plates, screws, and so on (Fig. 13.2g).

13.2.3 Graft Type

The graft types included osteoarticular in 31 cases (lower extremity 17, upper extremity 13, and pelvis 1), intercalary in 18 cases (lower extremity 18), composite with endoprosthesis in 20 cases (lower extremity 14, upper extremity 5, and pelvis 1), and hemicortical in 3 cases (lower extremity 2 and pelvis 1). For the osteoarticular and intercalary grafts, cement augmentation was used in recent cases to avoid collapse of the epiphysis and fracture (Fig. 13.3). For the composite

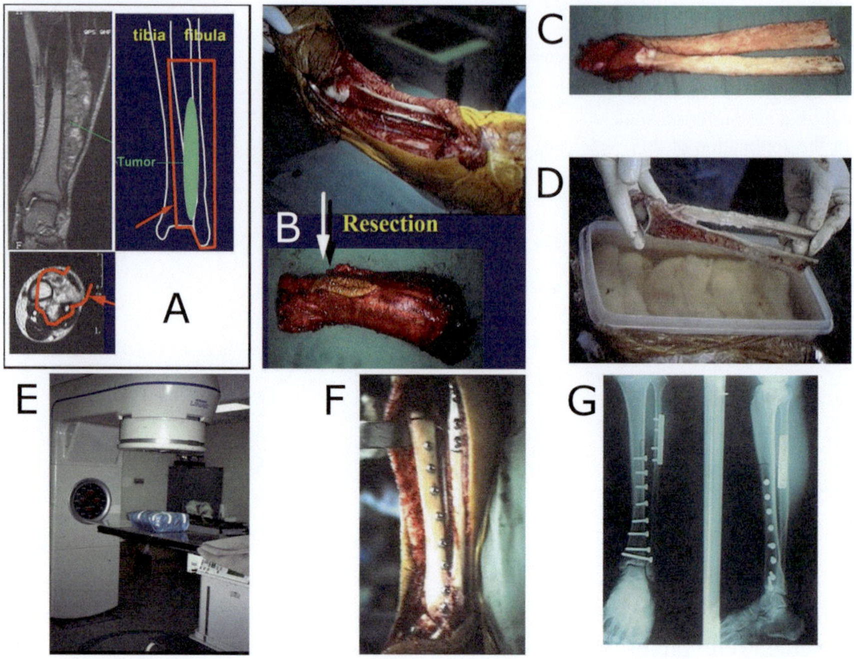

Fig. 13.2 Method of IORBG. (**a**) Wide resection of the tumor. The resection line can be planned in any way for this method. In this intraosseous tumor, the IORBG method was necessary for limb salvage. (**b**) Resected material and host. (**c**) The resected material was trimmed. The muscles were removed while preserving the ligaments. (**d**) The trimmed resected bone and ligaments were soaked in a plastic container filled with saline. (**e**) Irradiation to the whole container for 50 Gy at one time. (**f**) Reimplantation of the bone. Fixation could be done with screws, plates, rod, and so on. (**g**) XP after operation

graft, Link knee prosthesis was used for the lower limb and standard humeral head prosthesis was used for the humerus.

13.2.4 Analysis

Disease-specific survival rates, survival rates of the irradiated bone, and the reoperation-free survival rates were evaluated using the Kaplan-Meier method. The survival of the irradiated bone was considered from the date of implantation to the date of the last follow-up or to the removal of more than half of the bone because of complication or tumor recurrence. Reoperation procedures included any minor operation after the main surgery. The trend of IORBG graft types during the last 25 years was also reviewed and visualized. The NCI's Common Terminology Criteria for Adverse Events (CTCAE) version 4.0 was used for assessment of adverse events.

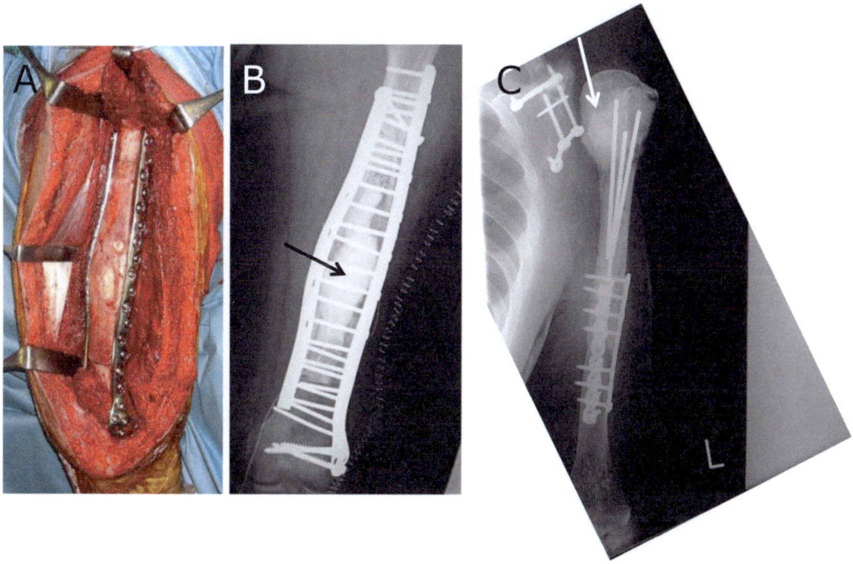

Fig. 13.3 Cement augmentation in intercalary (**a**, **b**) and osteoarticular (**c**) grafts. *White* and *black arrows* indicate the injected bone cement before implantation to the host bone. Note that the osteotomy areas were filled not with cement but with hydroxyapatite in order to achieve bone union

13.3 Results

13.3.1 Disease-Specific Survival and Local Control

The oncological results were CDF 56 cases, NED 6 cases, and DOD 10 cases at mean follow-up of 102 months (range: 12–299 months). Figure 13.4 shows the overall survival curve. The 5-year survival rate was 90 % and the 10-year survival rate was 81 %. There was one case of local recurrence outside the reimplanted bones. We underwent additional wide resection including the implanted irradiated bone and recurrence lesion and total femoral replacement. This case had no further recurrence and remained alive without disease at 19 years post-surgery.

13.3.2 Graft Survival According to the Graft Type

Figure 13.5 shows the survival rate of the irradiated bone according to the applied graft type. There was no significant difference between each graft type. There were only three cases of hemicortical graft, and one case got infected and the graft was removed. The 5-year survival rates were 72.3 % for the osteoarticular graft and 82.6 % for the intercalary graft. All composite grafts survived at mean follow-up of 88 months. The irradiated grafts were removed in 11 patients due to complications

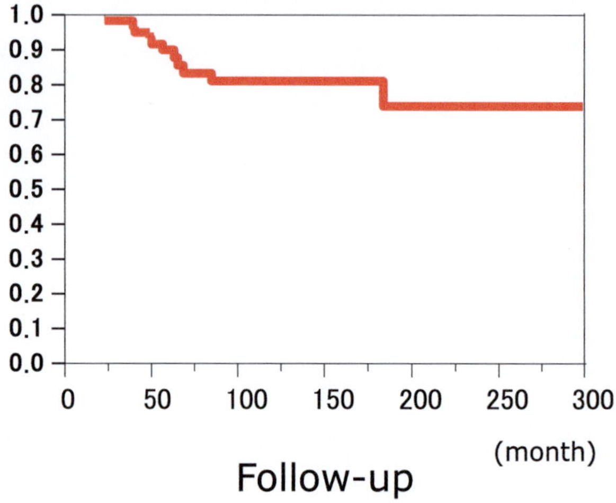

Fig. 13.4 Overall survival curve of 72 bone tumor cases. The 5-year survival rate was 90 % and the 10-year survival rate was 81 %

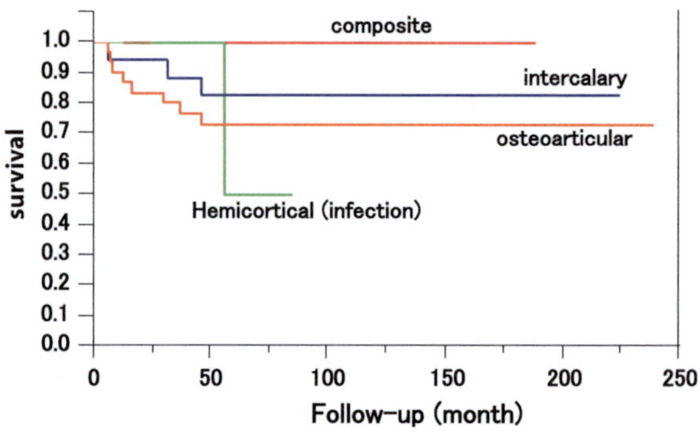

Fig. 13.5 Graft survival curve of 72 bone tumor cases according to graft types. "Survival" is defined as more than half of the graft remaining. The 5-year survival rate of each graft type was as follows: osteoarticular 72.3 %, intercalary 82.6 %, hemicortical 50 %, and composite graft 100 %

or local recurrences outside of the irradiated bone grafts. Eight of the 11 cases were osteoarticular grafts; hence, the survival curve of the osteoarticular grafts declined in a short time after the operation. The overall graft survival for all 72 cases was 81 % at 10 years as shown in Fig. 13.6

13.3.3 Complications

Table 13.2 shows the list of complications of IORBG. Infection was the most frequent (11 cases, 15 %) leading to severe complications, which affected seven osteoarticular, two intercalary, and two composite grafts. Surgical debridement was performed in nine cases corresponding to Grade 3 complication of the CTCAE. Antibiotics were administered in the other two cases. In 5 of the 11 cases, the grafts were removed. Collapse of the epiphysis occurred in nine cases of osteoarticular grafts. Five cases underwent observation without any further treatment because there were no pain and no functional disadvantages as shown in Fig. 13.7. The other

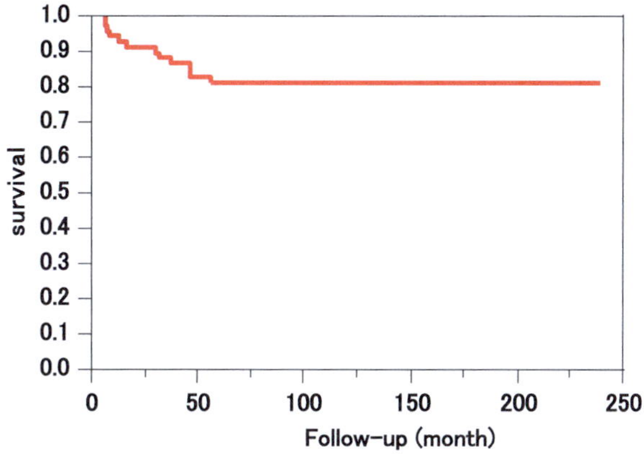

Fig. 13.6 Overall graft survival curve for all 72 bone tumor cases. The 10-year survival rate was 81 %

Table 13.2 Lists of complications of 72 cases

Graft related		
	Collapse	9
	Nonunion	7
	Fracture	6
	Resorption	1
	Dislocation	1
Operation related		
	Infection	11
	Recurrence[a]	1
	Neural palsy	2

[a]Outside of the graft

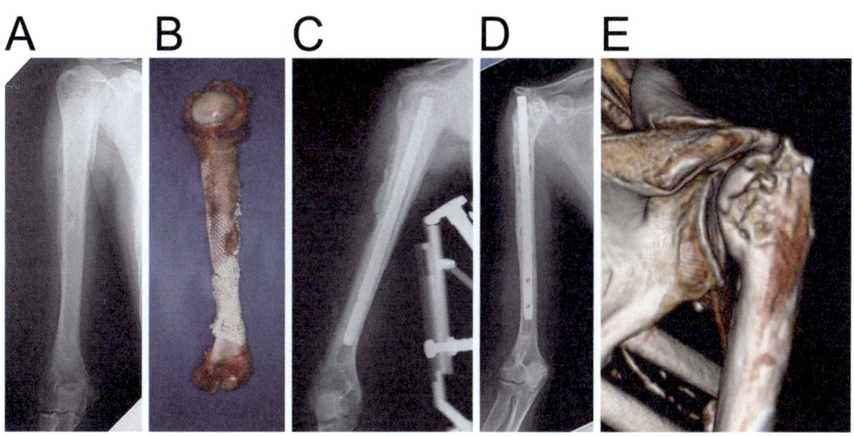

Fig. 13.7 Collapse of humeral head in an osteoarticular graft of the whole humerus. (**a**) Pre-operation XP. (**b**) Implanted irradiated bone. (**c**) Post-operation XP. (**d**) XP at 18 years later. Humeral head is collapsed but the irradiated distal humerus is still healthy. (**e**) 3D-CT shows that the articular surface of the glenohumeral joint is still preserved

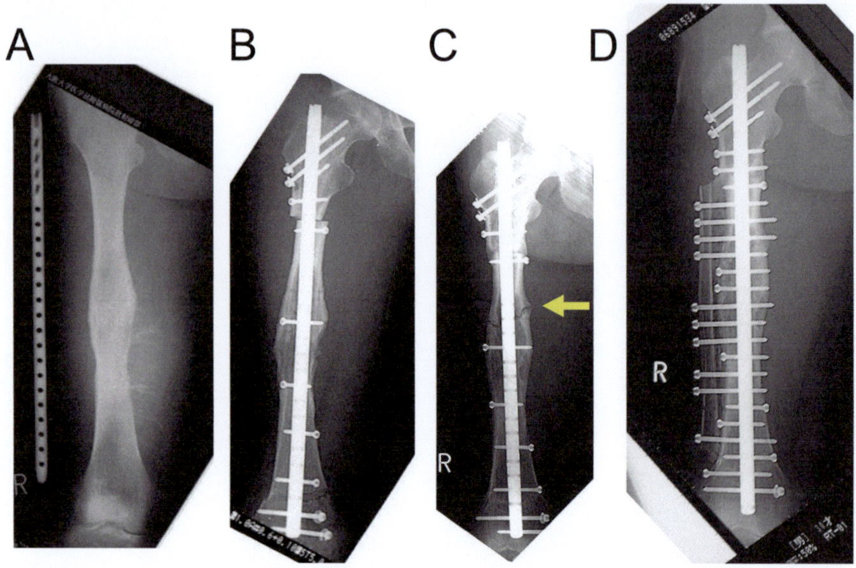

Fig. 13.8 A femoral intercalary graft with fracture at 3 years after initial operation. (**a**) Pre-operation XP. (**b**) Post-operation XP. (**c**) At 3 years post-operation, fracture occurred (*arrow*). (**d**) Free fibular graft was done, and it worked well after 10 years post-reoperation

four cases were treated surgically for partial replacement with prosthesis. Nonunion and fracture occurred mainly in the cases of intercalary graft cases. A femoral case treated with free fibular bone graft showed good function after reoperation (Fig. 13.8). As with this case, nonunion and fracture were salvaged by additional bone grafting with/without additional rigid fixation. Only 1 of 16 intercalary grafts required replacement with prosthesis because of nonunion. Overall, the reoperation rate was as high as 43 %. However, these reoperations due to complications occurred mostly during the short term compared with that of tumor knee prosthesis (Fig. 13.9). There were no Grade 4 or 5 complications.

13.3.4 Changes in Applied Graft Types During the Last 25 Years

Figure 13.10 shows the number of cases with changes in applied graft types. The number of osteoarticular grafts apparently decreased in the last 25 years. By comparison, the use of composite grafts increased. The numbers of intercalary and hemicortical grafts used did not change.

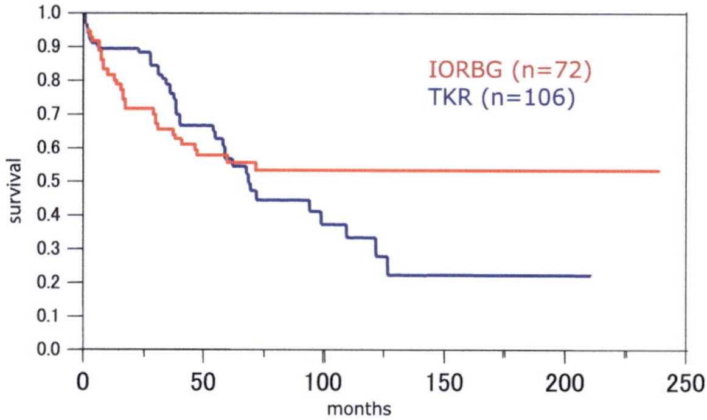

Fig. 13.9 Reoperation survival curve of 72 IORBG cases and 106 tumor knee prosthesis cases. *Red line* is survival curve of IORBG and *blue line* is that of prosthesis. Note the overlap of the reoperation-free survival curve of the two methods

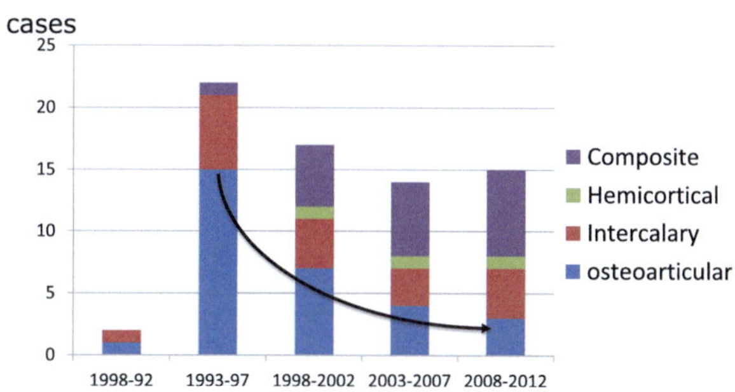

Fig. 13.10 Changes in applied graft types during the last 25 years. The frequency of application of the osteoarticular graft decreased dramatically over 25 years as shown by the arrow. In place of osteoarticular grafts, the use of the composite graft increased. The use of the intercalary and hemicortical grafts did not change

13.4 Discussion

For limb salvage surgery of osteosarcoma, prosthetic replacement is the most common and widely used method. However, prosthesis needs maintenance surgery for the wear of joint parts, loosening, stem breakage, and other complications. Amputation is sometimes required due to a severe complication, such as infection, after these maintenance surgeries [8, 9]. On the other hand, an allograft might be the most widely used biological reconstruction method in foreign countries after a wide resection for osteosarcoma [10]. However, the use of the allograft is difficult in Japan because of the availability of bone based on religious reason. Thus, the treated recycled bones, such as irradiated bone, pasteurized bone (see Chap. 14), and frozen bone (see Chap. 15), are mainly used in Japan. For these treated recycled bones, there are several advantages than allograft with regard to adaptation, disease transmission, availability, usability of attached ligaments, and immunological response. In contrast, the disadvantages of these treated recycled bones compared with prosthesis are problems of absorption and mechanical weakness, as with the allograft [11]. In IORBG, the collapse of the osteoarticular graft and fracture of the intercalary graft represent such conditions. The collapse of the osteoarticular graft was inevitable in our cases; hence, the number of applied decreased in the last 25 years and the application of composite graft increased instead. In particular, for children with growth plates, an osteoarticular graft is not suitable because the growth plate will slip. In this study, the use of the composite graft was shown to be increased with good results. However, we should be aware that this type of graft also requires maintenance surgery for the joint parts the same as prosthesis. For intercalary grafts, the reoperation frequency decreased with cement augmentation, dual plate fixation, and bone grafting, which strengthen the graft. Especially, intercalary graft with vascularized fibular graft showed the best result (Fig. 13.11). This case achieved a normal ADL and the plate could be removed. Although the overall reoperation rate was as high as 43 %, these reoperations due to

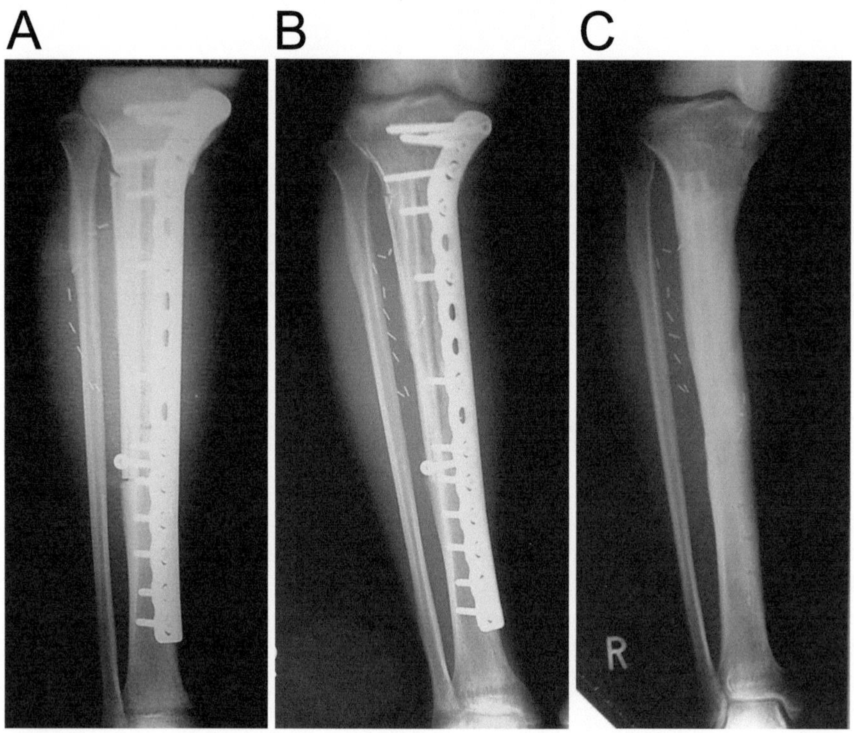

Fig. 13.11 Intercalary graft with vascularized fibular graft. (**a**) Post-operation XP. (**b**) XP at 6 months after operation. (**c**) XP at 65 months after the operation The plate could be removed

complications occurred rather in a shorter term compared with that of tumor knee prosthesis (TKR) (Fig. 13.9). The reoperation-free survival of IORBG overcomes that of TKR after 5 years. This is the advantage of biological reconstruction compared with prosthetic reconstruction, which requires maintenance surgery over the long term. Compared to the survivorship of prostheses of 35–71 % at 10 years reported in previous studies [9, 12, 13], the survivorship of irradiated bone of 81 % at 10 years is very attractive. The irradiated bone graft, once it has healed, is less troublesome compared with the prosthesis, particularly after long-term follow-up. Stable condition in the long term is the best advantage of IORBG. Another advantage of IORBG is the feasibility to reconstruct tendons, joints and small bones for which good prosthesis is not available. IORBG can be used to reconstruct any sites in the body, such as the hand, elbow, ankle, toe, tendons, and ligaments [6, 14].

In conclusion, the long-lasting stability of IORBG can be seen after 5 years, and the subsequent complication rate will decrease. The long-term effectiveness, safety, and reliability of irradiated bone grafting are advantages of IORBG as compared to prostheses, especially for the young patients with osteosarcoma who deserve a long survival period. However, we still need to create a maintenance-free reconstruction method for the knee joints instead of a composite graft.

Acknowledgment This study was supported in part by the Health and Labour Sciences Research Expenses for Commission, Applied Research for Innovative Treatment of Cancer from the Ministry of Health, Labour and Welfare (H26-084), and by the National Cancer Center Research and Development Fund (26-A-4).

References

1. Gatta G, Botta L, Rossi S, Aareleid T, Bielska-Lasota M, Clavel J, Dimitrova N, Jakab Z, Kaatsch P, Lacour B, Mallone S, Marcos-Gragera R, Minicozzi P, Sánchez-Pérez MJ, Sant M, Santaquilani M, Stiller C, Tavilla A, Trama A, Visser O, Peris-Bonet R, EUROCARE Working Group. Childhood cancer survival in Europe 1999–2007: results of EUROCARE-5 – a population-based study. Lancet Oncol. 2014;15(1):35–47.
2. Kudawara I, Aoki Y, Ueda T, Araki N, Naka N, Nakanishi H, Matsumine A, Ieguchi M, Mori S, Myoui A, Kuratsu S, Hashimoto N, Yoshikawa H. Neoadjuvant and adjuvant chemotherapy with high-dose ifosfamide, doxorubicin, cisplatin and high-dose methotrexate in non-metastatic osteosarcoma of the extremities: a phase II trial in Japan. J Chemother. 2013;25(1):41–8.
3. Morii T, Morioka H, Ueda T, Araki N, Hashimoto N, Kawai A, Mochizuki K, Ichimura S. Deep infection in tumor endoprosthesis around the knee: a multi-institutional study by the Japanese musculoskeletal oncology group. BMC Musculoskelet Disord. 2013;14:51.
4. Araki N, Myoui A, Kuratsu S, Hashimoto N, Inoue T, Kudawara I, et al. Intraoperative extracorporeal autogenous irradiated bone grafts in tumor surgery. Clin Orthop Relat Res. 1999;368:196–206.
5. Hayashi K, Araki N, Koizumi M, Suzuki O, Seo Y, Naka N, Isohashi F, Myoui A, Yoshioka Y, Teshima T, Ueda T, Yoshikawa H, Ogawa K. Longterm results of intraoperative extracorporeal irradiation of autogenous bone grafts on primary bone and soft tissue malignancies. Acta Oncol. 2015;54(1):138–41.

6. Ozaki R, Hamada K, Emori M, Omori S, Joyama S, Naka N, Tomita Y, Araki N. Limb salvage operation using intraoperative extracorporeal autogenous irradiated bone and tendon graft for myxoid liposarcoma on dorsum of foot. Foot (Edinb). 2010;20(2–3):90–5.
7. JOA musculoskeletal tumor committee and National Cancer Center, Bone tumor registry in Japan 2011.
8. Myers GJC, Abudu AT, Carter SR, Tillman RM, Grimer RJ. Endoprosthetic replacement of the distal femur for bone tumours: long-term results. J Bone Joint Surg Br. 2007;89:521–6.
9. Grimer RJ, Carter SR, Tillman RM, Sneath RS, Walker PS, Unwin PS, et al. Endoprosthetic replacement of the proximal tibia. J Bone Joint Surg. 1999;81:488–94.
10. Farfalli GL, Aponte-Tinao L, Lopez-Millán L, Ayerza MA, Muscolo DL. Clinical and functional outcomes of tibial intercalary allografts after tumor resection. Orthopedics. 2012;35:e391–6.
11. Wheeler DL, Enneking WF. Allograft bone decreases in strength in vivo over time. Clin Orthop Relat Res. 2005;435:36–42.
12. Tan PX, Yong BC, Wang J, Huang G, Yin JQ, Zou CY, et al. Analysis of the efficacy and prognosis of limb-salvage surgery for osteosarcoma around the knee. Eur J Surg Oncol. 2012;38:1171–7.
13. Myers GJC, Abudu AT, Carter SR, Tillman RM, Grimer RJ. Proximal tibia for bone tumours. J Bone Joint Surg Br. 2007;89:1632–7.
14. Omori S, Hamada K, Outani H, Oshima K, Joyama S, Tomita Y, Naka N, Araki N, Yoshikawa H. Intraoperative extracorporeal autogenous irradiated tendon grafts for functional limb salvage surgery of soft tissue sarcomas of the wrist and hand. World J Surg Oncol. 2015;13:179.

Biological Reconstruction for Extremity Osteosarcoma: Pasteurized Autogenous Bone Graft

14

Keisuke Ae

Abstract

A pasteurization method has been previously developed with the aim of enabling reconstruction using diseased bones following resection of malignant bone tumors. Using this method, bone containing tumor cells is heat-treated at 60 °C for 30 min to kill the tumor and then transplanted into the same patient at the same location. This approach has distinct advantages for initial strength, anatomical fitting to the defect of the affected bone, no disease transmission, and good accessibility, including economic efficiency.

We developed this pasteurization method and have used it in various graft forms since 1989. However, this method has been associated with pseudarthrosis in the short to middle term and bone resorption in the long term. Here we show its actual application and the results, with special focus on failure and long-term survival. Finally, we present an optimal indication for this method and clinical tips to reduce its failure.

Keywords

Pasteurization • Clinical application • Long-term results

14.1 Introduction

In the past, amputations were performed for treating malignant bone tumors, such as osteosarcomas. However, limb-sparing surgery has become mainstream today because of increased survival, thanks to advances in chemotherapy. In limb-sparing surgery, local curability is achieved by wide resection. It is then necessary to restore

K. Ae (✉)
Department of Orthopaedic Oncology, Cancer Institute Ariake Hospital of JFCR (Japanese Foundation for Cancer Research), 3-8-31 Ariake, Koto-Ward, Tokyo 135-8550, Japan
e-mail: keisuke.ae@jfcr.or.jp

T. Ueda, A. Kawai (eds.), *Osteosarcoma*, DOI 10.1007/978-4-431-55696-1_14

the motor function and support, which have been lost because of the resection of the diseased bone. In recent years, the local control rate for osteosarcomas has surpassed 90 % because of advances in preoperative chemotherapy and diagnostic imaging and improved surgical technique. This has meant that restoration of the function of the affected limb has become even more important.

Reconstruction of bone defects following resection of malignant bone tumors can be roughly classified into prosthetic reconstruction and biological reconstruction. Prosthetic reconstruction using an artificial joint is advantageous because it imparts excellent functionality soon after surgery, and the result is stable. However, artificial joints have disadvantages because there is always the risk of infection, and reoperation is unavoidable in the long term because of problems such as loosening, wear, metal fatigue, and damage, to name a few. For biological reconstruction, an autogenous bone graft is optimal for bone formation, but limitations include invasiveness at the donor site, loss of bone stock, and an inability to make up for large-volume bone loss. For these reasons, allografts have been used in Europe and the United States [1]. In Japan, on the other hand, because of cultural differences, an adequate bone bank system has not been established; therefore it is difficult to obtain the required allografts. As an alternative approach, methods for using regrafting of the recycled bone, by applying a devitalization process to excised bone that contains a tumor, have been developed [2]. Recycled bones include irradiated bone [3], autoclaved bone [4], heat-treated bone [5], and freeze-treated bone [6]. Each of these materials is expected to have high affinity for bone tissue, be incorporated into the recipient's metabolism and undergo remodeling, thus enabling a viable permanent graft.

A pasteurization method has been previously developed with the aim of enabling reconstruction using diseased bones following resection of malignant bone tumors. Using this method, bone containing malignant bone tumors is heat-treated at 60 °C for 30 min to kill the tumors and then transplanted into the same patient at the same location. Since the pasteurized bone is autogenous, it is safer to use because there is no risk of infection from a donor or rejection by the host immune system. It also has the advantage of being fully compatible with the graft bed. We previously developed this pasteurization method and have used it in the clinic since 1989. Herein, we explain the biology of pasteurized bone and present the results of its actual clinical application in patients with malignant bone tumors.

14.2 Biology of Pasteurized Bone

14.2.1 Oncological Safety

There are many reports regarding the effect of hyperthermia on tumors. Auersperg et al. studied cultured cells and reported that the temperature and time required to kill tumors differed, depending on the tumor cells [7]. We have previously performed basic research on transplantation using murine Mesh-A fibrosarcoma and B-16 melanoma-cultured cell lines, with a heating time of 30 min, and confirmed that the cells engrafted when the temperature was 43 °C, but not when it was 45 °C, 50 °C, 55 °C, or 60 °C. Later, Rong et al. used sarcoma tissue blocks and heat-treated swarm rat chondrosarcoma at 50 °C for 20 min or more and reported, using a histological approach, that the cells were completely killed [8]. Kode et al. heat-treated osteosarcoma tissues excised from humans at 60 °C for 40 min and compared them with a pasteurized bone model as the control [9]. Both in vivo and in vitro, the proliferative activity disappeared in the pasteurized group, and there was no engraftment or growth following xenografting or culture. We think that safety can be assured by heat-treating at 60 °C for 30 min, and in actual practice, we have never experienced a case of tumor recurrence following grafting of pasteurized bone.

14.2.2 Strength and Osteoconductivity of Pasteurized Bone

In the development of the pasteurization method, we investigated whether the strength and osteoconductivity of pasteurized bone were superior to those properties of conventionally used bone graft materials, for example, autoclaved bone and boiled bone. Regarding the osteoconductivity of autoclaved bone, Köhler et al. conducted experiments using rabbit ulnas [10]. They reported that pseudarthrosis was common when using autoclaved bone, and that the combined use of allogeneic bone matrix was necessary. Kreicbergs et al. reported that regrafted autoclaved bone remained necrotic over time [11]. With regard to bone strength, they also reported that the torsional strength decreased to 77 % and the hardness fell to 80 % when the autoclaving lasted for 20 min. Stroosma et al. used dog femora that had undergone boiling treatment and reported that replacement with new bone was delayed until more than 12 weeks after grafting [12].

Manabe et al. heat-treated rabbit iliac bones, regrafted them, and evaluated their osteoconductivity [13]. Grafted autoclaved bones were resorbed and did not show bone union with the graft bed, whereas pasteurized bones fused with the graft bed and were remodeled to new bone while maintaining the structure. Furthermore, pasteurized bone osteoconductivity was similar to that of fresh autogenous bone grafts. They also evaluated the mechanical strength of rat femora that had been heat-treated. They used the three-point bending and torsion test to compare fresh femora with femora that had been heat-treated for 30 min at 58 °C (pasteurization), 100 °C (boiling), and 120 °C (autoclaving). Pasteurized femora had identical strength to fresh femora, whereas the autoclaved and boiled bones showed significantly inferior strength. Histologically, the pasteurized bones showed neovascularization and infiltration of osteoblasts and were reported to be superior to the conventional heat-treated bones.

14.3 Clinical Application of Pasteurized Bones

14.3.1 Surgical Technique for Pasteurization

The excised bone specimens are processed on a sterilized table, away from the surgical field. The samples and defect are then prepared as follows:

(a) *Pretreatment of bones*: Soft tissues are used for evaluation of the surgical margin, so are removed from the bones en bloc. In the case of primary tumors in long bones, when necessary to evaluate the resected margin at the resected stump, a window of thin strips is opened in the cortex, and the intramedullary tissue is removed en bloc and used for evaluation of the resected margin.
(b) *Pasteurization*: Physiological saline is placed in a sterilized shaker-type thermostatic bath and heated. The device should be set at 65 °C in advance so that the temperature will not drop lower than 60 °C, even if a bone is immediately soaked in the bath. The bone is soaked and heat-treated for 30 min.
(c) *Bone grafting*: The form of the graft will differ depending on the state following bone excision and the objective of reconstruction. Graft types include osteoarticular graft, intercalary graft, inlay graft, composite graft matched with an artificial joint, or a pelvic graft to reconstruct the pelvic ring (Fig. 14.1).
(d) *Fixation method*: With an inlay graft, the graft bed is surrounded by fresh autogenous bone, and since the stability of the graft is good, fixation with only a screw is usually sufficient. An intercalary graft is prone to pseudarthrosis, so it is important to fix a strong bone junction and use an intramedullary nail and/or a double plate. In particular, at the junction of long bones, if there is an abundance of fresh cancellous bone, bone union is expected to be readily achieved. Therefore, in some cases, an autogenous bone graft should also be used at the junction.

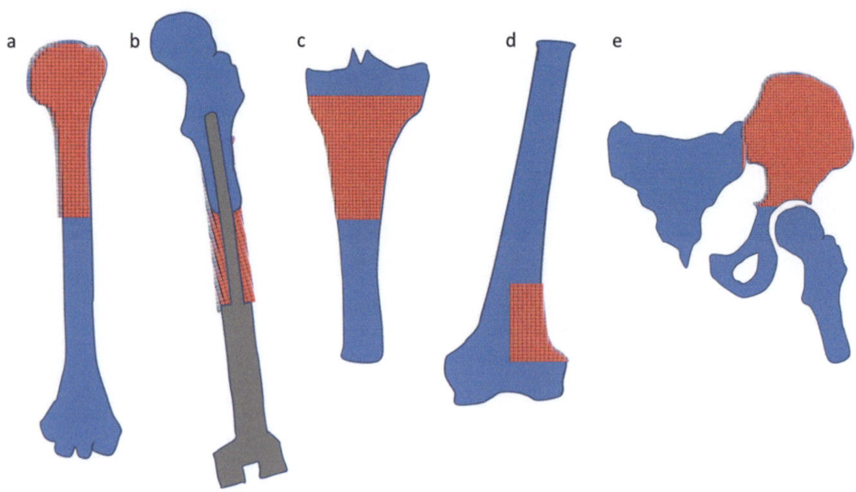

Fig. 14.1 Form of bone graft. (**a**) Osteoarticular graft, (**b**) composite graft, (**c**) intercalary graft, (**d**) inlay graft, (**e**) pelvic graft

(e) *Adjunct therapy*: The bed of the pasteurized bone may have poor blood flow after tumor resection because of loss of soft tissue. Alternately, not only the tumor in the pasteurized bone but also the bone tissue itself may have been devitalized, resulting in poor bone union and susceptibility to infection. For this reason, and in the hope of preventing infection and achieving early resumption of blood flow to the bone, it may be necessary to also use a cover consisting of a muscle flap or musculocutaneous flap having good blood flow, or a vascularized autogenous bone graft.

14.3.2 Clinical Results with Pasteurized Bones

14.3.2.1 Subjects

We have previously applied the pasteurization method for bone grafting to 32 patients with primary malignant tumors of bones between 1989 and 2014. From these patients, the subjects of this study were those who had been followed up for at least 1 year and those who were excluded because of complications within less than 1 year. In two patients, follow-up was discontinued at less than 1 year because of local recurrence, but they were excluded because the cause of recurrence was aside from the pasteurized bone. Four other patients died less than 1 year after the surgery and were excluded. As a result, 26 patients were excluded. The median duration of follow-up was 106.5 months (Table 14.1).

Mean patient age at the time of initial surgery was 21.6 years. Patient diseases included osteosarcoma (17), Ewing's sarcoma (5), chondrosarcoma (2), malignant fibrous histiocytoma (MFH) of bone (1), and lymphoma of bone (1). The mean long diameter of the diseased bones that were grafted after pasteurization was 15.3 cm, and the affected bone was the femur in 12 patients, tibia in 5, pelvis in 5, and humerus in 4. The graft method used was an osteoarticular graft in six patients (three proximal humeri, one distal femur, two proximal tibiae), with a mean long diameter of 17.1 cm; an intercalary graft in six patients (four femora, two tibiae), with a mean long diameter of 14.3 cm; an inlay graft in one patient (femur), with a long diameter of 5 cm; and a pelvic graft in five patients (P1 in one patient, P1-2 in one, P2-3 in one, and P1-3 in two), with a mean long diameter of 16.4 cm. A composite graft with a prosthesis was used in ten patients (one proximal femur, five distal femora, one proximal tibia, one proximal humerus, two pelvis), including four patients who underwent revision following collapse of an osteoarticular graft, with a mean long diameter of 16.0 cm.

14.3.2.2 Criteria for Assessing Treatment Results with Pasteurized Bone

The following criteria were used to assess the results of treatment using pasteurized bone:

Success: The pasteurized bone remains and shows movement of bone tissue and supporting function.

Table 14.1 Summary of patient data, form of graft, and result of functional evaluation of pasteurized bone

No.	Age	Diagnosis	Affected bone	Size of graft (cm)	Form of graft	Fixation	Autobone graft	Complication	Additional surgery	Period to union (month)	Radiographic evaluation of resorption
1	10	EWING	Femur	23.5	Osteoarticular	Intramedullary nail with cement	(–)	Infection, pseudarthrosis, resorption	TFR		Poor
2	16	EWING	Humerus	11	Osteoarticular	Plate and intramedullary nail with cement	Iliac bone	Pseudarthrosis	(–)		Poor
3	28	EWING	Humerus	19	Osteoarticular	Intramedullary nail with cement	Pedicled scapula and iliac bone	(–)	(–)	13	Poor
4	17	OS	Humerus	17	Osteoarticular	Intramedullary nail with cement	(–)	Infection, pseudarthrosis	Debri and LD flap		Poor
5	28	OS	Tibia	24	Osteoarticular	Intramedullary nail with cement	Iliac bone	Infection	Amputation	8	Fair
6	12	OS	Tibia	12	Osteoarticular	Intramedullary nail	Iliac bone	Infection, resorption		7	Poor
7	18	EWING	Humerus	14	Osteoarticular -> composite	Intramedullary nail with cement	Iliac bone	Resorption	Humeral head prosthesis	15	Poor
8	11	OS	Tibia	12.5	Osteoarticular -> composite	Intramedullary nail with cement	Iliac bone	Joint instability, resorption	TKR	4	Poor
9	11	OS	Femur	18	Osteoarticular -> composite	Intramedullary nail with cement	Iliac bone	Pseudarthrosis, infection	TKR -> amputation	6 m after 2nd op. with autobone graft	Good

10	13	OS	Femur	20	Osteoarticular -> composite	Intramedullary nail with cement	Iliac bone	Pseudarthrosis, joint instability, loosening	TKR->TFR	13 m after 2nd op. with autobone graft	Poor
11	61	LYMPHOMA	Femur	25	Composite	Femoral head prosthesis with cement fixation and plate	Iliac bone	Infection	Removal of prosthesis	12	Good
12	14	OS	Femur	16	Composite	TKA prosthesis with cement fixation	(–)	Pseudarthrosis, loosening	Rotation plasty		Poor
13	11	OS	Femur	4	Composite	TKA prosthesis without cement fixation and plate	(–)	(–)	(–)	12	Good
14	24	Paro.OS	Femur	10	Composite	TKA prosthesis with cement fixation	Femoral local bone	(–)	(–)	7	Fair
15	34	OS	Femur	6	Intercalary	Intramedullary nail	FVFG and iliac bone	Pseudarthrosis	Autobone graft	7	Fair
16	17	OS	Tibia	15	Intercalary	Intramedullary nail and plate	Iliac bone	Fracture, pseudarthrosis	Autobone graft and plate	6 m after 2nd op. with autobone graft	Good
17	5	OS	Femur	18	Intercalary	Plate	FVFG	Pseudarthrosis, resorption	Turnup plasty		Poor
18	31	OS	Tibia	16	Intercalary	Plate	FVFG and iliac bone	Infection	Removal of plate	6	Good
19	14	OS	Femur	24	Intercalary	Plate	FVFG and iliac bone	Pseudarthrosis	TFR		Fair

(continued)

Table 14.1 (continued)

No.	Age	Diagnosis	Affected bone	Size of graft (cm)	Form of graft	Fixation	Autobone graft	Complication	Additional surgery	Period to union (month)	Radiographic evaluation of resorption
20	37	CH.SA	Femur	7	Intercalary	Intramedullary nail and plate	Free fibula and iliac bone	(–)	(–)	8	Good
21	22	Peri.OS	Femur	5	Inlay	Plate	Iliac bone	(–)	(–)	3	Good
22	42	MFH	Pelvis	11	Pelvis P1	Plate and screw	Free fibula	Infection	Removal of screw and cement	10	Good
23	7	EWING	Pelvis	15	Pelvis P1-2	Plate	Free fibula	(–)	(–)	3	Poor
24	19	OS	Pelvis	20	Pelvis P1-3 with THA	Plate and wire	(–)	Infection, pseudarthrosis, loosening	THA revision	17	Poor
25	22	OS	Pelvis	20	Pelvis P1-3 with THA	Plate and screw	(–)	Infection	Removal of THA	8	Poor
26	39	CH.SA	Pelvis	16	Pelvis P2-3	Screw and wire	(–)	(–)	(–)	13	Good

Failure: The pasteurized bone was removed because of infection or resorption, or, if it remains, it does not function because of resorption and/or pseudarthrosis.

For patients who received an osteoarticular graft at the time of the initial surgery and in whom it was then reused as a composite graft at the time of re-surgery, the treatment result was assessed as "successful" if the pasteurized bone was functioning at the end.

14.3.2.3 Treatment Results with Pasteurized Bone Grafts

Bone union of the grafted bone was confirmed in 15 of the 26 patients following the initial surgery, with a union rate of 57.7 %. The median time required for union was 8 months. In the early surgeries, autogenous bone grafts were not used at the graft site, and pseudarthrosis was common. Later, we started to also use autogenous bone grafts, and the incidence of pseudarthrosis decreased.

The results of treatment using pasteurized bone grafts were analyzed as the success rate using the Kaplan-Meier method based on the results generated using the assessment criteria (Fig. 14.2). The success rate was 79.3 % after 5 years of follow-up and 58.4 % after 10 years. The cumulative success rate of pasteurized bone that remained and functioned was revealed in 27.3 % of cases and tended to decrease with time. However, this tendency differed as a function of the size of the grafted bone and the graft method. With regard to the graft size, the mean size was 12.2 cm in the successful group, which was significantly smaller than the mean of 18.5 cm in the failed group (Student's *t*-test: $P = 0.004$) (Fig. 14.3). Regarding the graft method (Fig. 14.4), there was a strong tendency for failure in the early post-graft period when using an osteoarticular graft for the reconstruction. At more than 2 years after the surgery, the number of functioning osteoarticular grafts had

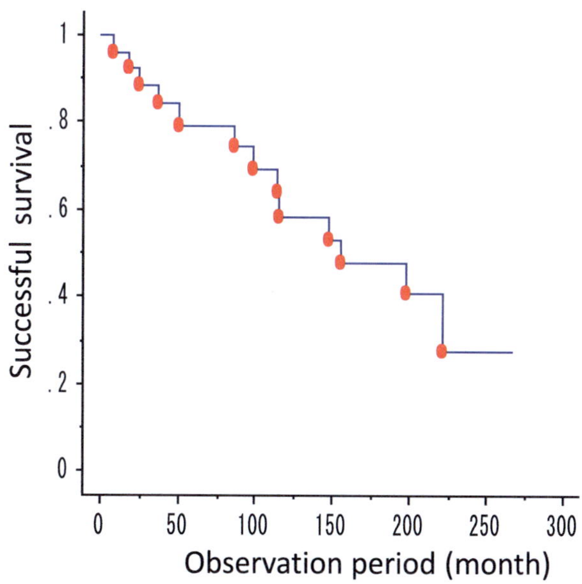

Fig. 14.2 Successful survival rate of all pasteurized bones. Failure was defined as graft removal or discontinued functioning due to absorption

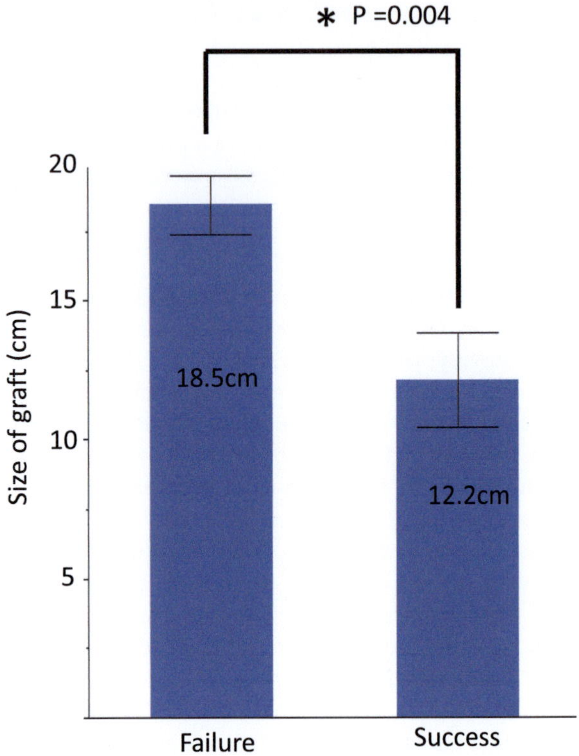

Fig. 14.3 Comparison of the size of pasteurized bone grafts between the failure group and success group

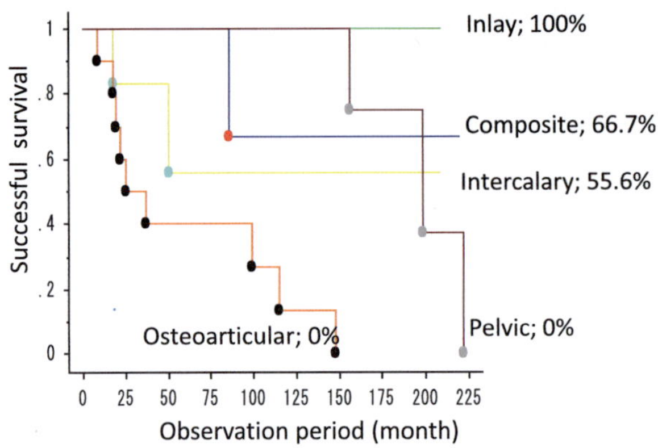

Fig. 14.4 Pasteurized bone survival classified by form of graft

decreased to half or less, and the cumulative rate became 0 %. When grafting pasteurized pelvis, there was a gradual tendency for failure in the long term, and the cumulative rate became 0 %. Stable long-term results can be expected with inlay (100 %), composite (66.7 %), and intercalary (55.6 %) grafts.

With regard to complications of the pasteurization method, we used the Kaplan-Meier method to analyze complication-free survival, with the need for additional surgery as the endpoint (Fig. 14.5). Overall, the complication-free survival rates

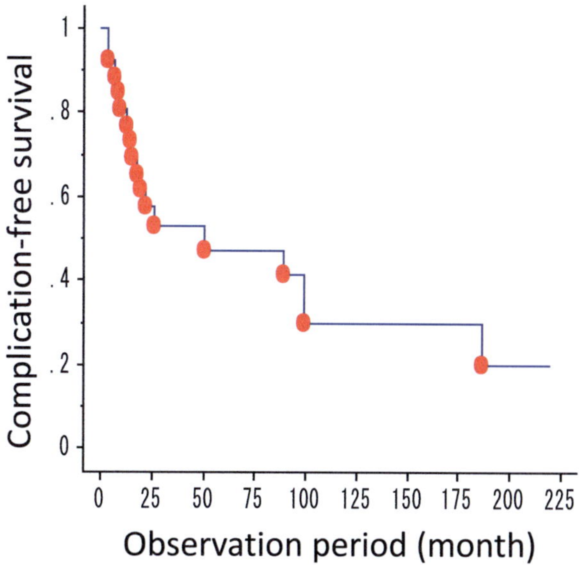

Fig. 14.5 Complication-free survival of all pasteurized bone grafts

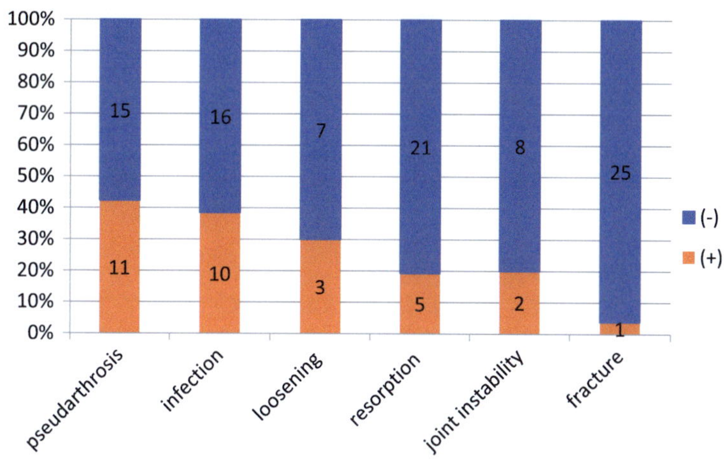

Fig. 14.6 Complications of all pasteurized bone grafts

were 80.8 % at 1 year, 57.4 % at 2 years, and 47.1 % at 5 years. The cumulative rate was 19.6 %, indicating a high incidence of complications requiring additional surgery. It is noteworthy that nearly half of the patients required additional surgery within 2 years after the initial reconstruction. The most common complications were pseudarthrosis and infection, with each occurring in about 40 % of the total patients (Fig. 14.6). Only one patient experienced fracture. The details of the results with each graft method are described below:

Osteoarticular graft (six cases)

Five patients failed because of infection and resorption. The one successful case had had a proximal humerus graft and was followed up for only 41 months, having died from disease. Two patients were followed up long term, more than 5 years, but both showed marked bone resorption. Another patient with a proximal humerus graft was followed up for 148 months, and the pasteurized graft was resorbed and had almost completely disappeared (Fig. 14.7). A patient

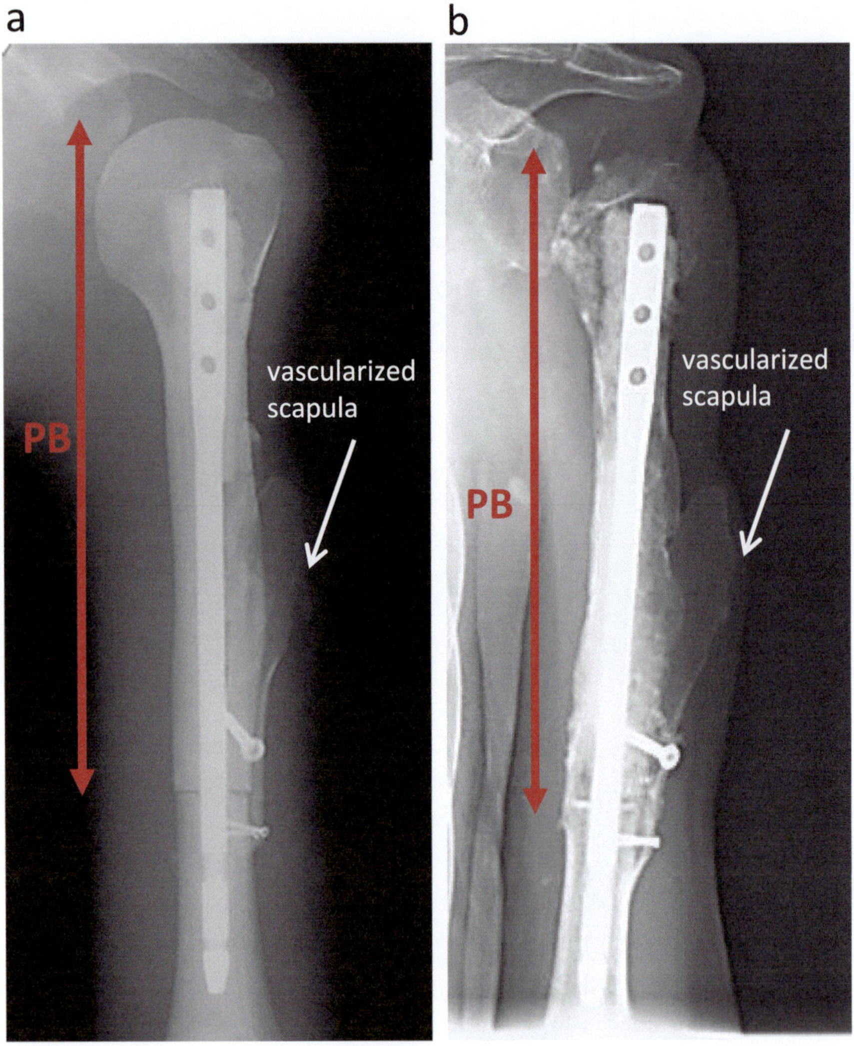

Fig. 14.7 Osteoarticular graft (case no.3). (**a**) Postoperative radiograph showing the pasteurized humerus fixed by an intramedullary nail with a vascularized scapula graft, (**b**) radiograph 12 years after surgery showing collapse of humeral head and absorption of proximal shaft except grafted scapula, (**c**) *PB* pasteurized bone

with a distal femur graft was followed up for 115 months, and total femur replacement (TFR) was performed because pseudarthrosis and resorption could not be controlled.

Composite graft (10 cases)

Additional surgery was needed in four patients because of complications of an osteoarticular graft, and the pasteurized bone was reused as a composite graft. In

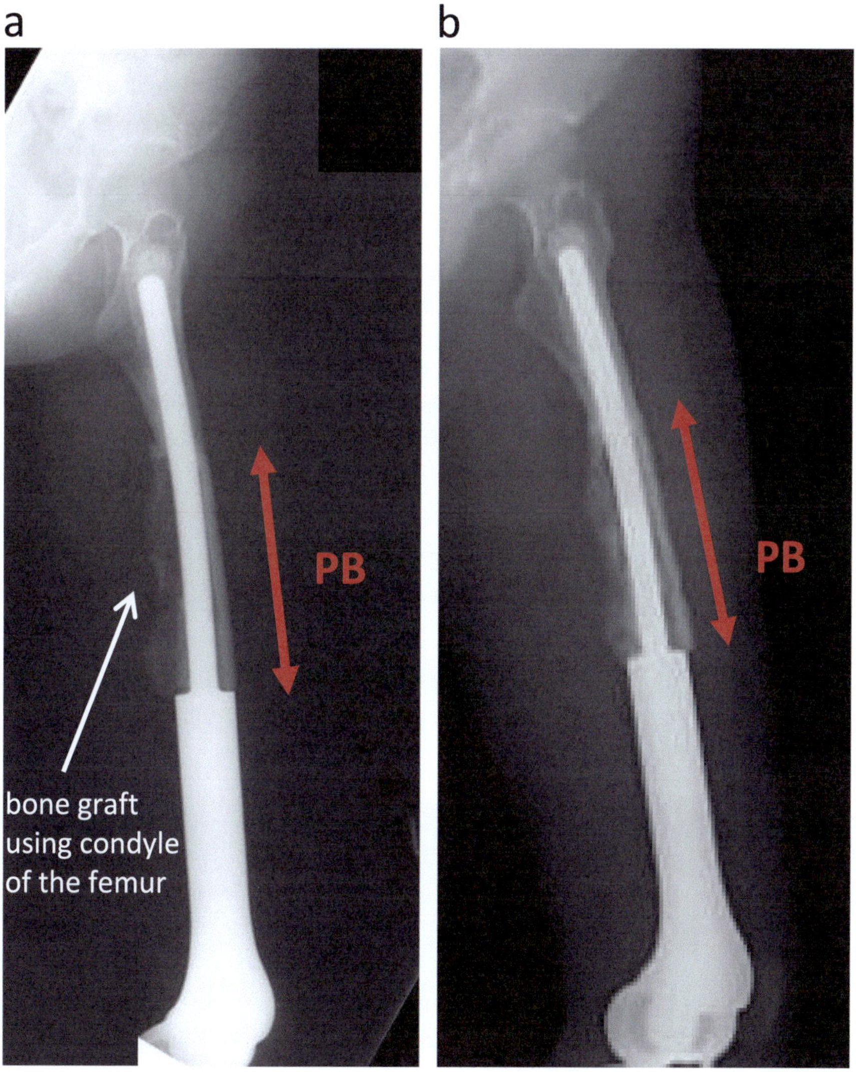

Fig. 14.8 Composite graft (case no. 14). (**a**) Postoperative radiograph showing a composite graft of a relatively short length (10 cm) of pasteurized bone with a total knee tumor prosthesis, (**b**) radiograph 18 years after surgery showing the pasteurized bone remaining without obvious resorption

two patients, total hip replacement (THA) was performed in conjunction with a pasteurized pelvic graft. Six patients underwent autogenous bone grafting at the junction. Five patients were assessed as successful, and all obtained union at the bone junction (Fig. 14.8). Three patients were assessed as failed, and the pasteurized bone was removed from each because of resorption, pseudarthrosis, loosening, and/or infection. Nine patients were followed up long term, at least 5 years; resorption was seen in seven, and five were assessed as failed.

Intercalary graft (six cases)

Autogenous bone grafting was performed in all six patients, and free vascularized fibula graft (FVFG) was also performed in four of those patients. Four patients were assessed as successful, and they all showed bone union. Two patients were assessed as failed, and both showed pseudarthrosis while one also showed bone resorption. Two of the successful patients were followed up long term, at least 5 years (209 months (Fig. 14.9) and 94 months), and neither showed bone resorption.

Inlay graft (one case)

This patient also underwent autogenous bone grafting using a small 5 cm bone piece. Union was achieved after 3 months, and no resorption was observed, even at 209 months after surgery (Fig. 14.10).

Pelvic graft (five cases)

All five patients achieved bone union. Later, three of these patients failed, and each had a history of irradiation. Two patients had an infectious complication

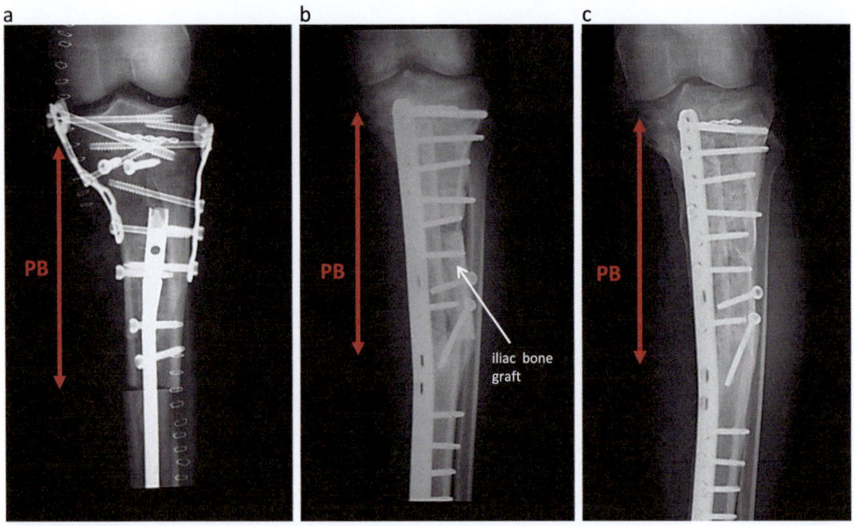

Fig. 14.9 Intercalary graft (case no.16). (**a**) Postoperative radiograph; (**b**) the pasteurized bone fractured in the distal end at 7 months postoperation. Radiograph shows the pasteurized bone after additional free iliac bone graft and refixation with a long plate; (**c**) radiograph 17 years after surgery showing no bone absorption

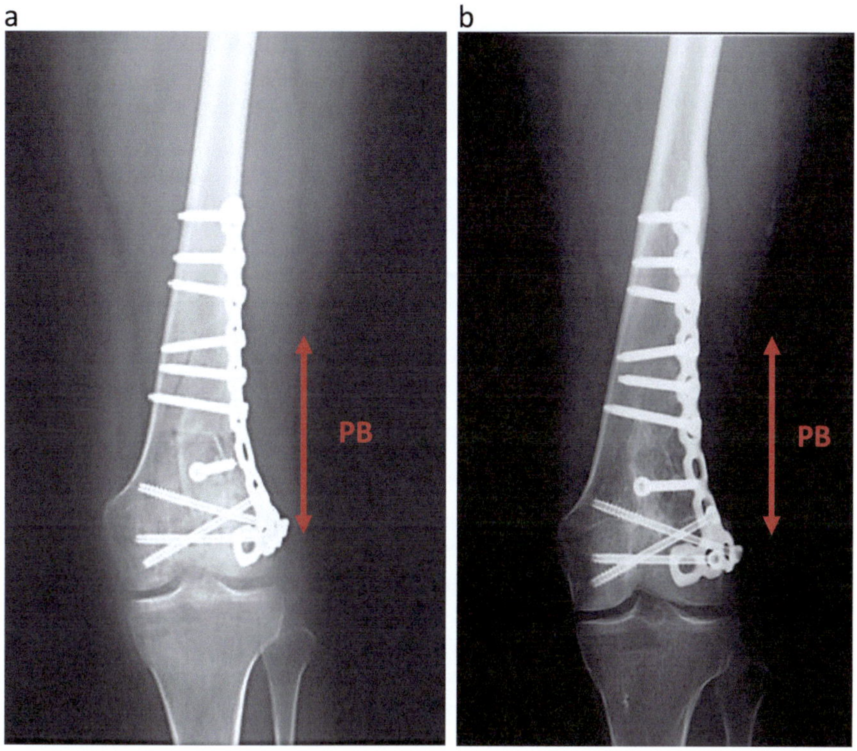

Fig. 14.10 Inlay graft (case no.21). (**a**) Postoperative radiograph, (**b**) radiograph 17 years after surgery showing no bone absorption

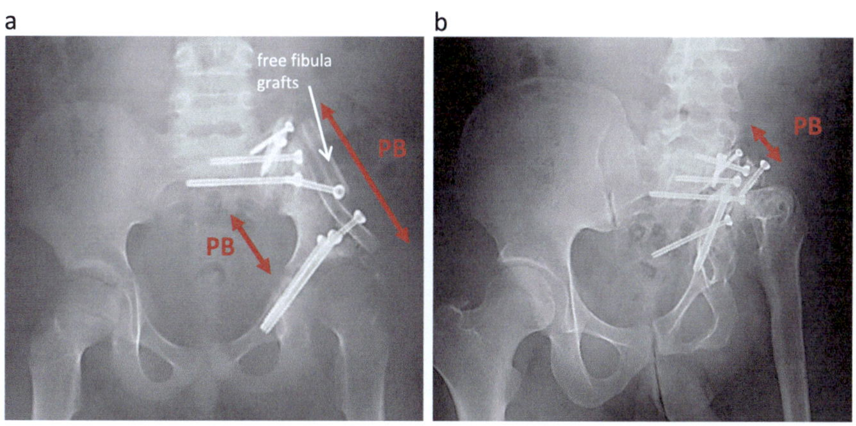

Fig. 14.11 Pelvic graft (case no.23). (**a**) Postoperative radiograph showing pasteurized bone graft with free fibula grafts, (**b**) radiograph 13 years after surgery showing massive absorption of grafted bone and shortening of affected limb

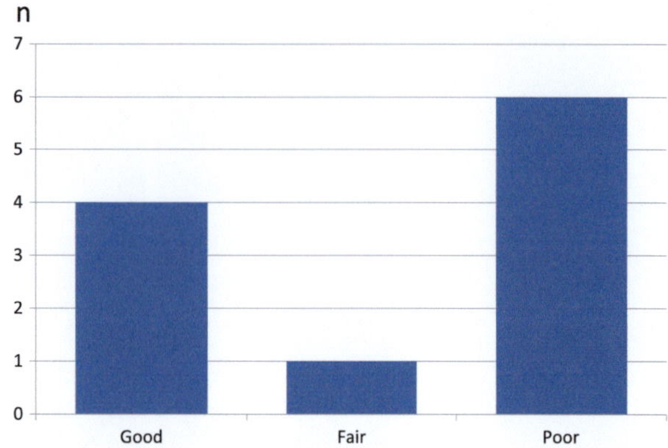

Fig. 14.12 Radiographic evaluation of pasteurized bone resorption over 10 years of observation

and were cases of a composite graft with THA. Four patients were followed up for at least 5 years, and resorption occurred in three (Fig. 14.11).

14.3.2.4 Resorption of Pasteurized Bone

The main reason that the function of pasteurized bone graft decreases with time is bone resorption that occurs over the long term. Bone resorption detected by radiographic evaluation of all patients showed 13 poor cases and 9 good cases. Even in cases of pasteurized bone grafts that lasted for 10 years or more, there were six poor cases and only four good cases (Fig. 14.12).

14.4 Conclusion

Pasteurized bones are necrotic bones. Since their initial strength is the same as that of normal bones, their supporting function is good. However, if they are reintegrated into the body's bone metabolism cycle, they are destined to be resorbed with time [14]. As a condition for reintegration into the bone metabolism cycle, the most important point is the supply of osteogenic cells as a result of bone union with the graft bed. However, for large grafts, it is often the case that bone union and revascularization is achieved only at the margin, so the supply of osteogenic cells does not reach the center portion and resorption occurs. It may be supposed that it is necessary for reperfusion and the supply of osteogenic cells to be established for the entire grafted bone, and that it is necessary to use a vascularized fibula graft and coverage using a muscle flap with good blood flow. Based on our experience to date with pasteurized bone grafts, we think that the indications for use of these grafts are as follows.

The optimal indication for use of pasteurized bone is the case of an inlay graft. Bone union can be readily attained because there is viable autogenous bone all around the graft bed, and integration into the surrounding bone metabolism and remodeling occurs easily. When used for intercalary grafts, the incidence of pseudarthrosis is high. However, if strong fixation at the bone junction is performed and a fresh autogenous bone graft is performed, bone fusion can be attained. The supply of osteogenic cells to the central portion of long grafts is insufficient, and for that reason, it is desirable to also use a free vascularized fibular graft and, in the case of large loss of soft tissue, to provide coverage with a muscle flap having good blood flow [15, 16]. In the case of composite grafts, one end is at the bone junction, while the other end is at the artificial joint junction, and the medullary cavity is occupied by the stem. Accordingly, since it is especially difficult to expect that the portion near the artificial joint junction will be integrated into the bone metabolism, resorption gradually takes place. However, because there is an intramedullary stem, stress is dispersed, and this type of graft is durable over a comparatively long time. Pelvic grafts entail a large soft tissue defect, resulting in a high risk of infection and susceptibility to resorption in the long term. Since the surgical time is long, the risk of infection is high, especially when using a composite with an artificial joint. We believe at present that pasteurized bone is not indicated for large grafts. In the case of osteoarticular grafts, one end is in soft tissue with no blood flow, and we could not expect blood vessels to infiltrate pasteurized bone. Pasteurized bone is also not indicated for load-bearing joints, since they collapse relatively soon. Even in the case of non-load-bearing joints, such as the humeral head, the indication for pasteurized bone is likely to be very limited since it would be resorbed in the long term.

References

1. Mankin HJ, Gebhardt MC, Jennings LC, Springfield DS, Tomford WW. Long-term results of allograft replacement in the management of bone tumors. Clin Orthop Relat Res. 1996;324:86–97.
2. Iwamoto Y, Sugioka Y, Chuman H, et al. Nationwide survey of bone grafting performed from 1980 through 1989 in Japan. Clin Orthop Relat Res. 1997;335:292–7.
3. Araki N, Myoui A, Kuratsu S, et al. Intraoperative extracorporeal autogenous irradiated bone grafts in tumor surgery. Clin Orthop Relat Res. 1999;368:196–206.
4. Khattak MJ, Umer M, Rasheed H, Umar M. Autoclaved tumor bone for reconstruction: an alternative in developing countries. Clin Orthop Relat Res. 2006;447:138–44.
5. Manabe J, Ahmed AR, Kawaguchi N, Matsumoto S, Kuroda H. Pasteurized autologous bone graft in surgery for bone and soft tissue sarcoma. Clin Orthop Relat Res. 2004;419:258–66.
6. Tsuchiya H, Sakurakichi K, Yamashiro, et al. Bone transport with frozen devitalized bone: an experimental study using rabbits and a clinical application. J Orthop Sci. 2004;9:619–24.
7. Auersperg N. Differential heat sensitivity of cells in tissue culture. Nature. 1996;209:415–6.
8. Rong Y, Sato K, Sugiura H, Ito T, Sakano S, Iwata H, Kimata K. Effect of elevated temperature on experimental swarm rat chondrosarcoma. Clin Orthop Relat Res. 1995;311:227–31.
9. Kode J, Taur P, Puri A, et al. Pasteurization of bone for tumour eradication prior to reimplantation – An *in vitro* and pre-clinical efficacy study. Indian J Med Res. 2014;139:585–97.
10. Kohler P, Kreicbergs A, Stromberg L. Physical properties of autoclaved bone. Torsion test of rabbit diaphyseal bone. Acta Orthop Scand. 1986;57:141–5.
11. Kreicbergs A, Kohler P. Diaphyseal reconstruction by autoclaved bone. Reimplantation experiments in rabbits. Acta Orthop Scand. 1987;58:61–5.
12. Stroosma OC, Klopper PJ, van den Hooff A. Boiled and unboiled detached autogenous bone fragments – an experimental study. Neth J Surg. 1986;38(4):112–7.

13. Manabe J. Experimental studies on pasteurized autogenous bone graft. Nihon Seikeigeka Gakkai Zasshi (J Jpn Orthop Assoc). 1993;67:255–66 (in Japanese).
14. Kubo T, Sugita T, Shimose S, et al. Histological findings in a human autogenous pasteurized bone graft. Anticancer Res. 2004;24(3b):1893–6.
15. Sugiura H, Yamamura S, Sato K, et al. Remodelling and healing process of moderately heat-treated bone grafts after wide resection of bone and soft-tissue tumors. Arch Orthop Trauma Surg. 2003;123:514–20.
16. Nishida Y, Tsukushi S, Wasa J, et al. Vascularized fibular flaps enhance histological repair in pasteurized autogenous bone graft. Ann Plast Surg. 2011;67:416–20.

Biological Reconstruction for Extremity Osteosarcoma: Liquid Nitrogen-Treated Tumor-Bearing Bone Graft

15

Hiroyuki Tsuchiya and Norio Yamamoto

Abstract

Reconstruction using liquid nitrogen-treated tumor-bearing bone has been utilized clinically since 1999 after its safety was confirmed by basic research. It provides several advantages: simplicity, osteoinduction, osteoconduction, short treatment time, optimal fit, sufficient biochemical strength, contagion-free, easy attachment of tendons and ligaments, and cryoimmunological activity. Time-dependent histological revitalization is also observed in frozen bone. There are two methods using liquid nitrogen-treated autografts: the pedicle freezing method and the free freezing method. The pedicle freezing method involves the dislocation of the joint proximal to the tumor or the use of osteotomy. The distal portion maintains continuity with the body in a pedicle form, and the affected bone is inverted and liquid nitrogen treatment is performed. The free freezing method involves resection and temporary removal of the affected bone and its treatment with liquid nitrogen. Satisfactory union can be achieved using liquid nitrogen-treated bone, and good clinical outcomes have been obtained in the midterm and long term without any case of recurrence from the treated bone. Reconstruction using liquid nitrogen-treated bone is a useful reconstruction method after resection of osteosarcoma.

Keywords

Biological reconstruction • Liquid nitrogen • Tumor-bearing bone • Pedicle freezing method • Free freezing method

H. Tsuchiya (✉) • N. Yamamoto
Department of Orthopedic Surgery, Graduate school of Medical Sciences, Kanazawa University, 13-1 Takaramachi, Kanazawa 920-8641, Japan
e-mail: tsuchi@med.kanazawa-u.ac.jp

T. Ueda, A. Kawai (eds.), *Osteosarcoma*, DOI 10.1007/978-4-431-55696-1_15

15.1 Introduction

Before the 1970s, the 5-year survival for osteosarcoma was approximately 10–20 % [1]. Its therapeutic outcomes improved greatly with the introduction of chemotherapy. Emergency amputation of the affected limb had been a common treatment for osteosarcoma until the introduction of chemotherapy. Today limb-sparing surgery has become a standard surgical method due to advancement in multidisciplinary treatment. In addition, efforts in biological reconstruction have actively been made not only to spare the limbs but also to improve the quality of life of patients and to better preserve the function of the limbs [2, 3].

There are various methods for reconstruction in limb salvage. Reconstruction using a tumor prosthesis is more commonly performed among these methods and is useful in the recovery of affected limb function in the early stages of treatment. However, a tumor prosthesis is an artificial object and its physiological repair does not occur in the body. Thus, the durability of artificial materials becomes a problem in the long term, and many patients inevitably undergo revision due to loose or damaged prostheses. Soft tissues such as muscles and ligaments play a major role in the function of the affected limb function. Since artificial materials are not expected to biointegrate into such soft tissues, a major problem is the reconstruction of soft tissue attachments.

Reconstruction of affected limbs using biological reconstruction has been sought to overcome the aforementioned problems. Such biological reconstruction uses materials such as distracted autologous bone, allogeneic bone, and treated autologous bone. In general, reconstruction is often performed using allogeneic bone. In Japan, allogeneic bone is difficult to obtain due to issues related to social and religious views. Thus, a biological reconstruction method has been used in which the patient's affected bone is treated and used for reconstruction. The treatments used to date include irradiation, autoclave treatment, and pasteurization. These treatment methods have issues such as requiring complicated techniques and temperature control and special devices. We sought to examine if affected bone can be subjected to cryotreatment and confirmed the safety and bone strength after such treatment [4, 5]. Subsequently in 1999, we began clinical application of tumor-bearing autografts treated with liquid nitrogen [6].

There are several favorable characteristics of liquid nitrogen treatment. It uses simple surgical techniques without complicated temperature control. There is optimal morphological fit because the treated bone itself is one's own, and bone strength is maintained after treatment. Satisfactory bone union and bone regeneration are expected to be achieved due to good osteoconduction and osteoinduction because proteins and enzymes are preserved in the bone. In addition, when liquid nitrogen treatment is used, re-suturing of soft tissues such as ligaments is simpler than for prosthesis, and there is satisfactory reattachment of ligaments and muscle tissues to the treated bone.

Over 100 cases to date have undergone this procedure in our hospital alone. Good clinical outcomes have been achieved without any case of recurrence from the treated bone itself. There have been reports on treated bone that regenerated into living bone. Histological studies have been performed on liquid nitrogen-treated bone excised due to complications such as postoperative infection. These studies have shown satisfactory bone union and bone regeneration in vivo in humans [7–9].

There are two methods using liquid nitrogen-treated autografts: the pedicle freezing method [10] and the free freezing method [6]. The pedicle freezing method involves the dislocation of the joint proximal to the tumor or the use of osteotomy. The distal portion maintains continuity with the body in a pedicle form, and the affected bone is inverted and liquid nitrogen treatment is performed. The free freezing method involves resection and temporary removal of the affected bone and its treatment with liquid nitrogen. Subsequently, it is returned to the body. To successfully perform these surgeries, surgeons need to prevent intraoperative tumor contamination and bone fracture during the freezing process and to achieve rigid fixation of the treated autograft during reconstruction. This paper discusses reconstructive surgeries using the pedicle freezing method and the free freezing method involving liquid nitrogen-treated autografts in osteosarcoma (malignant bone tumor) patients.

15.2 Pedicle Freezing Method

The pedicle freezing method is very useful to decrease the numbers of osteotomy site and to achieve favorable bone union (Fig. 15.1a–d) [11]. The exposure of the surgical field is performed in accordance with the principle for wide resection. Care

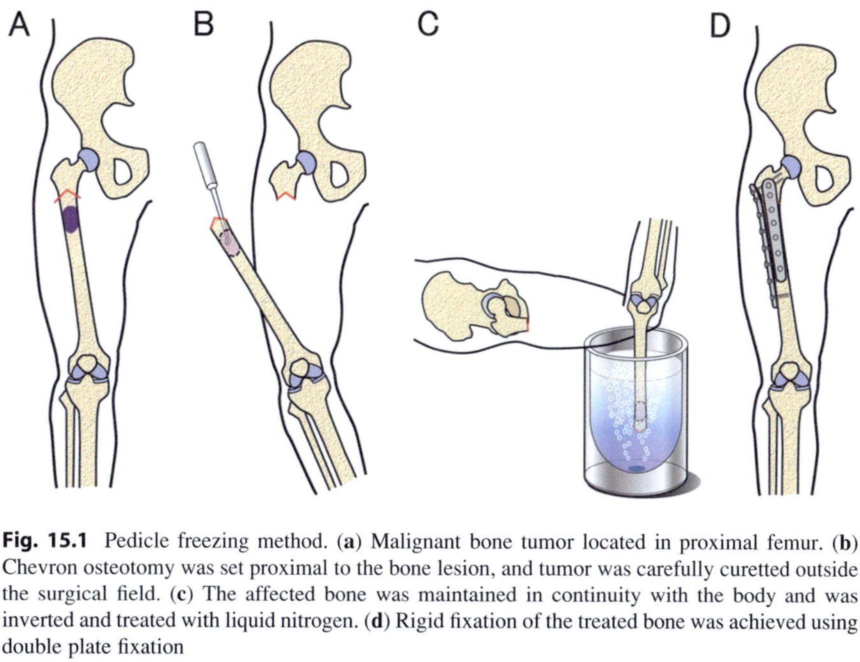

Fig. 15.1 Pedicle freezing method. (**a**) Malignant bone tumor located in proximal femur. (**b**) Chevron osteotomy was set proximal to the bone lesion, and tumor was carefully curetted outside the surgical field. (**c**) The affected bone was maintained in continuity with the body and was inverted and treated with liquid nitrogen. (**d**) Rigid fixation of the treated bone was achieved using double plate fixation

is taken to avoid exposure of the tumor, and the exposure of the surgical field is performed with excision of the biopsy tract and surrounding soft tissue attached to the tumor area. The osteotomy site is set at 2 cm proximal to the bone lesion, and chevron osteotomy is performed using tools such as a microsagittal saw. It is important to perform chevron osteotomy to prevent abnormal rotation during reconstruction and to increase the contact area for bone union. Bone is elevated from the osteotomy site. In the distal area, the soft tissue is detached from the bone up to approximately 5 cm distal to the site planned for freezing to prevent damage to normal soft tissue during liquid nitrogen treatment. An electrocautery knife or a surgical skin marker is used to mark the location that is planned to be immersed in liquid nitrogen. The site planned for freezing is elevated and then a tourniquet is applied to the affected limb. The use of a tourniquet is important to prevent bleeding during curettage and to prevent distant dissemination of tumor cells.

The base of the elevated bone is protected using cotton for cast padding or an Esmarch bandage, which is wrapped around the soft tissue to prevent damage to normal tissue when freezing. Two to three clean surgical sheets are passed through the pedicle, and the hole through which they are placed is closed using tape. The pedicle is tilted during curettage to enable the curetted tumor not to fall onto a sheet as much as possible. Carefully, curettage is performed and bone tunnels are created. This procedure is important to prevent fracture of the affected bone as blood and tumor tissue expand with freezing. Before the freezing process, a Kirschner wire can be used to place a few small holes into the bone that is to be treated. When the top surgical sheet that is passed through the pedicle is removed after curettage, the affected limb needs to be supported firmly so that the elevated bone does not contact the surrounding sheet. The basic materials needed for nitrogen treatment are a sterilized vacuum flask (Dewar flask) and liquid nitrogen. About 15–20 L of liquid nitrogen should be available, a volume sufficient to immerse the affected bone. The boiling point of liquid nitrogen is very low at −196 °C, and, thus, there is no concern about temperature control during the treatment. In the freezing procedure, it must be confirmed that the bone is immersed in liquid nitrogen up to the marked area while treating it in liquid nitrogen for 20 min. During this process, one should confirm that normal tissue does not freeze such as by placing one's fingers between the affected limb and the rim of the Dewar flask. After freezing, the treated bone is slowly removed from the Dewar flask by raising the operating table. The surgical sheet that has been passed through the pedicle is removed carefully. The bone is thawed at room temperature for 15 min and then thawed in 30 °C distilled water for about 15 min. If the bone defect caused by curettage of the tumor is large, it should be filled using autologous bone, artificial bone, or bone cement to maintain the strength of the treated bone.

Rigid fixation of the treated bone is achieved using double plate fixation or intramedullary nail-plate fixation while taking care not to cause rotation or create a gap in the osteotomy site. In the osteotomy site, bone union is promoted in the junction between the treated bone and host bone and in some cases by bone grafting at the junction. In pedicle freezing method, good bone union is achieved. The soft tissue is thought to be important in the stability of the joint and functional recovery of the affected limb. After fixation of the treated bone, the soft tissue is sutured to the attachment site that has been left as much as possible on the treated bone or it is reattached to the treated bone using screws with washers. A drain must always be placed. Subcutaneous suture is carefully performed and the wound is closed.

In the pedicle freezing method, the affected bone can be treated with liquid nitrogen by dislocation of the joint without osteotomy in some cases. In such cases, it is not necessary to wait for bone union, and weight-bearing walk can begin a few days after surgery. If both pedicle freezing method and free freezing method are indicated for a patient, we prefer the pedicle freezing method.

15.3 Free Freezing Method

The free freezing method is very useful in surgery such as when hemicortical resection is performed and when the lesion is near the articular surface (Figs. 15.2a–c). In the pedicle freezing method, it is difficult to precisely control the extent of the area to be frozen. The free freezing method avoids damage to the articular surface due to freezing. When freezing an area that includes the articular surface, chondrocytes die even though articular cartilage matrix is initially preserved. Thus, arthropathic changes occur over time. If freezing that includes the articular surface is desired, a useful method to be performed first is reconstruction using a composite graft, a combination of liquid nitrogen-treated bone and artificial joint or artificial head. For the treatment of articular surface, a patient consultation needs to be performed preoperatively regarding whether or not to use a two-stage approach in the future.

Hemicortical resection is indicated in cases where a malignant soft tissue tumor has invaded a part of the hemicortical cortex or in cases that have achieved

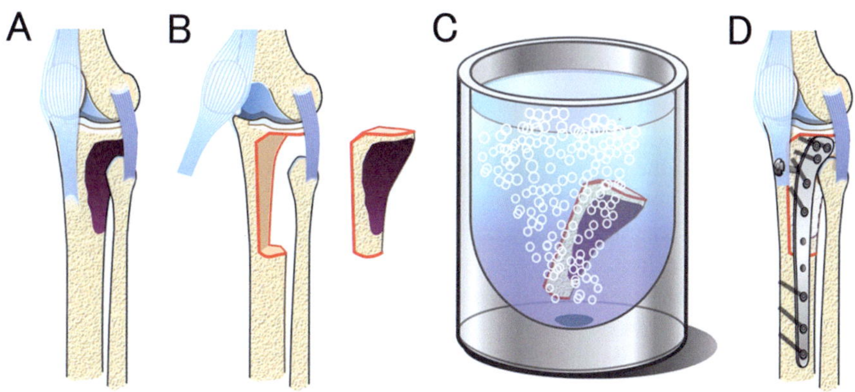

Fig. 15.2 Free freezing method. (**a**) Malignant bone tumor located in hemicortical proximal tibia. (**b**) Hemicortical resection was performed and articular surface was preserved. (**c**) Affected bone was temporarily removed and treated with liquid nitrogen. (**d**) Treated bone was returned to the original site and patella tendon was reattached

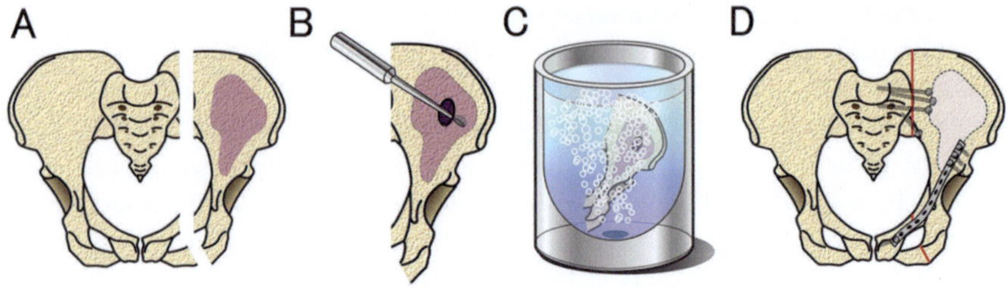

Fig. 15.3 Free freezing method. (**a**) Malignant bone tumor located in pelvis. (**b**) Hemipelvectomy was performed and tumor was curetted at another sterile table. (**c**) Resected bone was treated with liquid nitrogen. (**d**) Bone cavity was supplemented with antibiotic-loaded bone cement, and the treated bone was returned to the original site

complete response to chemotherapy even with a malignant tumor and in which the lesion is confined unilaterally in the bone. When hemicortical resection is used, satisfactory bone union tends to occur if the contact area of the treated bone to the host bone is large and rigid fixation of the treated bone is obtained. In particular, when the tumor is near the articular surface, hemicortical resection is a good surgical method [12]. It enables reconstruction with preservation of the articular surface and without the use of tumor prosthesis. Thus, postoperative function of the affected limb is nearly normal.

The free freezing method is also useful in reconstruction of the pelvic area where pedicle freezing cannot be performed (Figs. 15.3a–d).

15.4 Future of Reconstruction Using Liquid Nitrogen-Treated Bone

The procedure is simple in reconstruction using liquid nitrogen-treated bone. If surgeons learn small skills of these techniques, this procedure can be used in many institutions. However, surgeons need to be most cautious about a fracture when freezing the bone. That is, since the rate of expansion differs among different materials such as the bone, tumor, and blood, surgeons need to be very careful when freezing the bone. It is important to perform careful curettage of the tumor area or to create bone tunnels using a Kirschner wire to prevent a bone fracture. When surgeons become familiar with the procedure, bone fractures rarely occur. However, it is important to be prepared to use cable system or tumor prosthesis. Satisfactory union can be achieved using liquid nitrogen-treated bone, and good outcomes have been obtained in the midterm and long term. [13] These results suggest that there are factors that act favorably for bone union, including sufficient strength of the liquid nitrogen-treated bone in the early stages and optimal fit and a large contact area between the host bone and the reconstructed bone. In recent years, tumor immunity with the use of frozen tissue has gained interest, and more powerful immunotherapy used in combination with dendritic cell therapy is being developed [14, 15]. Reconstruction using liquid nitrogen-treated bone is a useful reconstruction method after resection of osteosarcoma.

References

1. Friedman MA, Carter SK. The therapy of osteogenic sarcoma- current status and thoughts for the future. J Surg Oncol. 1972;4:482–510.
2. Tsuchiya H, Tomita K, Mori Y, et al. Marginal excision for osteosarcoma with caffeine assisted chemotherapy. Clin Orthop Relat Res. 1999;358:27–35.
3. Kanazawa Y, Tsuchiya H, Nonomura A, et al. Intentional marginal excision of osteosarcoma of the proximal fibula to preserve limb function. J Orthop Sci. 2003;8:757–61.
4. Yamamoto N. Experimental study for reconstruction using liquid nitrogen treated tumor bearing bone. Juzen Gakkaishi. 2000;109:193–202.
5. Yamamoto N, Tsuchiya H, Tomita K. Effects of liquid nitrogen treatment on the proliferation of osteosarcoma and the biomechanical properties of normal bone. J Orthop Sci. 2003;8:374–80.
6. Tsuchiya H, Wan SL, Sakayama K, et al. Reconstruction using an autograft containing tumour treated by liquid nitrogen. J Bone Joint Surg (Br). 2005;87:218–25.
7. Sakayama K, Tsuchiya H, Fujibuchi T, Kidani T, Tanji N, Yamamoto H. Pathological findings of an autograft containing osteosarcoma treated by liquid nitrogen retrieved 2 years after implantation. J Orthop Sci. 2006;11:655–6.
8. Tanzawa Y, Tsuchiya H, Shirai T, Hayashi K, Yo Z, Tomita K. Histological examination of frozen autograft treated by liquid nitrogen removed after implantation. J Orthop Sci. 2009;14:761–8.
9. Yamamoto N, Inatani H, Shirai T, et al. Histological study on liquid nitrogen-treated tumor-bearing bone of the proximal femur excised eight years after transplantation. Low Temp Med. 2012;38:5–8.
10. Tsuchiya H, Nishida H, Srisawat P, et al. Pedicle frozen autograft reconstruction in malignant bone tumors. J Orthop Sci. 2010;15:340–9.
11. Shimozaki S, Yamamoto N, Shirai T, et al. Pedicle versus free frozen autograft for reconstruction in malignant bone and soft tissue tumors of the lower extremities. J Orthop Sci. 2014;19:156–63.
12. Chen WM, Wu PK, Chen CF, et al. High-grade osteosarcoma treated with hemicortical resection and biological reconstruction. J Surg Oncol. 2011;105:825–9.
13. Igarashi K, Yamamoto N, Shirai T, et al. The long-term outcome following the use of frozen autograft treated with liquid nitrogen in the management of bone and soft-tissue sarcomas. Bone Joint J. 2014;96-B:555–61.
14. Nishida H, Shirai T, Hayashi K, et al. Cryotreatment against metastatic renal cell bone tumour reduced multiple lung metastases. Anticancer Res. 2011;31:2927–30.
15. Nishida H, Yamamoto N, Tanzawa Y, et al. Cryoimmunology for malignant bone and soft-tissue tumors. Int J Clin Oncol. 2011;16:109–17.

Biological Reconstruction for Extremity Osteosarcoma: Distraction Osteogenesis Technique

16

Hidenori Matsubara and Hiroyuki Tsuchiya

Abstract

Prior to the 1970s, amputation or disarticulation was the standard treatment for malignant bone tumors in pediatric patients. Limb-sparing surgeries are now standard treatment due to multidisciplinary advancements in areas including radiological evaluation, chemotherapy, surgical techniques, implant technology, and tumor biology. Reconstruction methods of limb salvage include allograft, endoprostheses, and recycled autografts such as autoclaved bone and irradiated bone. However, limb function remains limited and deteriorates over time. When subsequent complications such as deep infection, fracture, and implant failure occur, it is likely that amputation or disarticulation will be eventually performed to solve problems. Therefore, biological reconstruction using distraction osteogenesis or frozen autograft was newly developed to obtain better limb function and reduce complications for bone tumor reconstruction. Our goal of limb-sparing surgery is the normalization of the affected limb in function and appearance. Based on this concept, we first performed and have been continuing biological reconstruction using a distraction osteogenesis technique and massive frozen tumor-bearing bone treated with liquid nitrogen.

In this chapter, we introduce our original biological reconstruction procedure using distraction osteogenesis for osteosarcoma according to our classification (Type I–VI) based on tumor site, size, and response to chemotherapy. Cases indicated for joint preservation with the distraction osteogenesis method should have tumors of Types I–IV according to our classification system, not more than 15 cm in length (resulting in a treatment time of less than 1 year), and with a good response to chemotherapy. Types V and VI are indicated for arthrodesis with distraction osteogenesis. The frozen autograft method can be applied to all types (in Chap. 15).

H. Matsubara • H. Tsuchiya (✉)
Kanazawa University Hospital, 13-1, Takara-machi, Kanazawa, Ishikawa 920-8641, Japan
e-mail: tsuchi@med.kanazawa-u.ac.jp

T. Ueda, A. Kawai (eds.), *Osteosarcoma*, DOI 10.1007/978-4-431-55696-1_16

Keywords
External fixator • Distraction osteogenesis • Bone transport

16.1 Introduction

There are various kinds of malignant bone tumors in pediatrics. Osteosarcoma is the most common primary malignant bone tumor in children. Prior to the 1970s, amputation or joint disarticulations were the standard treatment and the only choice of treatment. However, now over 90 % of osteosarcoma resections are limb-sparing surgeries due to advancements in chemotherapy, medical imaging, and implant technology [1–3]. Options for limb salvage reconstruction after wide resection include osteoarticular allografts, allograft prosthetic composites, recycled autograft, and modular or custom-made endoprostheses. However, the limb function often remains limited and deteriorates over time. Complications such as infections, nonunion of grafts, and bone resorption could eventually lead to amputation. Therefore, the aim of biological reconstruction is to achieve better limbs and almost normal limb function and to reduce complications.

We first performed transepiphyseal osteotomy and resected a malignant bone tumor followed by reconstruction using the distraction osteogenesis technique (DO method) [4–6] and massive frozen tumor-bearing bone treated with liquid nitrogen (LN method) [7, 8]. In this chapter, we introduce our original biological reconstruction procedures using DO method for osteosarcoma.

16.2 Indication

To facilitate decision-making for reconstruction in cases of juxta-articular osteosarcoma around the knee joint, we developed a new system for classifying tumor excision (Table 16.1, Fig. 16.1) [9]. Cases indicated for the DO method should have tumors of Types I–IV according to our classification system, no more than a 15 cm defect after the tumor resection (resulting in a treatment time of less than 1 year), and with a good response to chemotherapy. Theoretically, the DO method can be applied even in cases with Types V and VI tumors combined with arthrodesis. Currently, however, it has been replaced with the LN method (in Chap. 15). The LN method can be indicated in all cases. For chemotherapy responders, this enables preservation of the maximum amount of healthy tissue, such as soft tissue, growth plates, and joint surfaces, to provide excellent limb function [3].

Table 16.1 Resection types for reconstruction decision-making

Type I: Tumor at diaphyseal location or metaphyseal location over 2 cm far from the epiphyseal plate
Type II: Tumor at metaphyseal location extending to less than half of the epiphyseal growth plate
Type III: Tumor at metaphyseal location extending to the whole growth plate
Type IV: Metaphyseal tumor extending through the growth plate into part of the epiphysis at least 1 cm from the articular surface
Type V: Tumor extending into less than half of the epiphysis less than 1 cm away from the articular surface
Type VI: Tumor extending into more than half of the epiphysis less than 1 cm away from the articular surface

16.3 Surgical Techniques

16.3.1 Type I (Fig. 16.2)

In Type I, the tumor is diaphyseally or metaphyseally located over 2 cm far from the epiphyseal plate. The operative technique of the DO method consists of en bloc tumor excision with preservation of the epiphyseal plate and articular surface. An external fixator is applied and osteotomy is performed for postoperative bone transport. After docking bone transport, we usually perform bone graft at the docking site. Shortening-distraction is indicated if acute shortening is possible during the operation. Optional intramedullary nailing, if feasible, or plate conversion, are also used to shorten the external fixation time [4, 6].

16.3.2 Type II (Fig. 16.3)

In Type II, the tumor is located metaphyseally and extends to less than half of the epiphyseal growth plate. There is also a possibility of joint deformity due to unequal growth after reconstruction. The operative technique of the DO method consists of hemicortical en bloc tumor excision. An external fixator is applied, and proximal hemicortical osteotomy is performed for postoperative bone transport. Epiphysiodesis of the other side of the growth plate is one option to avoid future angular deformities for young patients. After docking bone transport, we usually perform a bone graft at the docking site. At that time, plate conversion is optionally used to shorten the external fixation time. If a deformity occurs in the future, correction with or without lengthening can be performed.

16.3.3 Type III (Fig. 16.4)

In Type III, the tumor is metaphyseally located and extends to the whole growth plate. Limb length discrepancies are anticipated in immature patients, which may

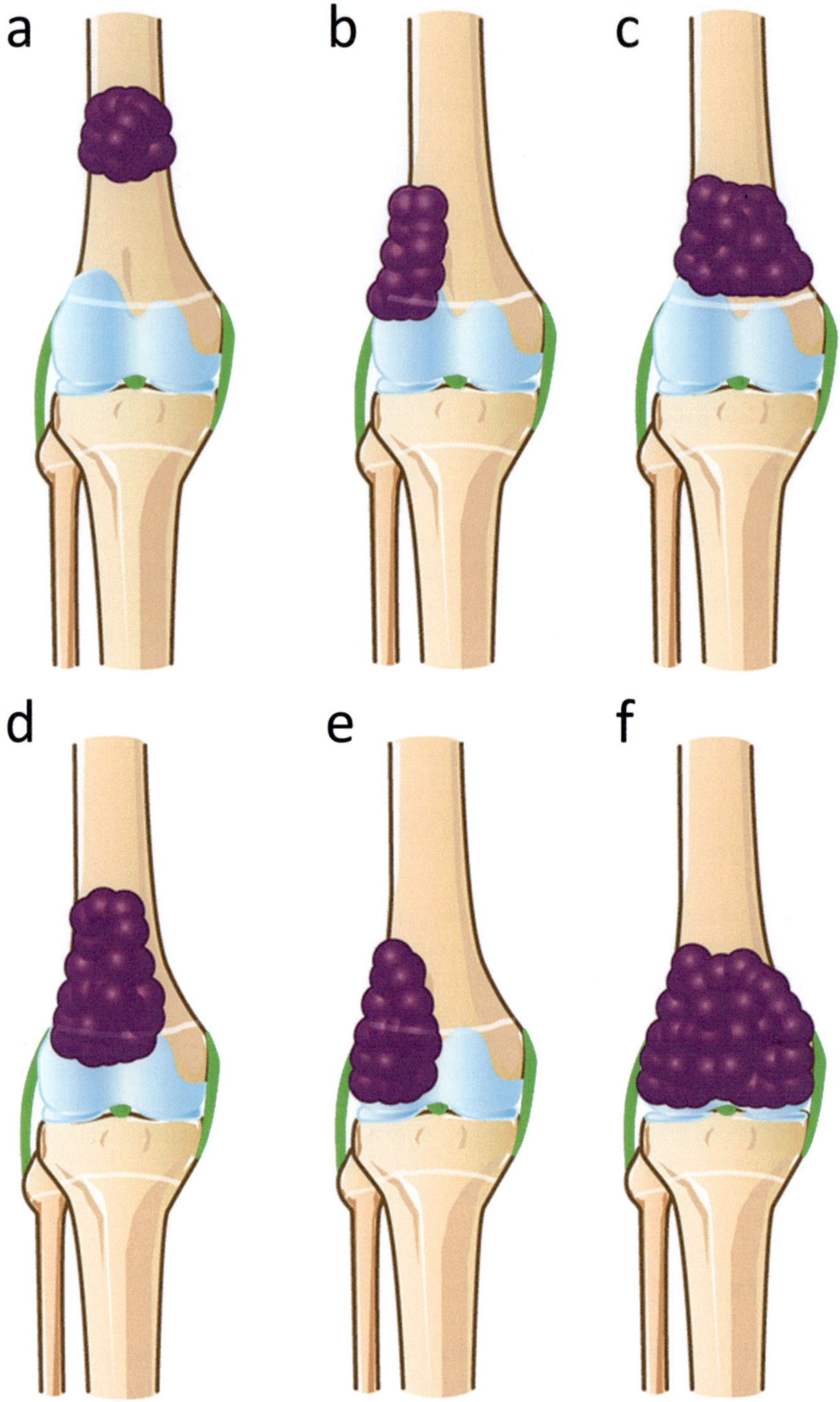

Fig. 16.1 Classification of tumor excision. (**a**) Type I. (**b**) Type II. (**c**)Type III. (**d**) Type IV. (**e**) Type V. (**f**) Type VI

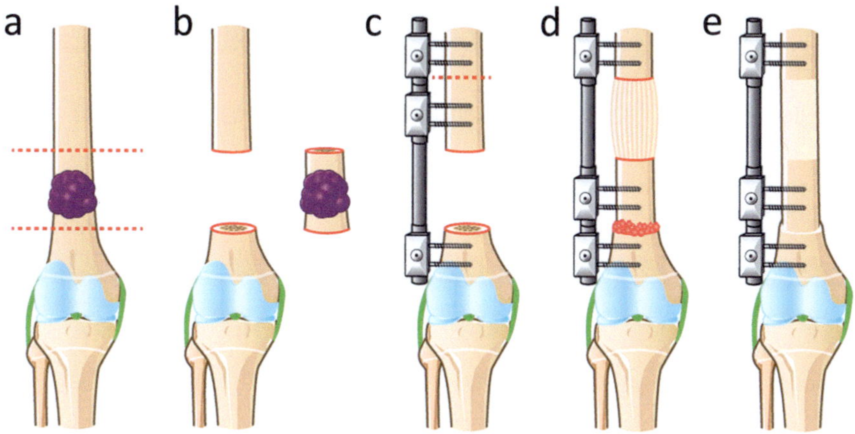

Fig. 16.2 Type I: surgical method. (**a**) Resection line. (**b**) Tumor resection. (**c**) Application of external fixator and osteotomy for lengthening. (**d**) Bone grafting at docking site. (**e**) After bone consolidation

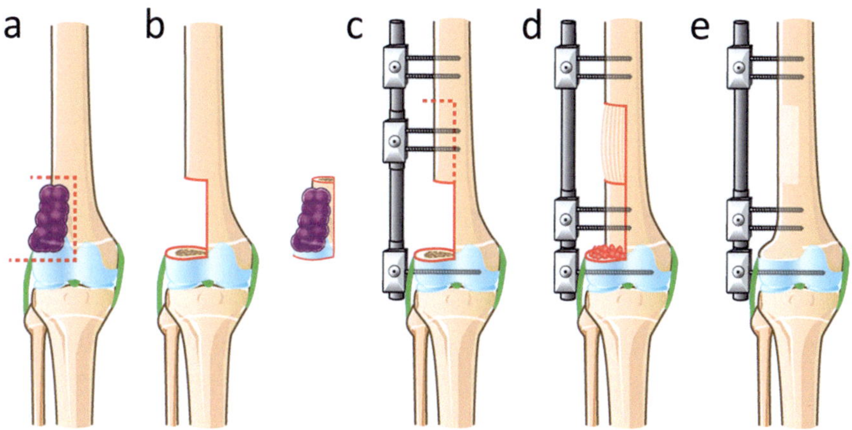

Fig. 16.3 Type II: surgical method. (**a**) Resection line. (**b**) Tumor resection. (**c**) Application of external fixator and osteotomy for lengthening. (**d**) Bone grafting at docking site. (**e**) After bone consolidation

be managed surgically if necessary. The operative technique of the DO method consists of transepiphyseal and intercalary en bloc tumor excision with the growth plate. Surgical technique is basically same as in the Type I DO method.

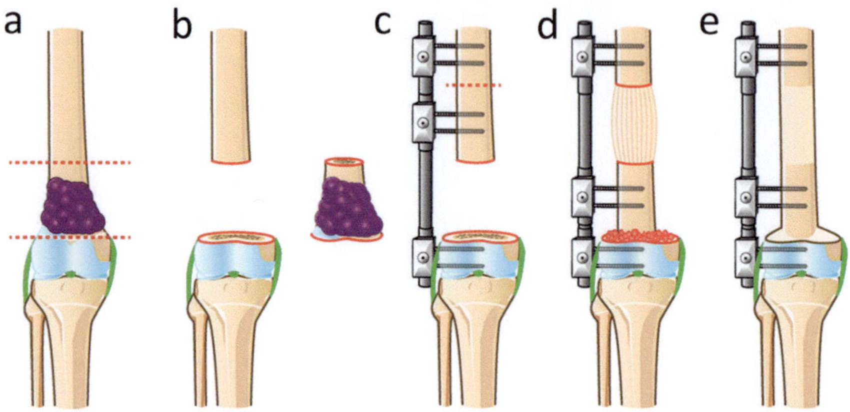

Fig. 16.4 Type III: surgical method. (**a**) Resection line. (**b**) Tumor resection. (**c**) Application of external fixator and osteotomy for lengthening. (**d**) Bone grafting at docking site. (**e**) After bone consolidation

16.3.4 Type IV (Fig. 16.5)

In Type IV, the tumor is metaphyseally located and extends to the whole growth plate into part of the epiphysis at least 1 cm away from the joint line. Limb length discrepancies are anticipated in immature patients, which may be managed surgically if necessary. The operative technique of the DO method consists of transepiphyseal and intercalary en bloc tumor excision with the growth plate and with preservation of the articular surface. The periarticular structure should be stabilized immediately to prevent joint contracture. If only a thin epiphysis or articular surface is preserved, a free bone cylinder should be taken from the diaphysis and fixed to the remaining epiphysis with a bone graft and a spike washer and screw, in order to stabilize and reconstruct the periarticular structure. The newly created diaphyseal defect is restored by bone transport. If feasible, optional plate conversion is also used.

16.3.5 Types V and VI (Fig. 16.6)

In Type V, the tumor extends into less than half of the epiphysis. In Type VI, the tumor extends into more than half of the epiphysis. There is no possibility of preservation of the original joint. There is a possibility of deformity and limb length discrepancy after reconstruction. Types V and VI are indicated for knee arthrodesis with distraction osteogenesis. However, the operations for these types are replaced by frozen autograft method with liquid nitrogen (in Chap. 15). The operative technique with DO consists of en bloc tumor excision with the growth plate and articular joint. An external fixator is applied and osteotomy is performed for postoperative bone transport. After docking bone transport, we usually perform

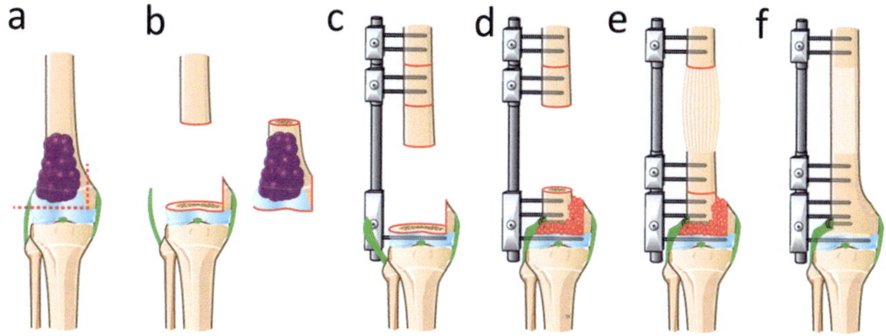

Fig. 16.5 Type IV: surgical method. (**a**) Resection line. (**b**) Tumor resection. (**c**) Application of external fixator and osteotomy for lengthening. (**d**) Reconstruction of periarticular structure with diaphyseal bone cylinder. (**e**) After docking. (**f**) After bone consolidation

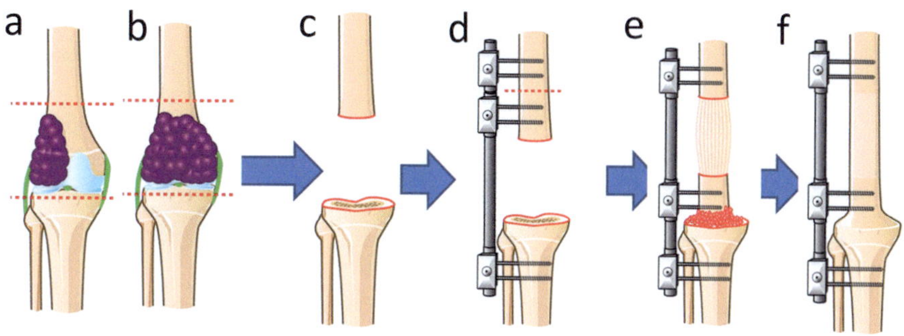

Fig. 16.6 Type V, VI: surgical method. (**a, b**) Resection line. (**c**) Tumor excision. (**d**) Application of external fixator and osteotomy for bone transport. (**e**) Bone grafting at docking site (knee arthrodesis). (**f**) After bone consolidation

bone graft at the docking site. Shortening-distraction is indicated if acute shortening is possible during the operation. Optional plate conversion is also used to shorten the external fixation time.

16.4 Example Cases

16.4.1 Case 1 (Fig. 16.7)

A 17-year-old boy presented with osteosarcoma of the proximal tibia. Neoadjuvant caffeine-potentiated chemotherapy was administered, and the clinical effect was a complete response with significant ossification of the soft tissue mass of the lateral tibia. We planned intercalary resection and reconstruction with the DO method (bone transport). After the operation, gradual lengthening was started and bone

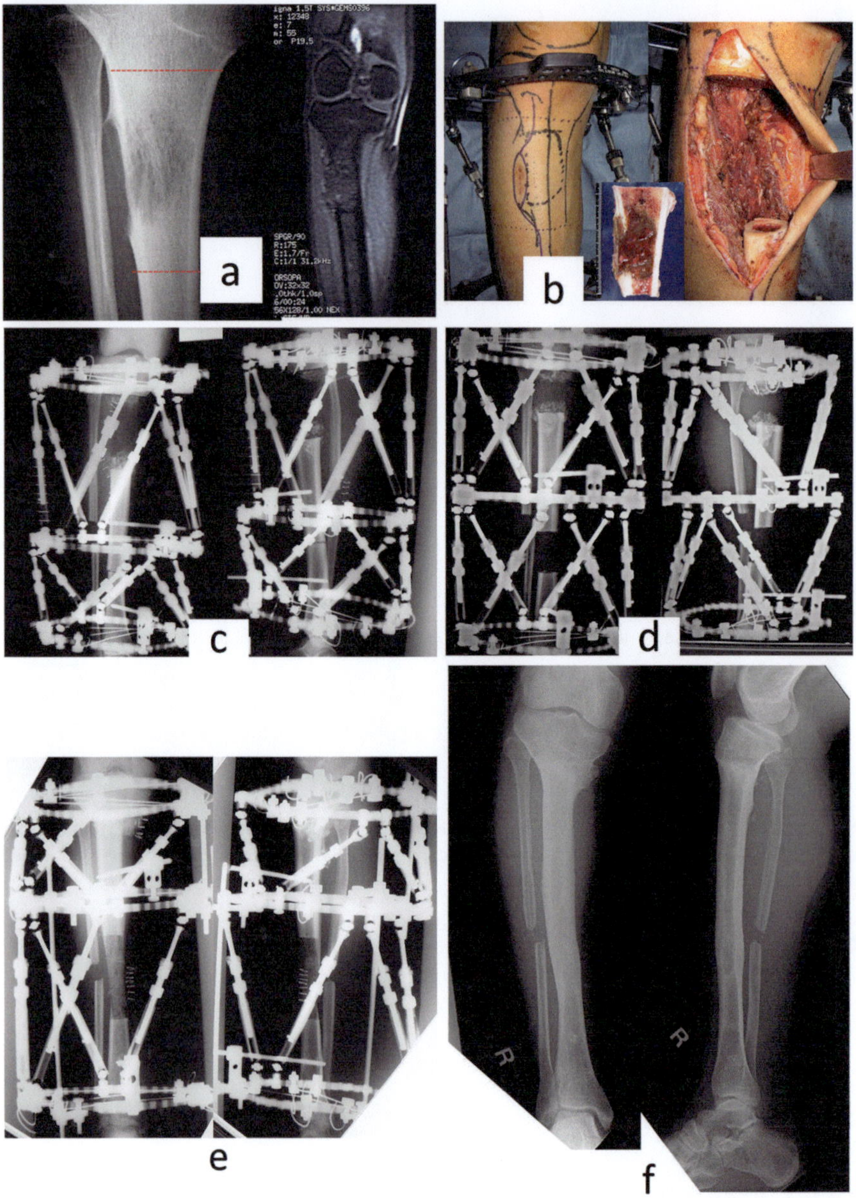

Fig. 16.7 Case (Type 1): A 17-year-old boy with an osteosarcoma of the proximal tibia. (**a**) Preoperative X-ray and MRI scan. Osteotomy line (*broken lines*). (**b**) After tumor resection with intercalary osteotomies. (**c**) X-ray after the operation. (**d**) X-ray during bone transport. (**e**) X-ray at the complication of docking of bone transporter. (**f**) X-ray at 26 months after the operation

Table 16.2 Advantages and disadvantages of DO method

Advantage	Disadvantage
Living bone regeneration	Lengthy external fixation
Sufficient strength	Patients burden
Biological affinity	Pin-track infection
Resistance against infection	Delayed consolidation
Life-long restored function	Delayed union of docking site

transporter docking was completed. As of the 26 month of follow-up, the patient is free of disease and can run without any pain.

16.5 Summary

In summary, we introduced limb salvage surgery for reconstruction after tumor resection using distraction osteogenesis, according to the tumor site, size, and response to chemotherapy. The advantages of the DO method include regeneration of living bone with sufficient strength and durability, biological affinity, resistance against infection, and lifelong restored function. The disadvantages include delayed union at the docking site and pin- or wire-tract infection, as well as the fact that the procedure is time-consuming (Table 16.2). Possible complications with the DO method include pin site infection managed with antibiotics or removal of pins, docking site nonunion or delayed union, and delayed consolidation of regenerated tissue treated with bone graft. There are two important points in obtaining better functional results when either method is selected: firstly, the surgeon should try to preserve the epiphysis if possible and secondly, it should be attempted to perform biological reconstruction as much as possible.

In the future, there may be greater use of biological reconstruction methods to obtain better and earlier functional results, because a natural limb is the best option. To achieve this, we have to aim to facilitate bone regeneration and revitalization much faster and to adopt biological soft tissue reconstruction, through advances in tissue engineering, such as with regard to osteogenic and angiogenic growth factors or with stem cell implantation.

References

1. Tomita K, Tsuchiya H. Intermediate results and functional evaluation of limb-salvage surgery for osteosarcoma: an intergroup study in Japan. J Surg Oncol. 1989;41(2):71–6.
2. Tsuchiya H, Tomita K. Prognosis of osteosarcoma treated by limb-salvage surgery: the ten-year intergroup study in Japan. Jpn J Clin Oncol. 1992;22(5):347–53.
3. Tsuchiya H, Tomita K, Mori Y, Asada N, Yamamoto N. Marginal excision for osteosarcoma with caffeine assisted chemotherapy. Clin Orthop Relat Res. 1999;358:27–35.

4. Tsuchiya H, Tomita K, Minematsu K, Mori Y, Asada N, Kitano S. Limb salvage using distraction osteogenesis. A classification of the technique. J Bone Joint Surg (Br). 1997;79 (3):403–11.
5. Tsuchiya H, Tomita K, Shinokawa Y, Minematsu K, Katsuo S, Taki J. The Ilizarov method in the management of giant-cell tumours of the proximal tibia. J Bone Joint Surg (Br). 1996;78 (2):264–9.
6. Tsuchiya H, Abdel-Wanis M, Kitano S, Sakurakichi K, Yamashiro T, Tomita K. The natural limb is best: joint preservation and reconstruction by distraction osteogenesis for high-grade juxta-articular osteosarcomas. Anticancer Res. 2002;22(4):2373–6.
7. Tsuchiya H, Wan SL, Sakayama K, Yamamoto N, Nishida H, Tomita K. Reconstruction using an autograft containing tumour treated by liquid nitrogen. J Bone Joint Surg (Br). 2005;87:218–25.
8. Tsuchiya H, Nishida H, Srisawat P, Shirai T, Hayashi K, Takeuchi A, et al. Pedicle frozen autograft reconstruction in malignant bone tumors. J Orthop Sci. 2010;15(3):340–9.
9. Tsuchiya H, Abdel-Wanis ME, Tomita K. Biological reconstruction after excision of juxta-articular osteosarcoma around the knee: a new classification system. Anticancer Res. 2006;26 (1B):447–53.

Limb-Saving Surgery Using In Situ Preparation (ISP) Method

17

Seiichi Matsumoto and Keisuke Ae

Abstract

Background: In situ preparation (ISP) makes it possible to intraoperatively prepare the neurovascular bundle and eventually evaluate the surgical margin without contamination of tumor cells. ISP was applied to locally advanced osteosarcoma of distal femur for limb salvage.

Methods: The tumor and femoral vessels are lifted en bloc from the surgical bed and separated from the operation field by the use of a vinyl sheet. The consistency of the vessels is preserved. The en bloc mass can be freely turned around and the femoral vessels are separated from the block through the nearest approach. The margin between the tumor and femoral vessels is evaluated and an additional procedure, such as alcohol soaking or distilled water soaking, is performed.

Results: Seven cases with locally advanced osteosarcoma of distal femur were operated on using this method. No local recurrences were found.

The advantage of ISP is no risk of contamination of tumor cells. Because there is no need of special equipment, this procedure can be easily done throughout the world.

Keywords

In situ preparation (ISP) • Osteosarcoma • Limb-salvage surgery

S. Matsumoto, M.D., Ph.D. (✉) • K. Ae, M.D., Ph.D.
Department of Orthopedic Oncology, Cancer Institute Ariake Hospital, 3-8-31 Ariake, Koto-ku, Tokyo 135-8550, Japan
e-mail: smatsumoto@jfcr.or.jp

T. Ueda, A. Kawai (eds.), *Osteosarcoma*, DOI 10.1007/978-4-431-55696-1_17

17.1 Background

When bone sarcomas occur near major neurovascular structures, preoperative images cannot always show the accurate relationship between the tumor and the structures. In cases of osteosarcoma of distal femur arising near femoral vessels, femoral vessels are sacrificed to ensure appropriate surgical margin and good curability, which however leads to poor functional results. On the other hand, the preservation of such vessels can result in an inappropriate margin. Therefore, accurate information about the relationship between the tumor and the surrounding tissue is required; however, such information cannot always be obtained even by using the most sophisticated imaging tools including MRI, CT scan, and angiography. Consequently, we tried a new surgical method, namely, in situ preparation (ISP), which was initially performed for soft tissue sarcoma. The ISP procedure makes it possible to intraoperatively prepare the nerve and vessels and eventually evaluate the surgical margin without tumor cell contamination. Furthermore, based on the determined surgical margin, an additional procedure can be carried out by soaking the surface of neurovascular structure with alcohol or distilled water in order to ensure curability.

17.2 Cases

From July 2002 to December 2010, 41 cases with distal femur osteosarcoma were operated on at our hospital. Among them, 7 cases underwent operation using the ISP procedure. All the 7 cases underwent limb-salvage surgery with an artificial knee joint.

17.3 Indication

Indication for this surgical method [1] was only for those cases with locally advanced tumors that are located close to major vascular structures (Fig. 1a, b). Cases showing occlusion of an artery were excluded from the ISP procedure. In these cases, the artery was sacrificed along with the tumor. Preoperative chemotherapy was performed in all cases.

17.4 Methods

The ISP procedure was carried out as follows: (1) At first, the tumor was excised en bloc, including the tumor and femoral artery and vein, to maintain an adequate wide margin. The continuity of vessels was preserved (Fig. 1d). (2) The en bloc mass was lifted from the surgical bed and then isolated from the surgical bed using a vinyl sheet (Fig. 1e) in order to prevent contamination from the next procedure. (3) At this point, the artery was clipped at the proximal site. The en bloc mass was turned around, and the nearest approach to the vessels was determined (Fig. 1f). (4) The vascular sheath was then split to release the vessels from the tumor. Small branches were ligated. This process made it possible to evaluate the surgical margin between the tumor and vessel. If the surface of the tumor was not exposed during this procedure, the resected mass was taken away from the operative field. The remaining structure, which covers the tumor surface, was evaluated apart from the operative field. At this time, the final evaluation of the surgical margin was decided. (5) Based on the final evaluation, we performed additional procedures:

(a) For an intralesional margin in which the tumor completely adheres to a vessel, we sacrificed the vessel.
(b) For a marginal margin and wide margin, one of the following additional procedures was employed: (1) soaking in distilled water for more than 5 min and (2) soaking in pure alcohol followed by distilled water.

17.5 Evaluation

The surgical margin was evaluated by using the evaluation method accepted by the Musculoskeletal Tumor Committee of the Japanese Orthopedic Association [2]. This method classifies surgical margins into four types, namely, curative, wide, marginal, and intralesional margins, depending on the distance between the surgical margin and the discolored area (reactive zone) just outside the tumor. A curative margin is defined as a margin 5 cm or more distant from the reactive zone, while a wide margin is a margin that is not sufficiently wide to be curative but it is still outside the reactive zone. A marginal margin is defined as a margin, which passes through the reactive zone, and an intralesional margin is a margin present within a lesion. In addition, fascia, joint capsules, cartilage, periosteum, retinaculum, tendon sheath, and vascular sheath are considered to be barriers and therefore judged to be equivalent to a definitive thickness of normal tissue. For instance, a margin outside a barrier with intervening normal tissue to the reactive zone would be converted to a margin distance of 5 cm, while a thinner barrier (such as muscle fascia of adult periosteum) would be regarded as 2 cm.

17.6 Results

Among the seven cases treated with the ISP procedure, no case recurred (Table 17.1) at a minimum follow-up period of 4 years and 4 months. Three patients died of disease, three patients remained disease free, and one patient (Case 5) was disease free for 4 years and 6 months after the first operation.

The evaluation of surgical margin between tumor and femoral artery was as follows: wide margin in six cases and marginal margin in one case. Femoral vein was sacrificed in three cases because of tumor thrombus or complete adhesion to the tumor.

Table 17.1 Summary of osteosarcoma treated with ISP

Age	Sacrifice vein	Vein graft	Tumor thrombus	Additional procedure	Outcome
59	–	–	–	Alcohol	CDF
15	+	+	+	Alcohol	DOD
15	–	–	–	Distilled water	DOD
11	–	–	–	Distilled water	CDF
13	+	+	+	Alcohol	NED
33	–	–	–	Distilled water	CDF
14	+	–	–	Distilled water	DOD

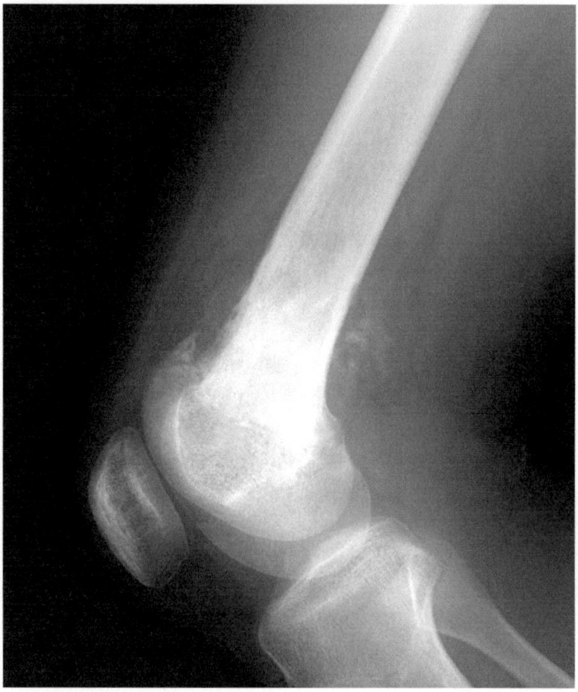

Fig. 17.1 Distal femur osteosarcoma: XP reveals bone destruction and periosteal reaction

In two of these three cases, femoral vein was grafted with an artificial vessel. As for the additional procedures, alcohol soaking was used in two cases, and soaking in distilled water only was performed in five cases.

In Case 5, an extraskeletal mass was adjacent to femoral vessels (Figs. 17.1 and 17.2). At the distal part of femoral vein, heterogeneous signal intensity suggested the existence of tumor thrombus; however, no calcification was found in the vein (Fig. 17.3). After intracapsular resection and cutting of the proximal femur (Fig. 17.4), the en bloc mass including tumor and femoral vessels was isolated with a vinyl sheet (Fig. 17.5). The consistency of femoral vessels was preserved. During the separation of femoral vein, a hard whitish mass was found in the vein. Since tumor thrombus was suspected, the femoral vein was sacrificed (Figs. 17.6

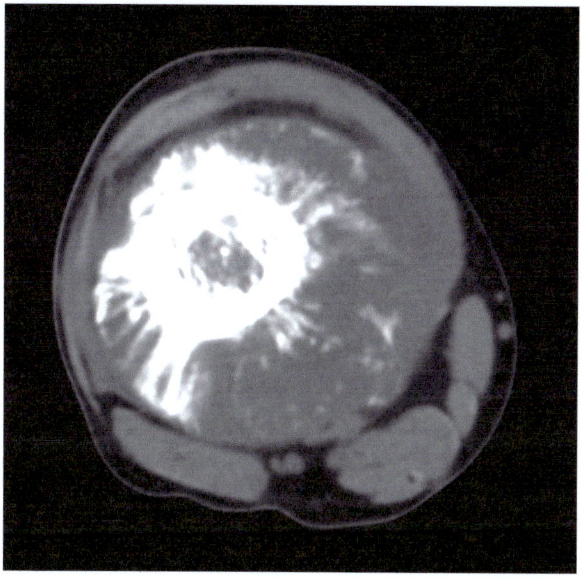

Fig. 17.2 Distal femur osteosarcoma: CT shows that the tumor is located close to femoral vessels

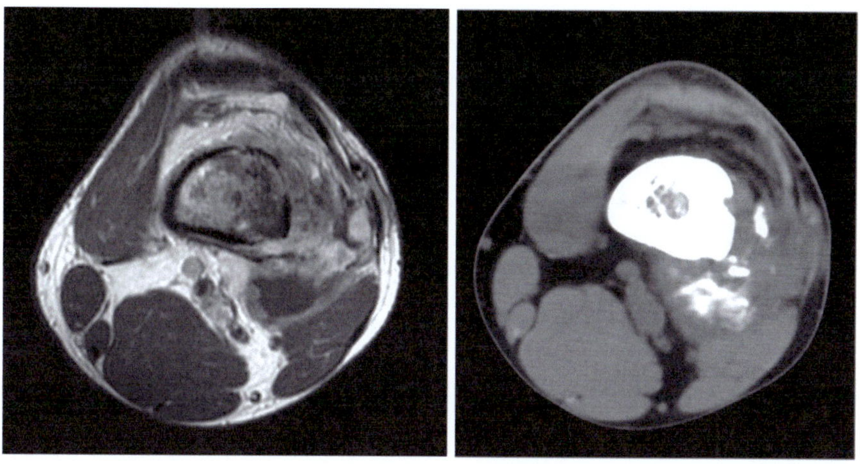

Fig. 17.3 Distal femur osteosarcoma: on Gd-enhanced MRI, heterogeneous lesion exists in femoral vein. On CT, there is no calcified lesion in the vein

and 17.7). Femoral artery was preserved. After the alcohol soaking of femoral artery, femoral vein was reconstructed with an artificial vessel (Fig. 17.8). Frozen section revealed that the hard mass was tumor thrombus. Bone defect was reconstructed using an artificial knee joint (Figs. 17.8 and 17.9). Lung metastases appeared 8 months after the operation. The removal of lung metastases was

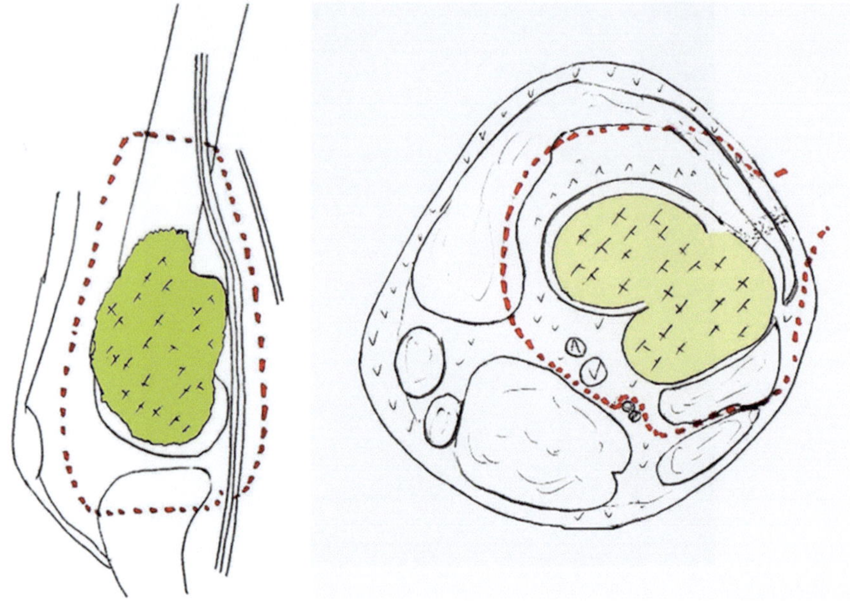

Fig. 17.4 Distal femur osteosarcoma: surgical line. The continuity of femoral vessels is preserved

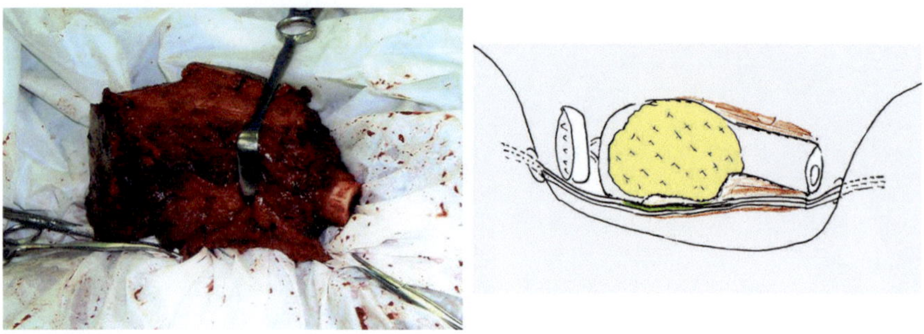

Fig. 17.5 Distal femur osteosarcoma: a vinyl sheet is used to separate the en block mass from surgical bed

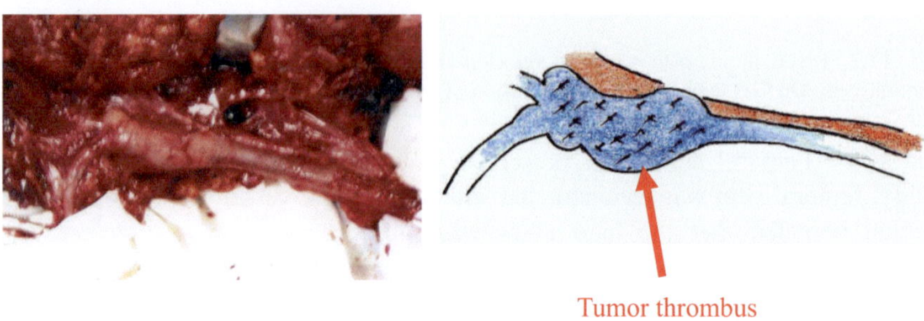

Fig. 17.6 Distal femur osteosarcoma: through the nearest approach, femoral vessel is approached. Inside the femoral vein, a hard mass is palpable, which suggests tumor thrombus

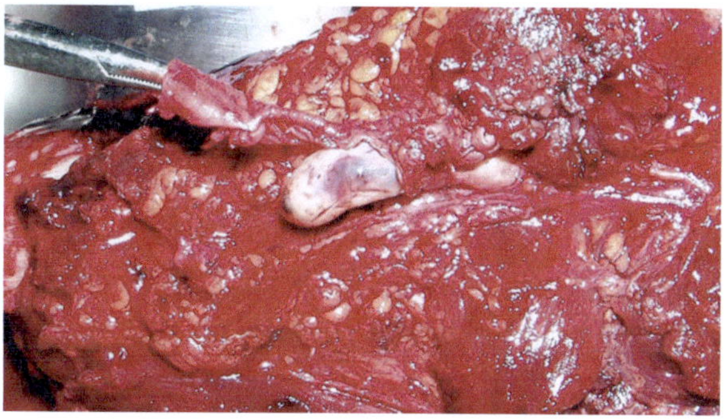

Fig. 17.7 Distal femur osteosarcoma: tumor thrombus is found in the femoral vein

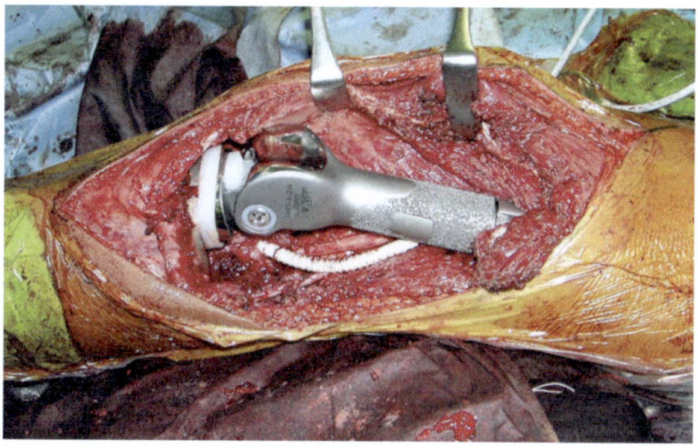

Fig. 17.8 Distal femur osteosarcoma: bone defect is reconstructed by tumor prosthesis

performed two times. Seven years and 6 months after the resection of primary lesion, this patient remained disease free.

17.7 Discussion

Tumor thrombus is the high risk factor of limb-salvage operation for osteosarcoma, but the preoperative diagnosis of tumor thrombus is not always easy. ISP was a very useful method to find tumor thrombus during operation. The advantage of ISP is no risk of tumor cell contamination. After the successful results of ISP for distal femur lesion, we applied ISP to other locations such as the proximal tibia, proximal humerus, and proximal fibula. There were also no local recurrences in these cases. Since there is no need of special facilities or equipment, this procedure can be easily performed all over the world.

In limb-saving surgery for the case with osteosarcoma near major vessels, there have been two options: (1) sacrifice and reconstruction of vessel and (2) dissection

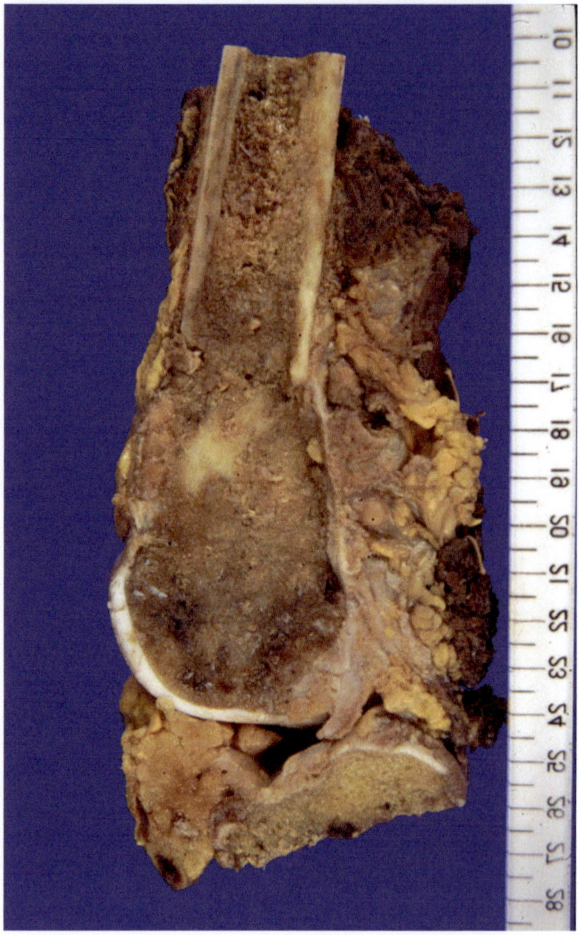

Fig. 17.9 Distal femur osteosarcoma: surgical specimen shows wide margin is achieved

alone. A removal of the nearby vessel with segmental grafting of vessel is the best option to ensure the safe surgical margin. However, the postoperative obstruction rate is slightly high around the mobile joint. Moreover, if an artificial vessel is used for arterial reconstruction, long-term postoperative anticoagulant therapy is necessary. These are disadvantages of segmental grafting. Even when simple dissection of major vessels from the operated tissue mass is attempted, the reactive zone might be exposed during dissection. Therefore, dissection of major vessels without transplantation and without tumor cell contamination would be an ideal procedure. In the ISP procedure, the location at which the major vessels are released from the tumor is completely isolated from the rest of the operative field. Thus, even if the tumor is exposed during these procedures and the major vessels are sacrificed with the tumor, the remaining operative field would not be contaminated by tumor cells. The advantages of ISP are as follows: (1) Intraoperative evaluation of surgical margin is possible without contamination of tumor cells. (2) Dissection of the major vessels is easily and quickly accomplished. This means that the en bloc mass connected only with vessel can be freely rotated, allowing the major vessels to be dissected through the nearest approach from the surface. This enables easy and quick dissection with the least possibility of contamination. If an artery is involved, temporary clamping of the artery at the proximal site can control bleeding and enables easy ligation of small branches. As for a vein, the wall is thin and there is a relatively high possibility of tumor thrombus, especially in high-grade sarcoma cases. Actually, in Case 5, preoperative images did not show the existence of tumor thrombus. If dissection of the vein does not go smoothly, sacrificing the vein might be a safer procedure. In fact, in four of our cases, the vein was sacrificed with the tumor. Reconstruction of the vein is suggested to the case with poor collateral blood flow. (3) Additional procedure can be applied when the surgical margin is found to be insufficient. The procedure includes alcohol soaking or distilled water soaking. ISP for sarcoma is suggested to the case in which only a small number of tumor cells possibly remains. The effects of alcohol to cancer cells were reported in many papers. Especially for hepatocellular carcinoma, percutaneous ethanol injection is very useful. While distilled water soaking can destroy red blood cells by osmotic pressure, its effect on tumor cells is unknown.

ISP is indicated at a location where the nerve and vessel can be dissected with enough length to elevate the tissue block and insert the sheet.

After the successful results of ISP for distal femur lesion, we applied ISP to other locations such as the proximal tibia, proximal humerus, and proximal fibula, and no local recurrences were found in these cases.

In conclusion, the ISP procedure has been shown to be a useful method to compensate for deficits at the time of preoperative diagnosis and can result in limb-saving operations without the need for transplantation. Moreover, no special facilities or equipment is required, and therefore, this procedure could be easily available all over the world.

References

1. Matsumoto S, Kawaguchi N, Manabe J, Matsushita Y. "In situ preparation": new surgical procedure indicated for soft-tissue sarcoma of a lower limb in close proximity to major neurovascular structures. Int J Clin. 2002;7:51–6.
2. Kawaguchi N, Ahmed AR, Matsumoto S, Manabe J, Matsushita Y. The concept of curative margin in surgery for bone and soft tissue sarcoma. Clin Orthop. 2004;419:165–72.

Part VI

Unresectable/Metastatic Disease

Carbon Ion Radiotherapy for Unresectable Osteosarcoma of the Trunk

18

Reiko Imai and Tadashi Kamada

Abstract

Osteosarcoma is a radioresistant tumor. There have been few reports on the effectiveness of radiotherapy for unresectable osteosarcoma using photon (X-ray) beams. Carbon ion beams have a unique physical advantage for avoiding irradiation of critical organs, and their biological effectiveness is higher than that of X-ray and proton beams. These specific characteristics are beneficial for the treatment of sarcomas. Carbon ion radiotherapy has thus been suggested as an effective local therapy for unresectable osteosarcoma of the trunk.

Keywords

Sarcoma • Charged particle therapy • Carbon ion radiotherapy

18.1 Introduction

The management strategy for osteosarcoma has changed dramatically in the last three decades [1, 2]. A combination of aggressive chemotherapy and limb preservation surgery is available as a treatment option for most patients with osteosarcoma, and the prognosis has considerably improved. Osteosarcoma of the trunk is rare, representing 6.3 % of all osteosarcomas [3]. Curative surgery has been the mainstay of local therapy for this disease; however, complete resection is sometimes difficult because of the location and extension of the tumor. In the Cooperative Osteosarcoma Study Group (COSS) study of 1,702 patients with high-grade osteosarcoma of the extremities and trunk, the 5-year overall survival rate for all patients was 67.3 %, whereas the survival rate among 107 patients who had tumors

R. Imai (✉) • T. Kamada
Research Center Hospital for Charged Particle Therapy, National Institute of Radiological Sciences, 4-9-1, Anagawa, Inage, Chiba 263-8555, Japan
e-mail: r_imai@nirs.go.jp

T. Ueda, A. Kawai (eds.), *Osteosarcoma*, DOI 10.1007/978-4-431-55696-1_18

of the trunk was only 34.2 % [3]. The COSS report also noted that the 5-year overall survival rate for patients undergoing complete surgical resection was 70.9 %, whereas that of those with macroscopic residual tumor after surgery was 15.7 % [3]. The prognosis remains poor in both incomplete surgery and unresectable cases [4–6].

Radiotherapy has been suggested as a possible alternative local therapy to surgery. However, there have been few reports on the effectiveness of radiotherapy for unresectable osteosarcoma using photon (X-ray) beams, because osteosarcoma is one of the most radioresistant tumors [7]. Charged particle therapy is another type of radiotherapy currently increasing in use worldwide. The particle beams used for cancer treatment are proton and carbon ion beams, which have a unique physical advantage called the Bragg peak. A charged particle penetrates the body and moves quickly, depositing an initial low dose of radiation. It then slows down and, finally, releases its maximum radiation dose at the end of its range, after which the dose falls off steeply, which is called the Bragg peak [8]. This special profile enables that a highly concentrated dose is distributed. The carbon ion beam (described below in Sect. 18.3) is one of the heavy particle beams and has another unique profile, which is its high biological effectiveness. Charged particle therapy makes the best use of these charged particle beams' special profiles to treat cancers.

18.2 History of Charged Particle Therapy

The first clinical application of proton beams was in 1954 at the University of California, Berkeley. The first patient to undergo charged particle therapy received pituitary irradiation to treat disseminated breast cancer [9]. Proton therapy then started in Uppsala in Sweden, Cambridge in the UK, Moscow in the USSR, and other facilities. In 1961, the Harvard Cyclotron Laboratory (HCL) and the Massachusetts General Hospital (MGH) collaborated to start proton therapy and have treated approximately 9,000 patients for 40 years [10]. In Japan, the National Institute of Radiological Sciences (NIRS) initiated proton therapy in 1979, and the University of Tsukuba launched the High Energy Accelerator Research Organization (KEK) using a synchrotron in 1983.

Between the 1950s and the 1970s, the main target for proton therapy was the pituitary; however, after the invention of computed tomography (CT) in 1972, in both the 1970s and 1980s, the tumors treated with protons were primarily choroidal melanomas, skull base tumors, and intracranial tumors. Only at the University of Tsukuba under the plans developed by Dr. Hirohiko Tsujii, deep-seated tumors in structures such as the lung, liver, esophagus, uterine cervix, and prostate, in addition to head and neck malignancies, were treated [11]. In 1990, a hospital-based proton facility was commissioned by James Slater at the Loma Linda University Medical Center in California.

Regarding heavy ion radiotherapy, in 1957, helium ion radiotherapy began at the Lawrence Berkeley National Laboratory (LBNL), and neon ion radiotherapy started in 1975. Until the laboratory closed in 1992, 2054 patients were treated with helium ion beams and 433 with neon ions [12, 13]. In 1977, carbon ion irradiation was used for the first time at the LBNL. In 1994, NIRS in Chiba, Japan, launched carbon ion radiotherapy using the world's first heavy ion accelerator complex, the Heavy Ion Medical Accelerator in Chiba (HIMAC), which was dedicated to medical use in a hospital setting. As of 2014, over 8000 patients were treated with carbon ion radiotherapy. In 1997, Gesellschaft für Schwerionenforschung (GSI) in Germany began clinical studies with carbon ion beams. After the close of the clinical department at GSI in 2009, Heidelberg Ion-Beam Center (HIT) launched the treatment. HIT was the first particle therapy facility in the world to use protons and carbon ions with a scanning beam delivery system. In Italy, the National Center for Oncological Hadrontherapy (CNAO) launched proton therapy in 2011 and carbon ion radiotherapy in 2012. As of 2014, there are eight centers providing carbon ion radiotherapy and 43 facilities with proton therapy machines worldwide. Among these facilities, four centers provide both carbon ion and proton therapy [14].

18.3 Carbon Ion Radiotherapy

As noted previously, carbon ion beams have a unique physical advantage called the Bragg peak. Carbon ion beams emit a low dose of radiation after penetrating the body and deliver their maximum dose at the end of their range, after which the dose drops sharply (Fig. 18.1). This pattern of irradiation facilitates delivery of an optimal radiation dose to the tumor while exposing critical organs surrounding the tumor to lower doses. In addition, the sharpness of lateral scattering of carbon ion beams is superior to that of proton beams, which is useful for avoiding high-dose irradiation of normal tissue close to the tumor. The lateral scattering is only 1.5 mm at a 20 cm depth in water for the carbon ion beams, hence, 6.5 mm for

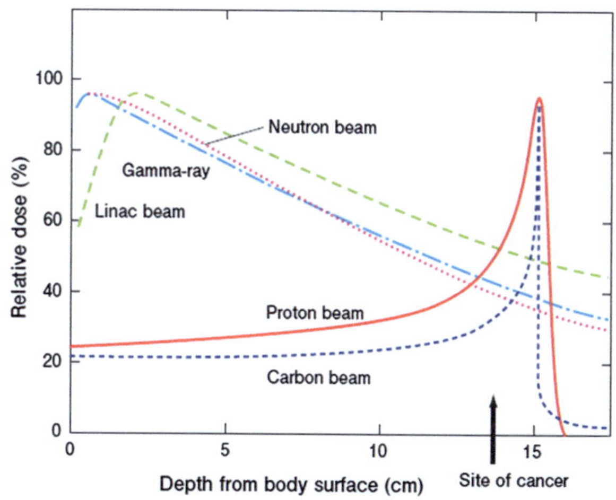

Fig. 18.1 Dose distribution of various radiations in the body. The neutron, X-ray, and gamma ray beams release their maximum radiation dose to tissues immediately after entering the body, whereas the proton and carbon ion beams penetrate the body and release low doses of radiation while traveling before releasing the maximum dose at the target site. The dose falls off steeply (Cited by Radiological Sciences 2007; 50: p51)

protons [15]. Another property that distinguishes carbon ion beams from photon and proton beams is their greater biological effectiveness. The biological effect of ionizing radiation is caused by damage to DNA depending on the ionization density produced along the radiation track. The average energy transferred per unit of length of the track is called linear energy transfer (LET). LET becomes larger as the weight of the particle increases and the particle goes into deeper sites of the body. Since LET in the peak of carbon beams is larger than that in photon and proton beams, its relative biological effectiveness (RBE) becomes two to three times greater than that of photon and proton beams. This RBE results in a biological benefit in killing cancer cells due to less recovery of the target cells from radiation damage. Tumor cells become more radioresistant in tissue environments with lower oxygen concentrations and in some phases of the cell cycle. A higher RBE is less dependent on the radiation effect on oxygen concentration in the tissue and less dependent on the cell cycle stage [15].

18.3.1 Carbon Ion Radiotherapy at NIRS

Carbon ion beams are generated from accelerators. The HIMAC at NIRS in Japan is the world's first heavy ion accelerator complex dedicated to medical use in a hospital setting. The accelerator system is composed of the injector at the ion source, linear accelerators, and a synchrotron. Carbon ion beams are accelerated to approximately 70–80 % of the speed of light and extracted for treatment. The accelerated energy of the beam available for treatment ranges from 290 to 430 MeV. The range of the 290 MeV carbon ion beam is approximately 15 cm in water, that of the 350 MeV beam is 20 cm, and that of the 400 MeV carbon ion beam is 25 cm. The beam lines are in fixed horizontal and vertical lines. A rotating gantry does not apply.

Two different systems of beam delivery are employed at NIRS. One is the passive beam delivery that has been used for 20 years, since the treatment started. To modulate the Bragg peak to conform to a target shape, the beam lines are equipped with a pair of wobbler magnets, beam scatters, ridge filters, multileaf collimators, and a compensation bolus. An appropriately sized ridge filter, which determines the size of the spread-out Bragg peak (SOBP), is selected in each port to adjust the irradiated field. Twelve different sizes of ridge filters cover the field size from 2 to 15 cm. The compensation bolus is fabricated for each patient to make the distal configuration of the SOBP similar to any irregular shape of the target volume. The collimator defines the margins of the target volume.

Another system is active beam delivery, which is a scanning system launched in 2010 at NIRS. The fixed horizontal and vertical beams are used in this system, as in the passive beam delivery. The delivery system does not use beam scatters, collimators, or a compensation bolus. Instead of using wobbler magnets, it employs scanning magnets to produce sophisticated beam control. It is more flexible and can make an irradiated field fitting the complex shape of a tumor [15]. Compared to passive delivery, active delivery generates fewer neutrons because the materials

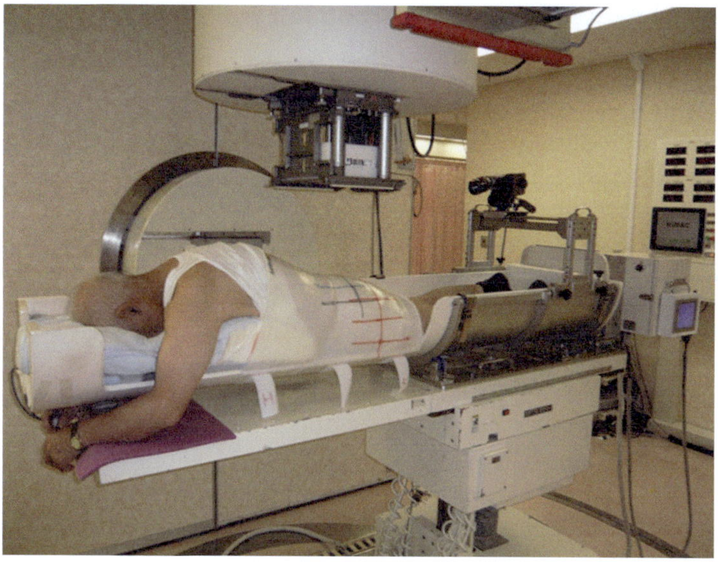

Fig. 18.2 A patient in the prone position in the treatment room. Patients are fixed using an immobilization device to the couch. It takes 30 min to examine the position on the images obtained in the room. Patients receive radiation for a few minutes. This photo shows irradiation in the vertical beam line

like bolus and collimators are not inserted in the beam line [16]. To ensure precise irradiation, tailor-made, body-fixed devices are prepared, and patients are positioned in customized cradles and immobilized with thermoplastic plates (Fig. 18.2). A set of 1-2.5-mm-thick CT images is taken with the immobilization devices for treatment planning. Respiratory gating of both the CT acquisition and the treatment is performed when indicated. A margin of 5 mm is usually added to the clinical target volume (CTV) to create the planning target volume (PTV) using a three-dimensional treatment planning system. When the tumor is located close to critical organs such as the spinal cord or bowel, the margin is reduced accordingly. The CTV is covered by at least 90 % of the prescribed dose [17]. Dose was expressed in gray equivalent (*GyE* = *carbon physical dose* [Gy] × *relative biologic effectiveness* [RBE]). Carbon ion radiotherapy is given once daily, 4 days a week (Tuesday to Friday). Patients with axial sarcomas are treated with more than three irregularly shaped ports. One port is treated in each session. At every treatment session, the patient's position is verified with a computer-aided, on-line positioning system. The patient is positioned on the treatment couch with the immobilization devices, and digital orthogonal x-ray television images are taken in that position and transferred to the positioning computer. They are compared with the reference image on the computer screen and the differences are measured. The treatment couch is then moved to the matching position until the largest deviation from the field edge, and the iso-center position is <2 mm [17].

18.3.2 Special Techniques in Carbon Ion Radiotherapy

18.3.2.1 Patch Combination Technique

Treatment of spinal and paraspinal tumors makes the best use of the characteristics of the charged particle beam, if the tumors are unresectable due to the high risk of sacrifice to the spinal cord. The radiation tolerance limit using photon beams to the spinal cord is generally 40–46 Gy in 20–25 fractions.

The "patch combination technique" is used when the tumors are both close to and surrounding the spinal cord. The target volume is divided into two segments, and each segment is treated by a separate radiation field using an anterior–posterior or posterior–anterior field and a right–left or left–right field. By using the sharp dose drop-off after the Bragg peak, the distal edge of one field is matched with the lateral edge of the second field. The combination of the two fields provides at least two varied patterns because the matching lines of the two fields where the lateral edge of one portal abuts the distal end of the stopping beam are utilized on alternating days to reduce potential dose inhomogeneity [18–20]. In the case of spinal sarcoma, by means of the patch technique, the dose distribution is doughnut shaped to avoid irradiation of the spinal cord (Fig. 18.3).

Irradiation of the spinal cord should be minimized. The dose constraint of the carbon ion beams directed in cross-sections involving the spinal cord is thought to be almost 30 GyE administered in 16 fractions, based on clinical experience at NIRS. As the incidence of radiation-induced myelopathy is quite rare, accumulation of more spinal sarcoma cases and further analysis of the relation between irradiated dose and adverse events are needed.

18.3.2.2 Inserting Spacers

In cases where the tumors are located close to or abutting the digestive tract, there is a high risk of adverse events related to irradiation of the digestive tract. To avoid excessive irradiation doses over the tolerance dose of the digestive tract, a spacer is

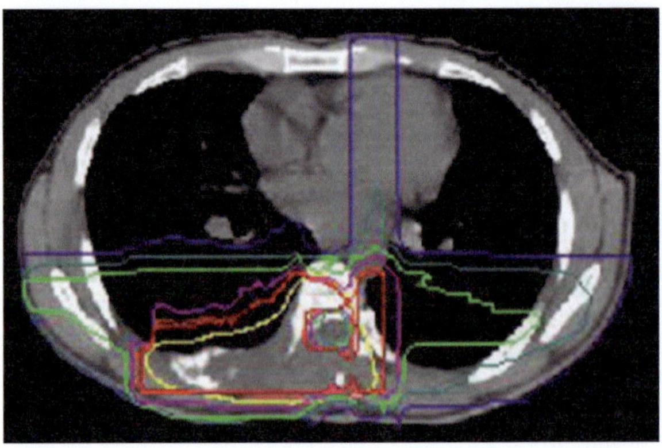

Fig. 18.3 Dose distribution in spinal sarcoma. This figure shows a tumor encompassing the spinal cord. The dose distribution was doughnut shaped to avoid irradiation of the spinal cord. This irradiation field uses the patch technique. The *red line* is 96 % of the total irradiation dose, *pink* is 70 %, *light green* is 50 %, and *deep green* is 30 %

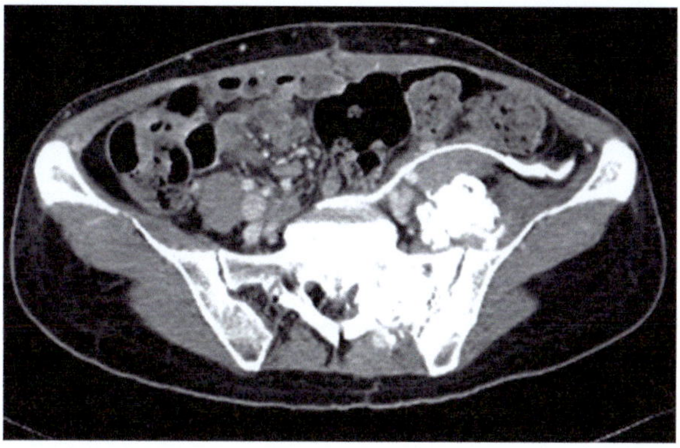

Fig. 18.4 Inserting a spacer between the bowels and a tumor. Creation of a space between the tumor and the bowels enables delivery of sufficient radiation to the tumor while avoiding adverse events in the bowels. The sheet is made from expanded polytetrafluoroethylene, which is an affinitive material to body tissues, and there is usually no need to remove it after irradiation. The inserted sheet was calcified

sometimes inserted. The surgical procedure involves placement of a spacer to separate the target tumor from the digestive tract before carbon ion radiotherapy [21]. The spacer is usually a sheet made from expanded polytetrafluoroethylene, which is affinitive to body tissues, and there is usually no need to remove it after irradiation (Fig. 18.4). Creating space between the tumor and digestive tract enables a sufficient dose of radiation to be applied to the tumor while avoiding adverse bowel events such as bloody discharge, perforation, and stenosis.

However, this surgical intervention has some risks. One is a risk of tumor progression. It usually takes >1 month to complete the surgery and move the patient to a hospital for carbon ion radiotherapy. During that period, the patients receive no antitumor therapy. After surgery to place the spacer, if the size of the tumor exceeds that which carbon ion radiotherapy can treat or if the tumor shows systemic spread, it will be impossible to undergo carbon ion radiotherapy. The risk is especially high in cases where the tumor either has a poor reaction to chemotherapy or grows rapidly, such as a high-grade sarcoma. Another risk is that of infection in the spacer. If infection occurs and spreads to the tumor, it can be difficult to control and the infection in the tumor is not suitable for carbon ion radiotherapy. Thus, a patient's risk of inserting a spacer should be examined well before the surgery.

18.3.3 Patient Eligibility

General eligibility criteria for carbon ion radiotherapy are shown in Table 18.1. Tumors directly invading critical organs such as the skin, digestive tract organs, and

Table 18.1 Major eligibility for carbon ion radiotherapy for bone and soft tissue sarcomas

Unresectable tumor (judged by surgeons)
Pathological confirmation as sarcoma
Gross measurable lesion
Lesion size less than a maximum of 15 cm
Expected positive long-term prognosis
No metal instrumentation in the treatment field
No infection in the treatment field
Accepting informed consent form

bronchus are excluded. Patients with metal instrumentation in the treatment area are also excluded because the metal implants cause artifacts on CT images for treatment planning, complicating determination of accurate dose distribution. It has also been reported that metal implantation was one of the causes of local failure after charged particle therapy [22]. If a patient with spinal sarcoma had previously undergone decompression surgery and metal instrumentation, the metal objects should be removed before initiating carbon ion radiotherapy.

At NIRS, carbon ion radiotherapy is performed only in accordance with protocols. There is no protocol for sarcomas with preplanned carbon ion radiotherapy combined with surgery, which means that pre- or post-carbon ion radiotherapy to support and complete surgical plans is not offered. For treating osteosarcomas of the extremities, which develop with a high incidence among younger generations, a paradigm based on a combination of surgery and chemotherapy has been well established to achieve a high control rate of tumors, and carbon ion radiotherapy is unlikely to outweigh their advantages. Irradiating bones affected by osteosarcomas can easily cause pathological fractures, and it is more difficult to restore function of irradiated bones by surgical intervention than it is to repair nonirradiated bones. In addition, as the majority of patients with limb osteosarcoma are children and adolescents, the validity of radiotherapy should be estimated carefully, considering late adverse events such as growth disturbances in the irradiated bone and second malignancies. Currently osteosarcoma of the extremities is not considered to be a good candidate for carbon ion radiotherapy.

18.4 Results of Carbon Ion Radiotherapy for Osteosarcoma

Since 1996, NIRS has used carbon ion radiotherapy for bone and soft tissue sarcomas and, as of March 2014, almost 1000 patients, including those receiving repeat treatment, have received carbon ion radiotherapy. Cases of osteosarcoma of the trunk comprised the third largest group at NIRS, following chordoma and chondrosarcoma cases. For unresectable osteosarcoma, carbon ion radiotherapy will be the mainstay of treatment, considering the survival benefits and adverse events noted below.

18.4.1 Survival and Local Control Benefits

Matsunobu et al. reported that patients with unresectable osteosarcomas of the trunk were treated at NIRS with carbon ion radiotherapy with or without chemotherapy between 1996 and 2009 in a Phase I/II study [23]. The patients had no systemic metastases before carbon ion radiotherapy. The median age at the time of initial referral was 41 years, ranging from 11 to 83 years. Seventy-four tumors were primary and four were metastatic. The tumor was located in the pelvis for 61 patients, the spinal and paraspinal areas (such as the spine and the ribs) for 15 patients, and other sites for 2 patients. The median applied radiation dose was 70.4 GyE (range, 52.8–73.6 GyE) in a total of 16 fixed fractions over 4 weeks. The median tumor diameter was 10 cm, and the median CTV was 510 cm^3 (range, 60–2,299 cm^3). Eleven patients had undergone previous surgical resection, including nine patients who underwent surgical resection and developed local recurrence and two patients who had residual tumors due to insufficient surgical resection. Sixty-one patients had received prior chemotherapy. The 5-year local control and 5-year overall survival rates were 62 % and 33 %, respectively. The literature reports a survival rate of $\leq$10 % for patients with unresectable osteosarcoma [4, 5, 24]. Therefore, carbon ion radiotherapy may provide a survival benefit for patients with unresectable osteosarcomas. Tumor volume was a prognostic factor for the survival and local control rate. Thirty-eight patients with a CTV <500 cm^3 had a 5-year overall survival rate of 46 % and a 5-year local control rate of 88 %, whereas 40 patients with a CTV >500 cm^3 had a 5-year overall survival rate of 19 % and a 5-year local control rate of 31 %.

18.4.2 Adverse Events and Functional Preservation

Regarding adverse events in the study by Matsunobu et al. with the exception of three patients who experienced severe skin/soft tissue complications requiring skin grafts, other severe toxicities such as bowel toxicity were not observed. Among the 78 patients, 12 patients survived for >5 years. Of nine patients who were continuously disease free for >5 years, eight could walk with or without the help of a cane, and six were not dependent on painkillers. One patient with acetabular osteosarcoma used a wheelchair in daily life but could walk short distances [23].

In cases of acetabular sarcoma, including osteosarcoma and other kinds of sarcomas, degeneration and deformity of the bone were sometimes observed after

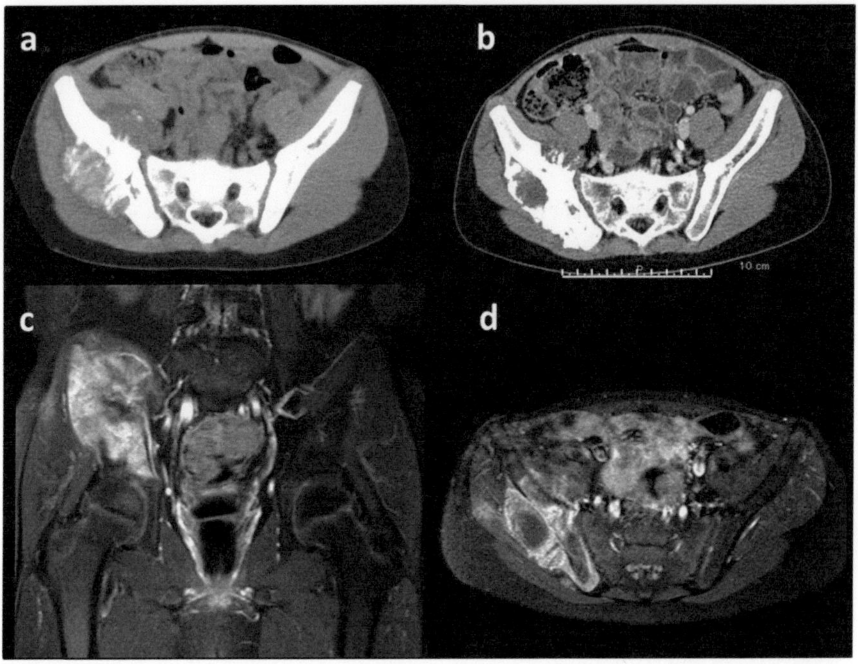

Fig. 18.5 Osteosarcoma of the right iliac bone. An 11-year-old boy with osteosarcoma of the right iliac bone. (**a**) Computed tomography (CT) image before chemotherapy. The tumor lies in the right iliac bone and had invaded the muscles. (**b**) CT image with contrast medium before carbon ion radiotherapy. (**c**) Coronal T1-weighted magnetic resonance image (MRI) with contrast medium before carbon ion radiotherapy. (**d**) Axial T1-weighted MRI with contrast medium before carbon ion radiotherapy

carbon ion radiotherapy, which caused pain, shortened legs, and walking disturbances (Figs. 18.5 and 18.6). In cases of sacral tumors involving sacral nerves, neurological events were sometimes observed after carbon ion radiotherapy. Sciatic nerve damage was related to symptoms such as numbness and pain, which sometimes required narcotic drugs for pain relief. The neurological damage was dependent on the irradiated volume of the nerve and the radiation dose, which can be challenging for physicians; osteosarcoma is a fatal disease for which the radiation dose should not be reduced (Fig. 18.7). In some cases of spinal tumors, Brown-Séquard syndrome was observed in one leg of unaffected side for >1 year after carbon ion radiotherapy [18].

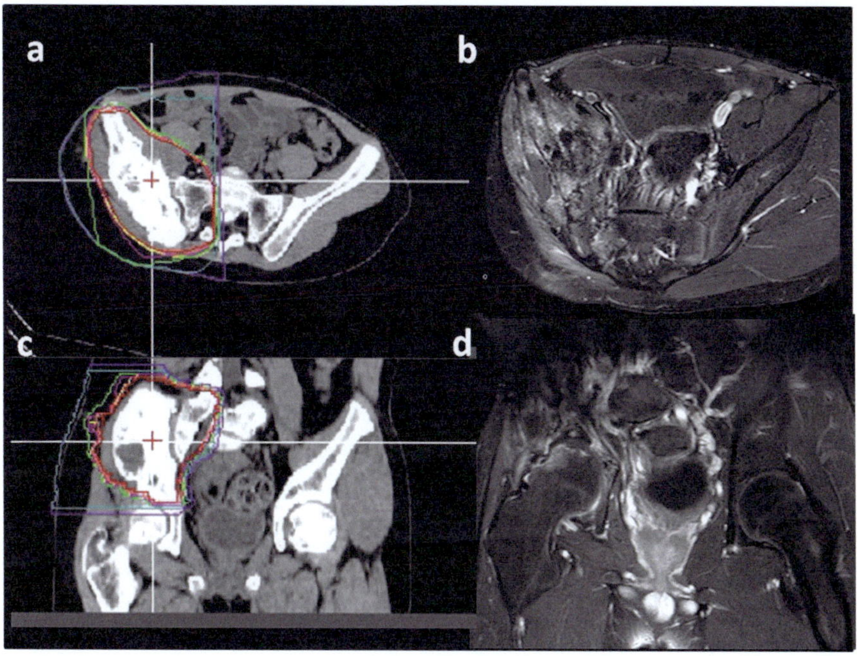

Fig. 18.6 Osteosarcoma of the right iliac bone. (**a**) The dose distribution of carbon ion radiotherapy. The *red line* is 96 % of the total irradiation dose, *pink* is 70 %, *light green* is 50 %, and *deep green* is 30 %. (**b**) Axial T1-weighted MRI with contrast medium 3 years after carbon ion radiotherapy. (**c**) Computed tomography images with coronal reconstruction of the dose distribution of carbon ion radiotherapy. (**d**) Coronal T1-weighted MRI with contrast medium 3 years after carbon ion radiotherapy. The acetabular bone is damaged

18.5 New Technology of Carbon Ion Radiotherapy

At HIT (the Heidelberg Ion-Beam Center), a rotating gantry has shown successful outcomes. It allows 360° rotation around the patient and facilitates selection of the optimal beam paths to the tumor. At NIRS, a compact heavy ion rotating gantry has been planned using superconducting technology. The plans suggest it will weigh 150 tons. NIRS will develop the quality of beams. A pencil beam will allow three-dimensional scanning irradiation using respiratory gating. The rotating gantry combined with pencil beam three-dimensional scanning will allow the use of intensity-modulated carbon ion radiotherapy for more accurate treatment. The further that technology develops, the safer and more precise irradiation will become.

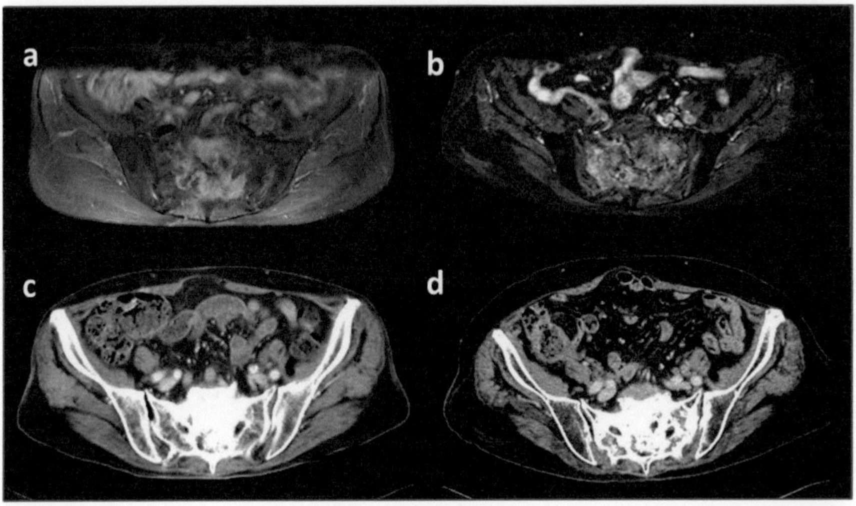

Fig. 18.7 Osteosarcoma of the sacrum. A 72-year-old woman with sacral osteosarcoma. (**a**) A T1-weighted MRI with contrast medium before carbon ion radiotherapy. The patient received chemotherapy before carbon ion radiotherapy. (**b**) A T1-weighted MRI with contrast medium 7 years after carbon ion radiotherapy. (**c**) Computed tomography image with contrast medium before carbon ion radiotherapy. (**d**) Computed tomography image with contrast medium 7 years after carbon ion radiotherapy. The patient could walk with a cane and her rectal and bladder functions were almost normal

References

1. Goorin AM, Schwartzentruber DJ, Devidas M, Gebhardt MC, Ayala AG, Harris MB, Helman LJ, Grier HE, Link MP, Pediatric Oncology Group. Presurgical chemotherapy compared with immediate surgery and adjuvant chemotherapy for nonmetastatic osteosarcoma: Pediatric Oncology Group Study POG-8651. J Clin Oncol. 2003;21:1574–80.
2. Eilber F, Giuliano A, Eckardt J, Patterson K, Moseley S, Goodnight J. Adjuvant chemotherapy for osteosarcoma: a randomized prospective trial. J Clin Oncol. 1987;5:21–6.
3. Bielack SS, Kempf-Bielack B, Delling G, Exner GU, Flege S, Helmke K, Kotz R, Salzer-Kuntschik M, et al. Prognostic factors in high-grade osteosarcoma of the extremities or trunk: an analysis of 1702 patients treated on neoadjuvant Cooperative Osteosarcoma Study Group protocols. J Clin Oncol. 2002;20:776–90.
4. Ozaki T, Flege S, Kevric M, Lindner N, Maas R, Delling G, Schwarz R, von Hochstetter AR, et al. Osteosarcoma of the pelvis: experience of the Cooperative Osteosarcoma Study Group. J Clin Oncol. 2003;21:334–41.
5. Ozaki T, Flege S, Liljenqvist U, Hillmann A, Delling G, Salzer-Kuntschik M, Jürgens H, Kotz R, et al. Osteosarcoma of the spine: experience of the Cooperative Osteosarcoma Study group. Cancer. 2002;94:1069–77.
6. Ferrari S, Palmerini E, Fabbri N, Staals E, Ferrari C, Alberghini M, Picci P. Osteosarcoma of the pelvis: a monoinstitutional experience in patients younger than 41 years. Tumori. 2012;98:702–8.

7. Hundsdoerfer P, Albrecht M, Rühl U, Fengler R, Kulozik AE, Henze G. Long-term outcome after polychemotherapy and intensive local radiation therapy of high-grade osteosarcoma. Eur J Cancer. 2009;45:2447–51.
8. Bragg WH, Kleeman R. On the ionization curves of radium. Philos Mag. 1904;S6:726–38.
9. Lawrence JH, Tobias CA, Born JL, McCombs RK, Roberts JE, Anger HO, Lowbeer BV, Huggins CB. Pituitary irradiation with high-energy proton beams: a preliminary report. Cancer Res. 1958;18:121–34.
10. Tsujii H. History of charged particle radiotherapy. In: Tsujii H, Kamada T, Shirai T, editors. Carbon-ion radiotherapy principles, practices, and treatment planning. Japan: Springer; 2014. p. 3–10.
11. Tsujii H, Tsuji H, Inada T, et al. Clinical results of fractionated proton therapy. Int J Radiat Oncol Biol Phys. 1993;25:49–60.
12. Castro JR, Saunders WM, Tobias CA, Chen GT, Curtis S, Lyman JT, Collier JM, Pitluck S. Treatment of cancer with heavy charged particles. Int J Radiat Oncol Biol Phys. 1982;8:2191–8.
13. Linstadt DE, Castro JR, Phillips TL. Neon ion radiotherapy: results of the phase I/II clinical trial. Int J Radiat Oncol Biol Phys. 1991;20:761–9.
14. Facilities in Operation. Particle Therapy Co-Operative Group. http://www.ptcog.ch/. Accessed Dec 2013.
15. Kamada T. The characteristic of carbon ion radiotherapy. In: Tsujii H, Kamada T, Shirai T, editors. Carbon-ion radiotherapy principles, practices, and treatment planning. Japan: Springer; 2014. p. 13–6.
16. Yonai S, Furukawa T, Inaniwa T. Measurement of neutron ambient dose equivalent in carbon-ion radiotherapy with an active scanned delivery system. Radiat Prot Dosim. 2014;161:433–6.
17. Kamada T, Tsujii H, Tsuji H, Yanagi T, Mizoe JE, Miyamoto T, Kato H, Yamada S, et al. Efficacy and safety of carbon ion radiotherapy in bone and soft tissue sarcomas. J Clin Oncol. 2002;20:4466–71.
18. Matsumoto K, Imai R, Kamada T, Maruyama K, Tsuji H, Tsujii H, Shioyama Y, Honda H, et al. Impact of carbon ion radiotherapy for primary spinal sarcoma. Cancer. 2013;119:3496–503.
19. Hug EB, Adams J, Fitzek M, De Vries A, Munzenrider JE. Fractionated, three-dimensional, planning-assisted proton-radiation therapy for orbital rhabdomyosarcoma: a novel technique. Int J Radiat Oncol Biol Phys. 2000;47:979–84.
20. Imai R, Kamada T, Tsuji H, Tsujii H, Tsuburai Y, Tatezaki S, Working Group for Bone and Soft Tissue Sarcomas. Cervical spine osteosarcoma treated with carbon-ion radiotherapy. Lancet Oncol. 2006;7:1034–5.
21. Fukumoto T, Komatsu S, Hori Y, Murakami M, Hishikawa Y, Ku Y. Particle beam radiotherapy with a surgical spacer placement for advanced abdominal leiomyosarcoma results in a significant clinical benefit. J Surg Oncol. 2010;101:97–9.
22. Rutz HP, Weber DC, Sugahara S, Timmermann B, Lomax AJ, Bolsi A, Pedroni E, Coray A, et al. Extracranial chordoma: outcome in patients treated with function-preserving surgery followed by spot-scanning proton beam irradiation. Int J Radiat Oncol Biol Phys. 2007;67:512–20.
23. Matsunobu A, Imai R, Kamada T, Imaizumi T, Tsuji H, Tsujii H, Shioyama Y, Honda H, et al. Impact of carbon ion radiotherapy for unresectable osteosarcoma of the trunk. Cancer. 2012;118:4555–63.
24. Kawai A, Huvos AG, Meyers PA, Healey JH. Osteosarcoma of the pelvis. Oncologic results of 40 patients. Clin Orthop Relat Res. 1998;348:196–207.

Treatment of Osteosarcoma Patients with Pulmonary Metastasis

19

Shintaro Iwata, Tsukasa Yonemoto, Hiroto Kamoda, and Takeshi Ishii

Abstract

The lung is the most common site of relapse from osteosarcoma. Several studies revealed that the patients with pulmonary metastases of osteosarcoma have a poor prognosis. This article aims to describe the current understanding of the characteristics, prognostic factors, and the local treatment strategy for pulmonary metastases of osteosarcoma.

Several clinical characteristics, such as a number or laterality of pulmonary nodules, location, or time interval from initial treatment, have been reported as potential prognostic factors for the patients with pulmonary metastases. Meanwhile, outcome of the patients with pulmonary metastases at initial presentation is not a dismal when the appropriate chemotherapy and thoracotomy are performed.

As a treatment factor, complete surgical resection of the pulmonary metastases is a most important predictor for survival of those patients, although the benefit of video-assisted thoracoscopic surgery or multiple thoracotomy is still controversial.

The number of published data available regarding the efficacy of radiotherapy in the treatment of pulmonary metastases is limited. Emerging techniques including stereotactic body radiotherapy and radiofrequency ablation could be an effective option of the treatment for unresectable metastatic lesion.

Keywords

Osteosarcoma • Pulmonary metastasis • Prognostic factor • Thoracotomy

S. Iwata • T. Yonemoto • H. Kamoda • T. Ishii (✉)
Division of Orthopaedic Surgery, Chiba Cancer Center, 666-2 Nitona-cho, Chuo-ku, Chiba 260-8717, Japan
e-mail: tishii@chiba-cc.jp

T. Ueda, A. Kawai (eds.), *Osteosarcoma*, DOI 10.1007/978-4-431-55696-1_19

19.1 Introduction

Although various attempts have been made to improve the outcome of the patients with osteosarcoma (OS), disease relapse remains the primary cause of mortality. The lung is the most common site of relapse from OS; almost 10 % of the patients showed the pulmonary metastases at diagnosis [1, 2], and 25–33 % of the patients who have achieved an initial complete remission of disease experienced pulmonary metastases [3, 4]. Several studies revealed that the patients with pulmonary metastases of OS have a poor prognosis (less than 30 %) [5–7]. Meanwhile, a growing body of evidence strongly suggests that the complete surgical remission of all metastases is the key to cure [2, 3, 5, 8–10].

This article aims to describe the current understanding of the characteristics, prognostic factors, and the local treatment strategy for pulmonary metastases of OS.

19.2 Characteristics of Pulmonary Metastases

It has been well established that the lung is the most common site among all metastatic relapse. Cooperative Osteosarcoma Study Group (COSS), which is one of the largest study groups for OS, reported that 81.4 % of 501 metastatic relapse occurred in the lung [3].

The number of the pulmonary nodules is a strong prognostic factor that has been repeatedly described in several reports (Table 19.1) [2–4, 6, 9–14]. Indeed, the number of the metastatic nodule is varied. COSS has reported that 145 (38.3 %) and 234 (61.7 %) patients have solitary and multiple nodules, respectively [8]. Majority of those reports emphasized the difference of impact on the survival between patients bearing solitary and multiple nodules [2, 3, 6, 8, 12], whereas some reports

Table 19.1 Summary of studies describing the number of the pulmonary nodules

Author (year)	*n*	Number of nodules	5-year OAS (%)	*P*	5-year EFS (%)	*P*
Kager (2003)	122	1	67	<.001	55	<.001
		2–5	24		19	
		6 –	19		2	
Hawkins (2003)	38	1	33[a]	.05	14[a]	.06
		2 –	17[a]		4[a]	
Bacci (2005)	202	1–2	–	–	44.1	<.005
		3 –			22.3	
Wu (2009)	91	1–2	56.5	.002	–	–
		3 –	21.3			
Iwata (2015)	71	1–3	33.9	.0079	17.2	.035
		4 –	17.2		12.1	

OAS Overall survival, *EFS* Event-free survival
[a]4-year OAS/EFS

supported the notion that smaller number of nodules (less than 3 [5, 13, 14] or 4 [9–11]) is a significant favorable prognostic factor. Recently, patients with only limited number of metastases have been recognized as an eligible for the local treatment, because they might achieve long-term survival or cure. These patients have been called "oligo-metastatic" by Hellman and Weichselbaum [15]. Therefore, a subset of the patients with smaller number of nodules as mentioned above might be regarded as oligo-metastatic OS patients and should be treated more aggressively.

Timing of occurrence of the pulmonary metastases has been reported to be a significant prognostic factor [11]. According to their results, the entire patients with the pulmonary metastases were divided into four groups: patients with the pulmonary metastases identified at the initial presentation, during pre- or postoperative chemotherapy, and after the completion of the treatment. They concluded that the patients with the pulmonary metastases identified after the completion of the treatment display a markedly better prognosis than any of the other patients ($P < .0001$). On the other hand, OS is known as a one of tumor subtype that the patients with pulmonary metastases at initial presentation (so-called M1 tumor) can be cured by an aggressive treatment. Bacci et al. described that 91 M1 patients underwent the complete surgical resection of all metastatic nodules and received systemic chemotherapy achieved a 5-year event-free survival rate of 27.4 % [16]. Yonemoto et al. also reported that the 5-year overall survival of nine M1 patients was 64.8 % with the complete removal of average 12.7 pulmonary nodules [17]. These data encourage us to make more effort to improve the survival of this patient group.

Laterality of the metastatic nodules is also considered to be an important prognostic factor [3, 4, 6, 8, 9]. Kempf-Bielack et al. found that 52.1 % of patients with the pulmonary metastases are unilateral and that is a favorable prognostic factor for survival as examined by uni- and multivariate analyses ($P < 0.001$) [3]. Interestingly, Bielack et al. described that the patients with unilateral metastases are associated with the development of the ipsilateral recurrences and postulated that some of those recurrences might be derived from the local recurrences of the incompletely removed pulmonary metastasis rather than new metastasis [8].

It has been described that the patients with an involvement of more than one lobe show a poorer outcome comparing to those with single lobe [14, 18]. Wu et al. demonstrated that 85.7 % of the patients with the pulmonary metastases have more than one lobe involved and their outcome is poorer among patients with more than one lobe (5-year survival; 27.0 % vs 56.5 %, $P = 0.006$) [14].

Metastatic location inside the lung (central or peripheral) is also one of the predictor for survival of those patients. Letourneau et al. strongly suggested an impact of the location of the pulmonary metastases in pediatric OS patients [19]. According to their results, the median overall survival after first pulmonary metastases was 1.06 years among the patients with the peripheral location as compared with 0.38 years in those with the central location ($P = 0.008$).

Table 19.2 Summary of studies describing the interval from the initial treatment to the metastatic relapse

Author (year)	n	Interval (months)	5-year OAS (%)	P	5-year EFS (%)	P
Ferrari (2003)	114	<=24	20	<.0001	–	–
		>24	60			
Chou (2005)	43	<24	23	<.05	–	–
		>24	53			
Bacci (2005)	202	<24	–	–	19.8	.0007
		>24			41.5	
Leary (2013)	110	<18	4.8[a]	<.0001	3.2[a]	<.0001
		>18	33.3[a]		23.4[a]	
Iwata (2015)	71	<=12	21.5	.017	11.7	.010
		>12	41.3		22.9	

OAS Overall survival, *EFS* Event-free survival
[a]10-year OAS/EFS

Time interval from the initial treatment to the metastatic relapse is a representative strong predictor for the outcome (Table 19.2). Bacci et al. examined the outcome of 235 patients with relapsed OS (80 % of those are pulmonary metastases) and demonstrated that the median interval from the initial treatment to the first relapse is 25.4 months (range, 3–135 months). Interestingly, the interval was longer in the patients showing a good response to chemotherapy compared to those of a poor responder (26.2 months and 24.2 months, $P < 0.04$) [4]. Based on the report from St. Jude children's research hospital, among the patients who achieved complete remission (CR) after relapse, the median interval from CR to the next relapse was shorter with the subsequent relapse [9]. Additionally, the interval from the initial diagnosis to the first relapse less than 18 months was correlated with poorer event-free and overall survivals after relapse ($P < 0.0001$). Similar observations showed that a longer interval to the relapse is associated with a better survival with a threshold of 12 months [10, 20], 18 months [8], and 24 months [5, 6, 13, 21].

Another striking clinical feature, pleural disruption by the pleural metastases, has been reported by COSS [3]. They defined a pleural disruption as pulmonary metastases caused by a contiguous growth into the pleural cavity, chest wall, diaphragm, or mediastinum or resulting in a malignant pleural effusion. The 5-year overall survival was 7 % or 25 % for the patients with or without pleural disruption by pulmonary metastases ($P < 0.0001$), respectively.

19.3 Surgical Treatment

As described, the complete surgical resection of the pulmonary metastases is a critical factor for the superior prognosis after the pulmonary relapse (Table 19.3) [2, 6, 8–10, 13, 21, 22], and the treatment without surgical CR never achieves a longer survival. Reported 5-year overall survival after the surgical CR of

Table 19.3 Summary of studies describing the complete surgical resection of the pulmonary metastases

Author (year)	*n*	Complete resection	5-year OAS (%)	*P*	5-year EFS (%)	*P*
Kager (2003)	122	Yes	39	<.0001	39	<.0001
		No	0		0	
Hawkins (2003)	38	Yes	33[a]	<.001	10[a]	N.A.
		No	0[a]		0[a]	
Chou (2005)	43	Yes	58	<.05	–	–
		No	0			
Bielack (2009)	249	Yes	32	<.0001	–	–
		No	0			
Leary (2013)	110	Yes	30.2[b]	<.0001	21.0[b]	<.0001
		No	0[b]		0[b]	
Iwata (2015)	71	Yes	30.6	<.0001	16.6	<.0001
		No	0		0	

OAS Overall survival, *EFS* Event-free survival, *NA* Not applicable
[a]4-year OAS/EFS
[b]10-year OAS/EFS

pulmonary relapse is ranging from 32 to 39 %, whereas that without surgical CR is ranging from 0 to 2 % [8, 13]. Leary et al. described that 41 out of 51 patients (80 %) with the unilateral pulmonary metastases and 12 out of 31 patients (39 %) bearing the bilateral pulmonary metastases underwent surgical CR, and this difference was statistically significant ($P = .0002$). Other factors involved in the achievement of surgical CR were age of patients, number of relapse nodule, recurrence-free interval, and the histologic response to preoperative chemotherapy [3, 4, 8].

Discrepancy between the number of radiographic pulmonary nodules and resected pulmonary metastases has been a common problem. Kayton et al. found that the preoperative evaluation of the pulmonary nodules by CT scan underestimates the pathologically proven metastatic nodules detected by surgeon in 35 % of thoracotomy [23]. On the other hand, Salah et al. described that 91 % of all resected nodules from the pulmonary metastatic OS patients are confirmed to be metastatic nodules, whereas the remaining 5 % and 3 % were inflammation and fibrosis, respectively, and 1 % contained benign lung tissue [22]. These observations raise a question whether the number of the pulmonary nodule found in the preoperative radiographic workup could be associated with the outcome of the patients with the pulmonary metastases.

The mode of surgery for the pulmonary relapse includes a wedge resection, lobectomy, and pneumonectomy. Although the preformed procedure is dependent on the distribution and number of nodules, approximately 80–85 % of the procedures contain a wedge resection, and lobectomy and pneumonectomy included are approximately 10–15 % and 5 %, respectively [4, 12, 19, 22]. Letourneau et al. demonstrated that the morbidity of a wedge resection is almost similar to that of lobectomy/pneumonectomy (9 % vs 8 %), and the statistical significance is not detectable between the median survivals of the patients undergoing a lobectomy and a wedge resection (0.61 years vs 1.14 years) [19].

From the viewpoint of less invasiveness, video-assisted thoracoscopic surgery (VATS) has been widely accepted as a useful method for resecting the pulmonary metastases. As Patrick et al. noted, VATS enables to provide a better visualization of the pleura as well as the pulmonary surface by magnification using optic system, and this system helps the surgeon to easily identify nodules on the pleural surface [24]. On the other hand, the disadvantage of VATS is that the surgeon is not able to directly palpate the nodule to identify much deeper lesions. To adequately address this issue, the preoperative localization of nodules by CT-guided needle hook wire placement [25], radioisotope marking [26], or intrathoracoscopic ultrasound [27] is utilized for the thoracoscopic surgery.

Since the complete resection of the pulmonary metastases of OS can be cured even when they are multiple [17], repeated surgery for the pulmonary metastases should be considered for the treatment of these patients. As described, the mean number of thoracotomy for the pulmonary metastases of OS as well as soft tissue sarcoma patients was ranging from 1.9 to 3.1, and the maximum number was 9 [28–30]. Iwata et al. performed retrospective analysis of 151 thoracotomies underwent in 71 patients with pulmonary metastases of OS and showed that first or second thoracotomy obtains significantly better post-relapsed survival comparing to third or more thoracotomy (3-years survival, 44.4 % vs 33.3 %, $P = .038$) [10].

19.4 Radiotherapy

Radiotherapy has not been accepted as a main option of the treatment for the pulmonary metastases of OS, since: (1) radiosensitivity of OS appears to be poor and (2) a large majority of OS patients is relatively young and would be able to receive major thoracotomy. The number of published data available regarding the efficacy of radiotherapy in the treatment of pulmonary metastases is limited.

Applying whole lung radiotherapy for pulmonary metastases of OS has never reached consensus, even in the palliative setting [31–33]. In addition, several authors failed to elucidate the advantage of prophylactic lung irradiation after thoracotomy, even these reports have a very small patient number and old description [31, 33].

Stereotactic body radiotherapy (SBRT) is a novel radiation treatment technique that enables highly focused as well as precise irradiation and also minimizes the surrounding normal lung parenchyma toxicity. Clinical benefit of SBRT for the pulmonary metastases from sarcomas has been emphasized recently. Yu et al. demonstrated the equivalence of the outcomes between the patients treated with SBRT for the pulmonary metastases from OS and those underwent surgery with a low frequency of toxicity such as pneumonitis [34]. They concluded that SBRT is an alternative treatment modality for the patients with the pulmonary metastases of OS, especially for those who are not tolerable to thoracotomy. Another group described the results of SBRT for the sarcoma patients with the pulmonary metastases including OS. Based on their results, their local control rate at 43 months was 94 %, and no patients experienced Grade 2–4 pneumonitis [35].

19.5 Radiofrequency Ablation

Since the multiple surgeries for the pulmonary metastases of OS have potential advantage for cure or prolonged survival, some thoracic surgeons have attempted to reduce patient's morbidity or hospital stay utilizing the minimally invasive treatment. Radiofrequency ablation (RFA) has been documented as an effective option of the treatment for unresectable lung cancer and the pulmonary metastases of colorectal cancer. RFA has been performed with the use of a percutaneously inserted electrode under the image guidance, which deposits heat energy to cause focal coagulation necrosis. So far, there are few reports showing the therapeutic outcome of RFA for the treatment of the pulmonary metastatic sarcoma patients. Nakamura et al. reviewed 20 patients with 89 pulmonary metastases from various sarcomas including OS. According to their result, patients with the complete ablation of all tumors had a 3-year survival rate of 59.2 % [36]. Additionally, Palussiere et al. described that disease-free survival after RFA for 47 pulmonary metastases from sarcomas including OS was 7 months, and 3-year survival rate was 65.2 %. The most frequent complication was a pneumothorax and observed in 68.7 % of the procedure [37].

19.6 Conclusion

Pulmonary metastasis has been considered to be a major cause of death for OS patients and the one who control the pulmonary metastasis can rule the OS. Nevertheless surgery has long been the mainstay of treatment in the pulmonary metastasis of OS, the outcome of the patients with the pulmonary metastasis of OS has been still unsatisfactory. With the advancement of research and technology, a novel strategy of treatment(s) and/or an innovative therapeutic method(s) for the pulmonary metastasis might be developed and gift much more benefit to the increasing number of patients with the pulmonary metastasis of OS.

References

1. Meyers PA, Heller G, Healey JH, Huvos A, Applewhite A, Sun M, et al. Osteogenic sarcoma with clinically detectable metastasis at initial presentation. J Clin Oncol. 1993;11(3):449–53.
2. Kager L, Zoubek A, Potschger U, Kastner U, Flege S, Kempf-Bielack B, et al. Primary metastatic osteosarcoma: presentation and outcome of patients treated on neoadjuvant Cooperative Osteosarcoma Study Group protocols. J Clin Oncol. 2003;21(10):2011–8. doi:10.1200/JCO.2003.08.132.
3. Kempf-Bielack B, Bielack SS, Jurgens H, Branscheid D, Berdel WE, Exner GU, et al. Osteosarcoma relapse after combined modality therapy: an analysis of unselected patients in

the Cooperative Osteosarcoma Study Group (COSS). J Clin Oncol. 2005;23(3):559–68. doi:10.1200/JCO.2005.04.063.
4. Bacci G, Briccoli A, Longhi A, Ferrari S, Mercuri M, Faggioli F, et al. Treatment and outcome of recurrent osteosarcoma: experience at Rizzoli in 235 patients initially treated with neoadjuvant chemotherapy. Acta Oncol. 2005;44(7):748–55. doi:10.1080/02841860500327503.
5. Bacci G, Ferrari S, Longhi A, Perin S, Forni C, Fabbri N, et al. Pattern of relapse in patients with osteosarcoma of the extremities treated with neoadjuvant chemotherapy. Eur J Cancer. 2001;37(1):32–8.
6. Hawkins DS, Arndt CA. Pattern of disease recurrence and prognostic factors in patients with osteosarcoma treated with contemporary chemotherapy. Cancer. 2003;98(11):2447–56. doi:10.1002/cncr.11799.
7. Meyers PA, Gorlick R. Osteosarcoma. Pediatr Clin N Am. 1997;44(4):973–89.
8. Bielack SS, Kempf-Bielack B, Branscheid D, Carrle D, Friedel G, Helmke K, et al. Second and subsequent recurrences of osteosarcoma: presentation, treatment, and outcomes of 249 consecutive cooperative osteosarcoma study group patients. J Clin Oncol. 2009;27(4):557–65. doi:10.1200/JCO.2008.16.2305.
9. Leary SE, Wozniak AW, Billups CA, Wu J, McPherson V, Neel MD, et al. Survival of pediatric patients after relapsed osteosarcoma: the St. Jude Children's Research Hospital experience. Cancer. 2013;119(14):2645–53. doi:10.1002/cncr.28111.
10. Iwata S, Yonemoto T, Iizasa T, Niibe Y, Kamoda H, Ishii T. Oligo-recurrence of osteosarcoma patients: treatment strategies for pulmonary metastases. Ann Surg Oncol. 2015 Jun 20. doi:10.1245/s10434-015-4682-1.
11. Tsuchiya H, Kanazawa Y, Abdel-Wanis ME, Asada N, Abe S, Isu K, et al. Effect of timing of pulmonary metastases identification on prognosis of patients with osteosarcoma: the Japanese Musculoskeletal Oncology Group study. J Clin Oncol. 2002;20(16):3470–7.
12. Briccoli A, Rocca M, Salone M, Bacci G, Ferrari S, Balladelli A, et al. Resection of recurrent pulmonary metastases in patients with osteosarcoma. Cancer. 2005;104(8):1721–5. doi:10.1002/cncr.21369.
13. Ferrari S, Briccoli A, Mercuri M, Bertoni F, Picci P, Tienghi A, et al. Postrelapse survival in osteosarcoma of the extremities: prognostic factors for long-term survival. J Clin Oncol. 2003;21(4):710–5.
14. Wu PK, Chen WM, Chen CF, Lee OK, Haung CK, Chen TH. Primary osteogenic sarcoma with pulmonary metastasis: clinical results and prognostic factors in 91 patients. Jpn J Clin Oncol. 2009;39(8):514–22. doi:10.1093/jjco/hyp057.
15. Hellman S, Weichselbaum RR. Oligometastases. J Clin Oncol. 1995;13(1):8–10.
16. Bacci G, Rocca M, Salone M, Balladelli A, Ferrari S, Palmerini E, et al. High grade osteosarcoma of the extremities with lung metastases at presentation: treatment with neoadjuvant chemotherapy and simultaneous resection of primary and metastatic lesions. J Surg Oncol. 2008;98(6):415–20. doi:10.1002/jso.21140.
17. Yonemoto T, Tatezaki S, Ishii T, Satoh T, Kimura H, Iwai N. Prognosis of osteosarcoma with pulmonary metastases at initial presentation is not dismal. Clin Orthop Relat Res. 1998;349:194–9.
18. Carter SR, Grimer RJ, Sneath RS, Matthews HR. Results of thoracotomy in osteogenic sarcoma with pulmonary metastases. Thorax. 1991;46(10):727–31.
19. Letourneau PA, Xiao L, Harting MT, Lally KP, Cox Jr CS, Andrassy RJ, et al. Location of pulmonary metastasis in pediatric osteosarcoma is predictive of outcome. J Pediatr Surg. 2011;46(7):1333–7. doi:10.1016/j.jpedsurg.2010.12.013.
20. Harting MT, Blakely ML, Jaffe N, Cox Jr CS, Hayes-Jordan A, Benjamin RS, et al. Long-term survival after aggressive resection of pulmonary metastases among children and adolescents with osteosarcoma. J Pediatr Surg. 2006;41(1):194–9. doi:10.1016/j.jpedsurg.2005.10.089.
21. Chou AJ, Merola PR, Wexler LH, Gorlick RG, Vyas YM, Healey JH, et al. Treatment of osteosarcoma at first recurrence after contemporary therapy: the Memorial Sloan-Kettering Cancer Center experience. Cancer. 2005;104(10):2214–21. doi:10.1002/cncr.21417.

22. Salah S, Fayoumi S, Alibraheem A, Massad E, Abdel Jalil R, Yaser S, et al. The influence of pulmonary metastasectomy on survival in osteosarcoma and soft-tissue sarcomas: a retrospective analysis of survival outcomes, hospitalizations and requirements of home oxygen therapy. Interact Cardiovasc Thorac Surg. 2013;17(2):296–302. doi:10.1093/icvts/ivt177.
23. Kayton ML, Huvos AG, Casher J, Abramson SJ, Rosen NS, Wexler LH, et al. Computed tomographic scan of the chest underestimates the number of metastatic lesions in osteosarcoma. J Pediatr Surg. 2006;41(1):200–6. doi:10.1016/j.jpedsurg.2005.10.024; discussion -6.
24. Partrick DA, Bensard DD, Teitelbaum DH, Geiger JD, Strouse P, Harned RK. Successful thoracoscopic lung biopsy in children utilizing preoperative CT-guided localization. J Pediatr Surg. 2002;37(7):970–3; discussion -3.
25. Parida L, Fernandez-Pineda I, Uffman J, Davidoff AM, Gold R, Rao BN. Thoracoscopic resection of computed tomography-localized lung nodules in children. J Pediatr Surg. 2013; 48(4):750–6. doi:10.1016/j.jpedsurg.2012.09.051.
26. Sugi K, Kaneda Y, Hirasawa K, Kunitani N. Radioisotope marking under CT guidance and localization using a handheld gamma probe for small or indistinct pulmonary lesions. Chest. 2003;124(1):155–8.
27. Gow KW, Saad DF, Koontz C, Wulkan ML. Minimally invasive thoracoscopic ultrasound for localization of pulmonary nodules in children. J Pediatr Surg. 2008;43(12):2315–22. doi:10.1016/j.jpedsurg.2008.08.031.
28. Chen F, Miyahara R, Bando T, Okubo K, Watanabe K, Nakayama T, et al. Repeat resection of pulmonary metastasis is beneficial for patients with osteosarcoma of the extremities. Interact Cardiovasc Thorac Surg. 2009;9(4):649–53. doi:10.1510/icvts.2009.212498.
29. Kandioler D, Kromer E, Tuchler H, End A, Muller MR, Wolner E, et al. Long-term results after repeated surgical removal of pulmonary metastases. Ann Thorac Surg. 1998;65(4): 909–12.
30. Suzuki M, Iwata T, Ando S, Iida T, Nakajima T, Ishii T, et al. Predictors of long-term survival with pulmonary metastasectomy for osteosarcomas and soft tissue sarcomas. J Cardiovasc Surg. 2006;47(5):603–8.
31. Burgers JM, van Glabbeke M, Busson A, Cohen P, Mazabraud AR, Abbatucci JS, et al. Osteosarcoma of the limbs. Report of the EORTC-SIOP 03 trial 20781 investigating the value of adjuvant treatment with chemotherapy and/or prophylactic lung irradiation. Cancer. 1988;61(5):1024–31.
32. Caldwell WL. Elective whole lung irradiation. Radiology. 1976;120(3):659–66. doi:10.1148/120.3.659.
33. Giritsky AS, Etcubanas E, Mark JB. Pulmonary resection in children with metastatic osteogenic sarcoma: improved survival with surgery, chemotherapy, and irradiation. J Thorac Cardiovasc Surg. 1978;75(3):354–62.
34. Yu W, Tang L, Lin F, Li D, Wang J, Yang Y, et al. Stereotactic radiosurgery, a potential alternative treatment for pulmonary metastases from osteosarcoma. Int J Oncol. 2014; 44(4):1091–8. doi:10.3892/ijo.2014.2295.
35. Mehta N, Selch M, Wang PC, Federman N, Lee JM, Eilber FC, et al. Safety and efficacy of stereotactic body radiation therapy in the treatment of pulmonary metastases from high grade sarcoma. Sarcoma. 2013;2013:360214. doi:10.1155/2013/360214.
36. Nakamura T, Matsumine A, Yamakado K, Matsubara T, Takaki H, Nakatsuka A, et al. Lung radiofrequency ablation in patients with pulmonary metastases from musculoskeletal sarcomas [corrected]. Cancer. 2009;115(16):3774–81. doi:10.1002/cncr.24420.
37. Palussiere J, Italiano A, Descat E, Ferron S, Cornelis F, Avril A, et al. Sarcoma lung metastases treated with percutaneous radiofrequency ablation: results from 29 patients. Ann Surg Oncol. 2011;18(13):3771–7. doi:10.1245/s10434-011-1806-0.

Part VII

Quality of Life

Long-Term Outcomes and Quality of Life (QOL) in Survivors of Pediatric and Adolescent Osteosarcoma

20

Tsukasa Yonemoto, Shintaro Iwata, Hiroto Kamoda, and Takeshi Ishii

Abstract

We investigated long-term outcomes (education, employment, marriage, fertility, multiple primary cancers, and psychosocial outcomes) and quality of life (QOL) in survivors of pediatric and adolescent osteosarcoma. In a limb-sparing group, the proportion of survivors who graduated from a university was significantly higher. There were few problems regarding employment. The marital rates were slightly lower in male survivors and in an amputation group. Recent chemotherapy affected male survivors' fertility. Of 162 patients, 13 had multiple primary cancers. When reviewing psychosocial outcomes, the incidence of posttraumatic stress symptom was low, and posttraumatic growth was marked. The QOL was satisfactory, excluding "physical functioning." The limb-sparing group was more adaptable to social life activities than the amputation group.

Keywords

Osteosarcoma • Quality of life (QOL) • Survivors

20.1 Introduction

Advances in multidisciplinary treatment for osteosarcoma have markedly improved treatment results, increasing the number of long-term survivors of pediatric and adolescent osteosarcoma. In osteosarcoma treatment, an era when the purpose of treatment was to cure the disease ended, and the postcure quality of life (QOL) has

T. Yonemoto (✉) • S. Iwata • H. Kamoda • T. Ishii
Division of Orthopaedic Surgery, Chiba Cancer Center, 666-2 Nitona-cho, Chuo-ku, Chiba 260-8717, Japan

Chiba Pediatric Orthopaedic Group (CPOG), Chiba, Japan
e-mail: tyonemot@chiba-cc.jp

T. Ueda, A. Kawai (eds.), *Osteosarcoma*, DOI 10.1007/978-4-431-55696-1_20

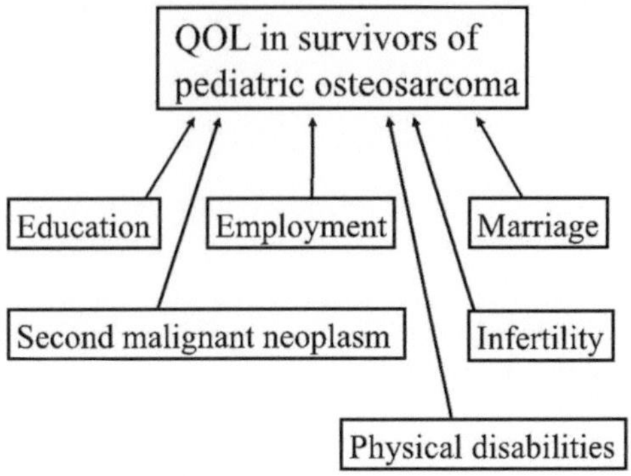

Fig. 20.1 QOL in survivors of pediatric osteosarcoma; various aspects and factors are involved in the QOL of long-term survivors of osteosarcoma. For QOL assessment, individual factors must be examined

been emphasized. However, few studies have examined the psychosocial outcome or QOL of long-term survivors of pediatric and adolescent osteosarcoma [1].

We conducted a study to comprehensively evaluate the QOL of long-term survivors of pediatric and adolescent osteosarcoma. As shown in Fig. 20.1, various factors are involved. To evaluate the QOL, individual factors must be investigated.

In this chapter, we introduce long-term outcomes (education, employment, marriage, fertility, multiple primary cancers, and psychosocial outcomes) and QOL in survivors of pediatric and adolescent osteosarcoma based on our study results [2–8].

20.2 Education and Employment

20.2.1 Our Report on Education [2]

In 41 survivors of pediatric and adolescent osteosarcoma who were treated in our hospital between 1976 and 1995, a questionnaire survey regarding education (returning to school, educational background) was conducted. In addition, they were divided into two groups based on affected limb conditions at the time of the survey: amputation (including rotationplasty) and limb-sparing groups. The results were compared between the two groups.

Of the 41 subjects, responses were obtained from 27 (response rate, 65.9 %). These consisted of 11 males and 16 females. The mean age at the initial presentation was 13.6 years. That at the time of the survey was 34 years. The amputation group consisted of 18 subjects, and the limb-sparing group consisted of 9. The mean interval from the completion of treatment was 218 months.

Of the 27 subjects, 19 could return to school, whereas 7 could not return. There was no description in 1. In 73.1 % (19/26), it was possible to return to the former school. The educational background was senior high school in 12 subjects and university in 13. There was no description in 2. Of these subjects, 52 % (13/25) graduated from a university, being similar to the proportion of Japanese who graduate from a university (45 %). In the limb-sparing group, the proportion of

Table 20.1 Status of education

Final education level	Amputation group (18 patients)	Limb-sparing group (9 patients)
University	5	5
College	1	2
High school	11	1
No mention	1	1

Reference [2]

survivors who graduated from university was significantly higher, suggesting that affected limb conditions influence education (Table 20.1, published from Reference [2] based on approval).

20.2.2 Other Reports on Education

Nagarajan et al. reported that the education level was lower in an amputation group [9]. Novakovic et al. indicated that there was no difference in the education level between survivors and their siblings [10]. These results were similar to those of our study.

20.2.3 Our Report on Employment [2]

We investigated employment (occupation, annual income) in the above 27 survivors of pediatric and adolescent osteosarcoma. There were 18 clerical workers, four technicians, one sales worker, and two housewives. There was no description in 2. Of these, 72 % (18/25) had clerical jobs. The mean annual income was 4,010,000 yen, being similar to that of Japanese businessmen (4,280,000 yen). There was no difference in the mean annual income between the amputation and limb-sparing groups. In Japan, laws for the handicapped have been implemented, and there were few problems regarding survivors' employment.

20.2.4 Other Reports on Employment

Nagarajan et al. reported that the employment rates were higher in survivors who had received high-level education and male survivors, and that there was no difference in the employment rate between amputation and limb-sparing groups [9]. Hays et al. indicated that there were few financial problems in pediatric cancer patients [11]. In our study, there were also few problems regarding survivors' employment. Nicholson et al. reported that there was no difference in the employment rate between survivors and their siblings [12]. On the other hand, Novakovic et al. emphasized that the employment rate in survivors was significantly lower [10].

20.3 Marriage and Fertility

20.3.1 Our Report on Marriage [3, 4]

In 62 survivors of pediatric and adolescent osteosarcoma who were treated in our hospital between 1976 and 2002, a questionnaire survey regarding marriage was conducted. Of these, responses were obtained from 46 (response rate, 74.2 %). We investigated the marital rate (number of married survivors/total number of survivors) in the 46 survivors. In addition, they were divided into two groups: amputation and limb-sparing groups. The marital rate was examined in each group. As controls, it was investigated in 52 siblings.

Overall, the marital rate was 63.0 % (29/46). In the siblings, it was 63.5 % (33/52) (Table 20.2, Reference [4]). The marital rates were slightly lower in male survivors and in the amputation group, although there were no significant differences.

Table 20.2 Summary of marital rate

	Marital rate	*p*-Value
Total		
Patients	63.0 % (29/46)	
Siblings	63.5 % (33/52)	>0.999
Patients		
Males	55.0 % (11/20)	
Females	69.2 % (18/26)	0.369
Amputation group	60.0 % (15/25)	
Limb-sparing group	66.7 % (14/21)	0.762
Males in amputation group	45.5 % (5/11)	
Females in amputation group	71.4 % (10/14)	0.241
Males in limb-sparing group	66.7 % (6/9)	
Females in limb-sparing group	66.7 % (8/12)	>0.999
Siblings		
Males	63.0 % (17/27)	
Females	64.0 % (16/25)	>0.999
Males		
Patients	55.0 % (11/20)	
Siblings	63.0 % (17/27)	0.765
Females		
Patients	69.2 % (18/26)	
Siblings	64.0 % (16/25)	0.771

Reference [4]

20.3.2 Other Reports on Marriage

Nagarajan et al. reported that the marital rate in female survivors was higher than in male survivors, and that the marital rate in survivors was lower than in their siblings. In addition, they indicated that there was no difference in the marital rate between amputation and limb-sparing groups [9]. Our study also showed that the marital rate was lower in male survivors. Novakovic et al. reported that in survivors, the marital rate was lower than in their siblings, and that the number of divorces was greater [10]. On the other hand, Nicholson et al. indicated that there was no difference in the marital rate between survivors and their siblings [12]. In our study, there was also no difference in the marital rate between survivors and their siblings.

20.3.3 Our Report on Fertility [3, 4]

In 29 survivors who were married, we investigated the fertility rate (number of survivors raising a child/number of married survivors). They were divided into two groups: MC group in which moderate-dose chemotherapy was performed between 1976 and 1986 and IC group in which intensive-dose chemotherapy was performed between 1987 and 2002. The fertility rate was examined in each group. As controls, it was investigated in 33 siblings.

Overall, the fertility rate was 58.6 % (17/29). In the siblings, it was 81.8 % (27/33). In male survivors, the fertility rate was slightly lower (Table 20.3, Reference [4]). In particular, the fertility rate in male survivors in the IC group was significantly lower than in male siblings ($p = 0.018$), suggesting that recent intensified chemotherapy for osteosarcoma affects male survivors' fertility.

20.3.4 Other Reports on Fertility

Williams et al. reported that ifosfamide influenced fertility [13]. Longhi et al. indicated that ifosfamide-related infertility was more frequent in males [14]. The influence of chemotherapy on fertility is an important issue for long-term survivors; this should be further reviewed in the future.

20.4 Multiple Primary Cancers

20.4.1 Our Report on Multiple Primary Cancers

We investigated the incidence of multiple primary cancers in 162 patients with osteosarcoma who were treated in our department between 1976 and 2009, with an age of 30 years or younger on initial presentation. Nine patients with second malignant neoplasms following osteosarcoma were assigned to Group A. Four

Table 20.3 Summary of fertility rate

	Fertility rate	*p*-Value	
Total			
Patients	58.6 % (17/29)		
Siblings	81.8 % (27/33)	0.055	
Patients			
Males	36.4 % (4/11)		
Females	72.2 % (13/18)	0.119	
MC group	52.9 % (9/17)		
IC group	16.7 % (1/6)	0.703	
Siblings			
Males	76.5 % (13/17)		
Females	87.5 % (14/16)	0.656	
Males			
Patients	36.4 % (4/11)		
Siblings	76.5 % (13/17)	0.053	
Females			
Patients	72.2 % (13/18)		
Siblings	87.5 % (14/16)	0.405	
Male patients in MC group	60.0 % (3/5)		
Male siblings	76.5 % (13/17)	0.585	
Female patients in MC group	71.4 % (5/7)		
Female siblings	87.5 % (14/16)	0.557	
Male patients in IC group	16.7 % (1/6)		
Male siblings	76.5 % (13/17)	0.018	*
Female patients in IC group	72.7 % (8/11)		
Female siblings	87.5 % (14/16)	0.371	

Reference [4]
MC group: moderate-dose chemotherapy group
IC group: intensive-dose chemotherapy group
*Statistically significant (Fisher's exact probability test)

patients with osteosarcoma as a second malignant neoplasm were assigned to Group B. We examined the clinical features of these 13 patients.

In Group A, second malignant neoplasms were diagnosed as breast carcinoma in four patients, acute myelogenous leukemia in two, a malignant phyllodes tumor in one, ovarian carcinoma in one, and small intestine carcinoma in one. Ages at the development of second malignant neoplasms ranged from 14 to 34 years (mean, 25.9 years). Intervals from the development of osteosarcoma until that of second malignant neoplasms ranged from 3 to 16 years (mean, 9.6 years) (Table 20.4).

In Group B, first malignant neoplasms were diagnosed as adrenocortical cancer in one patient, malignant teratoma in one, Ewing's sarcoma in one, and retinoblastoma in one. Ages at the time of the development of the first malignant neoplasms ranged from 0 to 10 years (mean, 3 years). Intervals from the development of the

Table 20.4 Multiple primary cancers in patients with pediatric osteosarcoma

		First malignant neoplasm (FMN)		Interval from FMN to SMN (years)	Second malignant neoplasm (SMN)		Age at final follow-up (years)	Outcome
	Sex	Age (years)	Diagnosis		Age (years)	Diagnosis		
Group A								
1	F	12	Osteosarcoma of femur	3	15	Acute myelogenous leukemia	15	DOD
2	M	7	Osteosarcoma of tibia	7	14	Acute myelogenous leukemia	14	DOD
3	F	12	Osteosarcoma of femur	9	21	Malignant phyllodes tumor	22	DOD
4	F	29	Osteosarcoma of ulna	3	32	Breast carcinoma	46	NED
5	F	13	Osteosarcoma of femur	16	29	Breast carcinoma	43	NED
6	F	19	Osteosarcoma of sacrum	5	24	Ovarian carcinoma	24	DOD
7	F	19	Osteosarcoma of tibia	15	34	Small intestine carcinoma	36	DOD
8	F	20	Osteosarcoma of humerus	13	33	Breast carcinoma	34	NED
9	F	16	Osteosarcoma of femur	15	31	Breast carcinoma	31	NED
Group B								
1	F	0	Adrenocortical carcinoma	10	11	Osteosarcoma of femur	23	NED
2	F	2	Malignant teratoma of sacrum	12	14	Osteosarcoma of femur	27	NED
3	M	10	Ewing's sarcoma of humerus	5	15	Osteosarcoma of femur	17	NED
4	M	0	Retinoblastoma	34	34	Osteosarcoma of femur	36	DOD

NED no evidence of disease, *DOD* died of disease

first malignant neoplasms until that of osteosarcoma ranged from 5 to 34 years (mean, 15.3 years) (Table 20.4).

In most patients in Groups A and B, high-dose anticancer drugs were used to treat the first malignant neoplasms. Anticancer treatment may have been involved in the development of the second malignant neoplasms. Li-Fraumeni syndrome is known to be in the same cancer family as osteosarcoma. Of our 13 patients, two had Li-Fraumeni syndrome.

20.4.2 Other Reports on Multiple Primary Cancers

Malkin et al. reported that germ cell mutations of the *p53* tumor suppressor gene were etiologically involved in the pathogenesis of Li-Fraumeni syndrome and that the incidence of breast cancer was high [15]. According to Turaka et al.. osteosarcoma was observed in three patients in a chart review of 245 patients with retinoblastoma [16]. Goldsby et al. indicated that the incidence of second malignant neoplasms increased with the follow-up period [17]. In the future, the incidence of multiple primary cancers in osteosarcoma patients may further increase. Strict long-term follow-up may be necessary.

20.5 Psychosocial Outcomes

20.5.1 Our Report on Psychosocial Outcomes [6]

In 55 survivors of pediatric and adolescent osteosarcoma who were treated in our hospital, a questionnaire survey regarding psychosocial outcomes was conducted. To evaluate psychosocial outcomes, the following questionnaires were used: For family function assessment, the Family APGAR [18] was used. For social support assessment, the SSQ-S and SSQ-N [19] were used. For posttraumatic stress symptom assessment, the IES-R [20] was used. For posttraumatic growth assessment, the PTGI [21, 22] was used. Subsequently, multiple regression analysis was performed using the IES-R and PTGI as dependent variables. Independent variables included the sex, age at diagnosis, affected limb condition (amputation/preservation), Family APGAR, SSQ-S, and SSQ-N.

Of the 55 survivors, responses were obtained from 30 (response rate, 54.5 %). They consisted of 16 in whom amputation was performed and 14 in whom the affected limb was spared. The mean Family APGAR score was 7.97, suggesting high-level family function. The mean SSQ-N and SSQ-S scores were 4.03 and 5.02, respectively, being similar to those in healthy adults. The mean IES-R score was 9.70; posttraumatic stress symptom was not frequent. The mean PTGI score was 51.8, being markedly higher than in Japanese university students (33.9). Posttraumatic growth was marked (Table 20.5, Reference [6]). In the survivors of osteosarcoma, the incidence of posttraumatic stress symptom was low, and posttraumatic growth was marked.

Table 20.5 Psychosocial outcomes (Reference [6])

	Mean	Standard deviation
Family APGAR	7.97	2.99
SSQ-S	5.02	1.04
SSQ-N	4.03	1.81
IES-R	9.70	9.71
PTGI	51.80	18.54

Multiple regression analysis with the IES-R as a dependent variable showed that only the Family APGAR was a significant independent variable. High-level family function reduced the survivors' posttraumatic stress symptom.

Multiple regression analysis with PTGI as a dependent variable showed that the age at diagnosis, affected limb condition, and SSQ-N were significant independent variables. In patients of an advanced age and those after amputation, posttraumatic growth was marked. Social support led to the survivors' posttraumatic growth.

20.5.2 Other Reports on Psychosocial Outcomes

Bressound et al. reported that a low-level family function was associated with posttraumatic stress symptom [23]. Nicholson et al. indicated that survivors' psychosocial outcomes were favorable [12]. Michel et al. suggested that a prospective outcome occurs after pediatric cancer and that it is promoted by appropriate counseling [24]. We reported that not only survivors but also their parents showed posttraumatic stress disorder or posttraumatic growth [7]. In the future, psychosocial care for survivors may be important.

20.6 Evaluation of Quality of Life (QOL)

20.6.1 Evaluation Methods of QOL

To evaluate the affected limb function of survivors of pediatric and adolescent osteosarcoma, the Musculoskeletal Tumor Society score (MSTS score) [25], Toronto Extremity Salvage Score (TESS) [26], Functional Mobility Assessment (FMA) [27], and Reintegration to Normal Living Index (RNLI) [28] are used. For QOL assessment, the Short Form-36 (SF-36) [29], TNO-AZL Questionnaire for Adult's Quality of Life (TAAQOL) [30], TNO-AZL Child Quality of Life (TACQOL) [31], Bt-DUX [32], and Utrecht Coping List for Adolescents (UCL-A) [33] are used. For the details of respective evaluation methods, refer to the references.

20.6.2 Our Report on QOL [8]

In 59 survivors of pediatric and adolescent osteosarcoma who were treated in our department between 1976 and 2000, a questionnaire survey regarding QOL was conducted. Of these survivors, responses were obtained from 33 (response rate, 55.9 %).

We evaluated the survivors' QOL using the SF-36 consisting of eight subscales [29]. On global QOL assessment, the "physical functioning" score was markedly lower than the national standard value. However, the scores for the other seven subscales were higher than national standard values (Fig. 20.2, Reference [8]). The survivors' QOL was satisfactory, excluding "physical functioning."

We compared the QOL between limb-sparing and amputation groups ($n = 14$ and 19, respectively). In the former, the "social functioning" score was significantly higher ($p = 0.023$). There were no significant differences in the other seven subscales. In our study, the limb-sparing group was more adaptable to social life activities than the amputation group; the QOL was higher.

20.6.3 Relationship Between Affected Limb Function and QOL

We examined the relationship between the affected limb function and QOL in long-term survivors of pediatric and adolescent osteosarcoma. We evaluated the survivors' limb function using a Musculoskeletal Tumor Society score (MSTS score) [25] and investigated the correlation between the MSTS score and SF-36.

There were positive correlations among three subscales: "physical functioning," "bodily pain," and "social functioning." However, there were no correlations among the other five subscales. Furthermore, there was a positive correlation between the MSTS score and "physical component summary" of SF-36. However, there was no correlation between this score and "mental component summary" of SF-36, suggesting that the QOL cannot be evaluated based on the affected limb

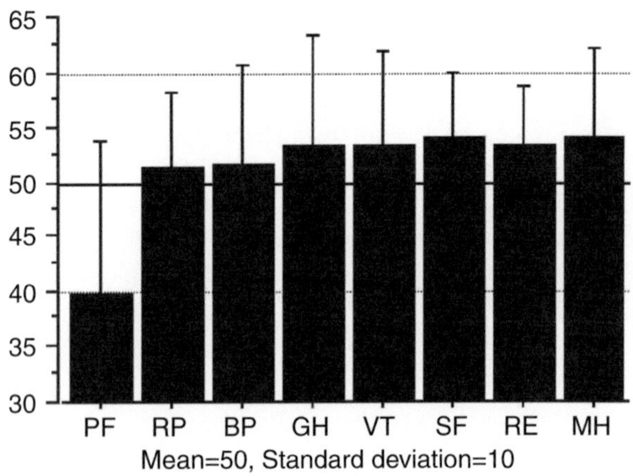

Fig. 20.2 QOL evaluated using SF-36. The "physical functioning (PF)" score was lower than the national standard value, but the scores for the other seven subscales were higher than the standard values. *PF* physical functioning, *RP* physical role, *BP* bodily pain, *GH* general health perceptions, *VT* vitality, *SF* social functioning, *RE* emotional role, *MH* mental health

function only. It was shown that a favorable affected limb function did not always lead to a good QOL.

20.6.4 Other Reports on QOL

Nagarajan et al. reported that most survivors of bone tumors were adaptable to their environments using the RNL [34]. Koopman et al. also examined the QOL using the TAAQOL, TACQOL, and UCL-A and indicated that survivors were adaptable after treatment, and that there were no long-term emotional or social problems [33]. On the other hand, Ness et al. emphasized that survivors of osteosarcoma were less active than their siblings, requiring positive support [35].

Zahlten-Hinguranage et al. reported that the long-term QOL was similar between limb-sparing and amputation groups [36]. In our study, the limb-sparing group was more adaptable to social life activities than the amputation group; the QOL was higher. Forni et al. and Veenstra et al. indicated that the QOL of patients who underwent rotationplasty was high using the SF-36 [37, 38].

Thus, many studies have suggested that survivors' QOL is relatively favorable. However, the survivor-supporting system is not sufficient, as reported by Ness et al. [35]. In the future, it may be necessary to positively support survivors.

20.7 Epilogue

It is difficult to standardize the results of our study for the following reasons: This was a retrospective study; the number of patients was small; and the data were obtained from a single institution. However, our study may provide clues to QOL improvement in survivors of pediatric and adolescent osteosarcoma. Lastly, issues to be improved in the future are presented.

20.7.1 Issue 1

Recent intensified treatment for osteosarcoma showed good results, but raised a new issue, male infertility. Strategies to resolve this issue must be established.

20.7.2 Issue 2

It is expected that the incidence of second malignant neoplasms in survivors of osteosarcoma will increase. Strict long-term follow-up is necessary.

20.7.3 Issue 3

Survivors of osteosarcoma show mental growth after treatment. The survivors' QOL was satisfactory, excluding "physical functioning." However, social support is still insufficient; total care must be intensified.

Acknowledgments The authors thank Dr. Shin-ichiro Tatezaki and Dr. Kiyoko Kamibeppu, for their invaluable advice. The authors also thank the members of the Chiba Cancer Center and the Chiba Pediatric Orthopaedic Group (CPOG), for their encouragement.

References

1. Nagarajan R, Clohisy DR, Neglia JP, et al. Function and quality-of-life of survivors of pelvic and lower extremity osteosarcoma and Ewing's sarcoma: the childhood cancer survivor study. Br J Cancer. 2004;91:1858–65.
2. Yonemoto T, Ishii T, Takeuchi Y, et al. Education and employment in long-term survivors of high-grade osteosaroma: a Japanese single center experience. Oncology. 2007;72:274–8.
3. Yonemoto T, Tatezaki S, Ishii T, et al. Marriage and fertility in long-term survivors of high grade osteosarcoma. Am J Clin Oncol. 2003;26:513–6.
4. Yonemoto T, Ishii T, Takeuchi Y, et al. Recently intensified chemotherapy for high-grade osteosarcoma may affect fertility in long-term male survivors. Anticancer Res. 2009;29:763–7.
5. Yonemoto T, Tatezaki S, Ishii T, et al. Multiple primary cancers in patients with osteosarcoma: the influence of anticancer drugs and genetic factors. Am J Clin Oncol. 2004;27:220–4.
6. Yonemoto T, Kamibeppu K, Ishii T, et al. Psychosocial outcomes in long-term survivors of high-grade osteosaroma: a Japanese single-center experience. Anticancer Res. 2009;29:4287–90.
7. Yonemoto T, Kamibeppu K, Ishii T, et al. Posttraumatic stress symptom (PTSS) and posttraumatic growth (PTG) in parents of childhood, adolescent and young adult patients with high-grade osteosarcoma. Int J Clin Oncol. 2012;17:272–5.
8. Yonemoto T, Ishii T, Takeuchi Y, et al. Evaluation of quality of life (QOL) in long-term survivors of high-grade osteosaroma: a Japanese single center experience. Anticancer Res. 2007;27:3621–4.
9. Nagarajan R, Neglia JP, Clohisy DR, et al. Education, employment, insurance, and marital status among 694 survivors of pediatric lower extremity bone tumors: a report from the childhood cancer survivor study. Cancer. 2003;97:2554–64.
10. Novakovic B, Fears TR, Horowitz ME, et al. Late effects of therapy in survivors of Ewing's sarcoma family tumors. J Pediatr Hematol Oncol. 1997;19:220–5.
11. Hays DM, Landsverk J, Sallan SE, et al. Educational, occupational, and insurance status of childhood cancer survivors in their fourth and fifth decades of life. J Clin Oncol. 1992;10:1397–406.
12. Nicholson HS, Mulvihill JJ, Byrne J. Late effects of therapy in adult survivors of osteosarcoma and Ewing's sarcoma. Med Pediatr Oncol. 1992;20:6–12.
13. Williams D, Crofton PM, Levitt G. Does ifosfamide affect gonadal function? Pediatr Blood Cancer. 2008;50:347–51.
14. Longhi A, Macchiagodena M, Vitali G, et al. Fertility in male patients treated with neoadjuvant chemotherapy for osteosarcoma. J Pediatr Hematol Oncol. 2003;25:292–6.
15. Malkin D, Li FP, Strong LC, et al. Germ line p53 mutations in a familial syndrome of breast cancer, sarcomas, and other neoplasms. Science. 1990;250:1233–8.

16. Turaka K, Shields CL, Meadows AT, et al. Second malignant neoplasms following chemoreduction with carboplatin, etoposide, and vincristine in 245 patients with intraocular retinoblastoma. Pediatr Blood Cancer. 2012;59:121–5.
17. Goldsby R, Burke C, Nagarajan R, et al. Second solid malignancies among children, adolescents, and young adults diagnosed with malignant bone tumors after 1976: follow-up of a Children's Oncology Group cohort. Cancer. 2008;113:2597–604.
18. Smilkstein G, Ashworth C, Montano D. Validity and reliability of the family APGAR as a test of family function. J Fam Pract. 1982;15:303–11.
19. Furukawa TA, Harai H, Hirai T, et al. Social support questionnaire among psychiatric patients with various diagnoses and normal controls. Soc Psychiatry Psychiatr Epidemiol. 1999;34:216–22.
20. Horowitz M, Wilner N, Alvarez W. Impact of event scale: a measure of subjective stress. Psychosom Med. 1979;41:209–18.
21. Tedeschi RG, Calhoun LG. The posttraumatic growth inventory: measuring the positive legacy of trauma. J Trauma Stress. 1996;9:455–71.
22. Taku K, Calhoun LG, Tedeschi RG, et al. Examining posttraumatic growth among Japanese university students. Anxiety Stress Coping. 2007;20:353–67.
23. Bressoud A, Real del Sarte O, Stiefel S, et al. Impact of family structure on long-term survivors of osteosarcoma. Support Care Cancer. 2007;15:525–31.
24. Michel G, Taylor N, Absolom K, et al. Benefit finding in survivors of childhood cancer and their parents: further empirical support for the benefit finding scale for children. Child Care Health Dev. 2010;36:123–9.
25. Enneking WF, Dunham W, Gebhardt MC, et al. A system for the functional evaluation of reconstructive procedures after surgical treatment of tumors of the musculoskeletal system. Clin Orthop Relat Res. 1993;286:241–6.
26. Davis AM, Wright JG, Williams JI, et al. Development of a measure of physical function for patients with bone and soft tissue sarcoma. Qual Life Res. 1996;5:508–16.
27. Marchese VG, Rai SN, Carlson CA, et al. Assessing functional mobility in survivors of lower-extremity sarcoma: reliability and validity of a new assessment tool. Pediatr Blood Cancer. 2007;49:183–9.
28. Wood-Dauphinee SL, Opzoomer MA, Williams JI, et al. Assessment of global function: the reintegration to normal living index. Arch Phys Med Rehabil. 1988;69:583–90.
29. Fukuhara S, Ware JE, Kosinski M, et al. Psychometric and clinical tests of validity of the Japanese SF-36 health survey. J Clin Epidemiol. 1998;51:1045–53.
30. Fekkes M, Kamphuis RP, Ottenkamp J, et al. Health-related quality of life in young adults with minor congenital heart disease. Psychol Health. 2001;16:239–50.
31. Theunissen NC, Vogels TG, Koopman HM, et al. The proxy problem: child report versus parent report in health-related quality of life research. Qual Life Res. 1998;7:387–97.
32. Bekkering WP, Billing L, Grimer RJ, et al. Translation and preliminary validation of the English version of the DUX questionnaire for lower extremity bone tumor patients (Bt-DUX): a disease-specific measure for quality of life. J Surg Oncol. 2013;107:353–9.
33. Koopman HM, Koetsier JA, Taminiau AH, et al. Health-related quality of life and coping strategies of children after treatment of a malignant bone tumor: a 5-year follow-up study. Pediatr Blood Cancer. 2005;45:694–9.
34. Nagarajan R, Mogil R, Neglia JP, et al. Self-reported global function among adult survivors of childhood lower-extremity bone tumors: a report from the Childhood Cancer Survivor Study (CCSS). Cancer Surviv. 2009;3:59–65.
35. Ness KK, Leisenring WM, Huang S, et al. Predictors of inactive lifestyle among adult survivors of childhood cancer: a report from the childhood cancer survivor study. Cancer. 2009;115:1984–94.
36. Zahlten-Hinguranage A, Bernd L, Ewerbeck V, et al. Equal quality of life after limb-sparing or ablative surgery for lower extremity sarcomas. Br J Cancer. 2004;91:1012–4.

37. Forni C, Gaudenzi N, Zoli M, et al. Living with rotationplasty–quality of life in rotationplasty patients from childhood to adulthood. J Surg Oncol. 2012;105:331–6.
38. Veenstra KM, Sprangers MA, van der Eyken JW, et al. Quality of life in survivors with a Van Ness-Borggreve rotationplasty after bone tumour resection. Eur J Surg Oncol. 2000;73:192–7.

MIX
Papier aus verantwortungsvollen Quellen
Paper from responsible sources
FSC® C105338

If you have any concerns about our products,
you can contact us on
ProductSafety@springernature.com

In case Publisher is established outside the EU,
the EU authorized representative is:
Springer Nature Customer Service Center GmbH
Europaplatz 3, 69115 Heidelberg, Germany

Printed by Libri Plureos GmbH
in Hamburg, Germany